T0180477

Gametes – the oocyte

Cambridge Reviews in Human Reproduction

SERIES EDITORS

Professor J. G. Grudzinskas, Dr J. L. Yovich, Professor J. L. Simpson,
Professor T. Chard

This major new series on human reproduction provides a comprehensive and integrated review of the reproductive process. The first six volumes concentrate on the essential reproductive events leading up to birth. The series provides a synthesis of the scientific, clinical and physiological elements of the reproductive process. Each volume focuses on a well-defined aspect of reproduction and provides a multidisciplinary though self-contained review.

Each volume is prepared by an international and authoritative team of writers involving many of the world's leading experts. The series is edited to the highest standard to insure an integrated and uniformly high level of presentation. An important feature of the series is the inclusion of high-quality line illustrations.

The series provides an essential source of information for all trainees in obstetrics, gynaecology, andrology and reproductive medicine and will also be of interest to reproductive biologists and geneticists, physiologists and endocrinologists.

Titles in the series:
THE UTERUS
GAMETES – THE SPERMATOZOON

Gametes – The Oocyte

Edited by

J. G. GRUDZINSKAS
The Royal London Hospital, London, UK

and

J. L. YOVICH
PIVET Medical Centre, Perth, Australia

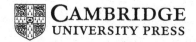

CAMBRIDGE
UNIVERSITY PRESS

Published by the Press Syndicate of the University of Cambridge
The Pitt Building, Trumpington Street, Cambridge CB2 1RP
40 West 20th Street, New York, NY 10011-4211, USA
10 Stamford Road, Oakleigh, Melbourne 3166, Australia

First published 1995

A catalogue record for this book is available from the British Library

Library of Congress cataloguing in publication data

Gametes : the oocyte / edited by J.G. Grudzinskas and J.L. Yovich.
   p.   cm. — (Cambridge reviews in human reproduction)
Includes index.
ISBN 0-521-47490-6 (hardback). — ISBN 0-521-47995-9 (pbk.)
1. Ovum—Physiology. 2. Ovulation—Regulation. I. Grudzinskas,
J. G. (Jurgis Gedimines) II. Yovich, John. III. Series.
[DNLM: 1. Oocytes. 2. Ovulation—physiology.   WQ 205 G1926 1995]
QM611.G35   1995
612.6′2—dc20
DNLM/DLC
for Library of Congress 94-42701 CIP

ISBN 0 521 47490 6 hardback
ISBN 0 521 47995 9 paperback

Transferred to digital printing 2004

Contents

Editors' preface

The aim of this book is to provide a complete and up-to-date account of the physiology, endocrinology and biochemistry of the oocyte, with particular emphasis on the human and on the relationship of clinical abnormalities to ovarian function. The book begins with a detailed account of the evolution of the oocyte, an extraordinary perspective of events leading to our present state of knowledge of the human oocyte by Colin Austin. The molecular and cellular aspects of oocyte development are detailed by Roger Gosden's group, whilst Gerry Schatten's team deals with the organizational and dynamic events during maturation and fertilization. The genetic aspects of oocyte function are considered by Michelle Plachot whilst genetic control of ovarian development is reviewed by Joe Leigh Simpson. A full review of the mechanisms of ovulation including endocrine and paracrine regulation are addressed by Roger Gosden, Stephen Downs, David Baird and Markku Seppälä's group. Oocyte transport (Croxatto and Villalón) and conditions which affect oocyte quality (Homburg and Shelef) together with clinical disorders (Michael Hull) and then treatment (John Yovich) are examined in detail. Paterson and Aitken highlight the role of the zona pellucida in oocyte function and Al-Hasani and Diedrich review progress on storage of human oocytes. Finally, in a provocative essay, Rob Jansen reflects on the bioethical issues and challenges resulting from research on human oocytes and its current clinical implications.

J. G. Grudzinskas
and J. L. Yovich
March 1995

Contributors

R. J. AITKEN
MRC Reproductive Biology Unit, 37 Chalmers Street, Edinburgh EH3 9EW, UK

S. AL-HASANI
Department of Obstetrics & Gynaecology, Medical University of Lubeck, Ratzeburger Alle 160, D-23538, Lubeck, Germany

C. R. AUSTIN
47 Dixon Road, Buderim, Qld 4558, Australia

D. T. BAIRD
Department of Obstetrics & Gynaecology, 37 Chalmers Street, Edinburgh EH3 9EW, UK

M. BOWNES
Institute of Cell & Molecular Biology, University of Edinburgh, Edinburgh EH3 9EW, UK

M. BRÄNNSTRÖM
Department of Obstetrics & Gynaecology, University of Götenborg, Sweden

H. B. CROXATTO
Laboratorio de Endocrinologia, Facultad de Ciencias Biologicas, Universitad Catolica de Chile, Casilla 114-D, Santiago, Chile

K. DIEDRICH
Department of Gynaecology & Obstetrics, Medical University of Lubeck, Ratzeburger Allee 160, D-23538, Lubeck, Germany

S. M. DOWNS
Department of Biology, Marquette University, 530 N. 15th Street, Milwaukee WI 52233, USA

R. G. GOSDEN
Division of Obstetrics & Gynaecology, University of Leeds School of Medicine, D floor, Clarendon Wing (LGI), Belmont Grove, Leeds LS2 9NS, UK.

J. G. GRUDZINSKAS
Department of Obstetrics & Gynaecology, Holland Wing, The Royal London Hospital, London E1 1BA, UK

R. HOMBURG
9 Hatomer Street, Ramat Ilan, Givat Schmuel, 51905, Israel

M. G. R. HULL
Dept Obstetrics & Gynaecology, Bristol Maternity Hospital, Southwell Street, Bristol BS2 8EG, UK

R. P. S JANSEN
Sydney IVF, 187 Macquarie Street, Sydney, NSW 2000, Australia

P. O. JANSON
Department of Obstetrics & Gynaecology, University of Götenborg, Sweden

W. L. LEDGER
Nuffield Department of Obstetrics & Gynaecology, John Radcliffe Hospital, Oxford OX3 9DU, UK

C. NAVARA
Department of Zoology, University of Wisconsin-Madison, 1117 West Johnson Street, Madison, WI 53706, USA

M. PATERSON
MRC Reproductive Biology Unit, 37 Chalmers Street, Edinburgh EH3 9EW, UK

M. PLACHOT
Laboratoire de Fecondation *In Vitro* de la Biologie de la Reproduction, Hôpital Necker, Paris, France

G. SCHATTEN
Department of Zoology, University of Wisconsin-Madison, 1117 West Johnson Street, Madison, WI 53706, USA

M. T. SEPPÄLÄ
Department of Obstetrics & Gynaecology, Helsinki University Central Hospital, Haarthaninkatu 2, Helsinki SF-00290, Finland

M. SHELEF
Infertility Unit, Golda Medical Centre, Petah Tikva 49372, Israel

C. SIMERLY
Department of Zoology, University of Wisconson-Madison, 1117 West Johnson Street, Madison, WI 53707, USA

J. L. SIMPSON
Department of Obstetrics & Gynaecology, Baylor College of Medicine, One Baylor Plaza, Houston, Texas, 77030-3498, USA

M. VILLALÓN
Unidad de Reproduccion y Dessarrollo, Facultad de Ciencas Biologicas, P. Universitad Catolica de Chile, Casilla 114-D, Santiago, Chile

G.-J. WU
Department of Zoology, University of Wisconsin-Madison, 1117 West Johnson Street, Madison, WI 53706, USA. *Present address*: Department of Obstetrics & Gynaecology, No. 8, 3rd Sec. Ting-Chou Road, Taipei, Taiwan 100

J. L. YOVICH
PIVET Medical Centre, 166 Cambridge Street, Leederville, Perth, W. Australia 6007

1

Evolution of human gametes–oocytes

C. R. AUSTIN

Evolution in outline

Remarkably enough, fossil relics of pre-metazoan unicellular life are recognizable as far back as the period between 3900 and 3400 Myr (million years ago) (Strother, 1989). Though their systematic status is unknown, the spheres and filaments that are visible in the rocks are thought to be the remains of prokaryotes, which would have required the support of firm cell walls, and in some instances these organisms could have been cyanobacteria. Undoubted stomatolite remains date from about 3000 Myr, and many more instances of presumed early organisms, including eukaryotes, are evidenced from about 1500 Myr onwards. Consistently with this estimate, de Duve (1991) maintains that the transition from prokaryote to eukaryote must have taken about 2000 Myr. Representatives of most invertebrate phyla were already established by the start of the Cambrian era 1600 Myr, and pre-Cambrian rocks were subjected to such temperatures and pressures that useful fossil evidence of complex organisms there is scarce (Table 1).

Modern blue-green algae, similar to those responsible for stromatolite formations, reproduce asexually by means of spores, as well as sexually with ciliated gametes, but there does not appear to be evidence relating to gametes of any kind in the fossil record; of course, it is quite possible that multiplication in the early forms took place without the involvement of gametes. Consequently (as with 'Evolution of human gametes – spermatozoa' in 'The Spermatozoon'), the course of evolution of eggs or macrogametes of man and other species must be inferred from the taxonomic relationships of whole organisms, as revealed in fossil relics or by the detailed study of existing forms.

Valentine & Erwin (1987) proposed that the impressive Cambrian 'explosion' in animal forms was possible because the genetic programme of animals was then more flexible. As evolution proceeded, successful genetic sequences became 'locked in', so that the possibilities of change progressively diminished. However,

Table 1. *Evolution in outline* (approximate dates for the first
appearance of many living forms)

(Earth began	4500 Myr)
Prokaryotes	3900–3400
Invertebrates	3400–1500
Stromatolites	3000
Plant life	2500
Eukaryotes	1500
First vertebrates	500–600
Tetrapods	425
Amphibians	370
Reptiles	320
Mammals (primitive)	220
Mammals (modern groups)	150
Primates	65
(Extinction of dinosaurs and radiation of mammals)	64
Primitive apes (*Propliopithecus*)	38–24
Primate radiation	26–7
Hominidae	15–5
Australopithecus afarensis	4
Homo erectus	3–1.5
'African Eve'	0.2

this situation could be changed dramatically by major catastrophies, and the mass extinction which terminated the era of the dinosaurs about 64 Myr allowed reptiles, birds and mammals to radiate. Ohno (1985) has argued much along the same lines, namely that evolution is, in effect, 'a continuous series of irrevocable commitments', the first of which was the adoption of three base triplets as codons for protein synthesis. Each new commitment reduced the range of future possibilities, and so variation became increasingly restricted, and progressively each apparent innovation is in fact attributable to a modified gene. With something of the order of 150 000 genes in mammals, and the prospects of interactions between genes and between their induced characters, the possible range of responses would be sufficient to account for the remarkable diversity of animal and plant life.

As to the origins of man himself, the evidence is really quite abundant (see, for example, Campbell, 1979). The first identifiable primates (admittedly recognizable from evidence of continuity rather than morphology) are represented by fossils found in strata dating back to the start of the Tertiary period, about 65 Myr. More abundant relics occur in the Paleocene (65–54 Myr), some 60 genera being recognized, grouped in eight families (the three most primitive genera were rodent-like and later became extinct). Approaching 38 Myr, the fossils represent more advanced forms, resembling contemporary lemurs and tarsiers. During the Oligocene (38–26 Myr), primitive monkey forms are recognizable and some very primitive apes, labelled *Parapithecus*. More distinctive forerunners of apes were *Aelopithecus*, an ancestral gibbon, and *Aegyptopithecus* phyletic to modern great apes. There was also *Propliopithecus* which was possibly ancestral to the hominids. During the Miocene (26 Myr to as recently as 7 Myr), the fossil record reveals 50 species in 20 genera of large primates, including *Dryopithecus fontani*, a species of large ape that was notably numerous. Also relatively abundant among the Miocene relics are entities classed as *Hominidae*, which separated from the ape stock between 15 and 5 Myr. Notable members of this group were *Ramapithecus* and *Kenyapithecus*. Then, about 4 Myr, the Australopithecine series began, exhibiting the highly significant innovation of erect stance and bipedal progression; the earliest representative was *A. afarensis*, of which an unusually complete collection of bones has been made. Finally, the apparent forerunner of modern man emerged in the form of *Homo erectus*, between 3 and 1.5 Myr, the bones being accompanied by crude stone tools.

Modern biochemical technology has produced a large body of evidence that is broadly confirmatory of the archaeological data. Thus the indications from amino acid sequencing, restriction mapping of mitochondrial DNA, sequencing of mitochondrial and genomic DNA and analysis of the globin gene complex all put the period of separation of human and chimpanzee stocks at between 5 and 10 Myr.

The most recent advancement for the human race could have resulted from the acquisition of the power of speech, and there are reasons to believe that this occurred in a group of Australopithecines in Africa about 200 000 years ago. The evidence rests on analyses that have been made of mitochondrial DNA in 147 living individuals from five geographic populations, the results being interpreted to show this time and place of the probable common origin (Cann, Stoneking & Wilson, 1987).

Diverse ways of multiplying

Quite an impressive variety of methods is employed by living organisms to multiply their kind (or by man to multiply other creatures) and a number of these is set out in Table 2. The first four systems listed do not involve gametes, but are included here as they could well represent procedures that were preliminary to the evolution of gametes. In many instances, species depend on more than one method (as, for example, both sexual reproduction and 'identical' twinning

Table 2. *Reproductive strategies*

	Description	Species
Binary fission	Whole-body division into two parts	Protozoa to identical twinning in mammals
Multiple fission	Whole-body division into many parts	Protozoa to identical twinning in mammals
Autogamy	Twin daughter cells unite	Protozoa, e.g., *Actinophrys sol*
Endogamy	Union of descendants of one cell after several divisions	Protozoa, e.g. *Paramecium aurelia*
Syngamy	Union of specialized sex cells after meiosis	
	(a) Union in the same individual	*Dicyema* and other hermaphrodites, e.g. *Serranus, Sagus*
	(b) Union in different individuals	Mammals and others
Parthenogenesis		
Cyclical	Parthenogenesis and sexual reproduction alternating	Rotifers, aphids, *Daphnia*
Arrhenotoky	Production of haploid males (ameiotic)	*Hymenoptera,* turkeys
Thelytoky		
Apomictic	Production of haploid females (ameiotic)	Cockroaches, *Pyknocelis*
Automictic	Ditto but with meiosis and fusion of nuclei	*Lacerta* and *Cnemidophorus* spp.
Deuterotoky (or amphitoky)	Production of both sexes without mating but with meiosis	
Gynogenesis	Females produce young after mating but without syngamy	*Poecilia* (Amazon molly) and *Poeciliopsis*
Androgenesis	*Development with only paternal chromosomes*	
	Experimental:	Various animals
	Natural:	Human hydatidiform mole
Paedogenesis	Reproduction by larvae within mother	Gall flies, midges
Artificial	Development from eggs stimulated by heat, cold, acid, needle prick, etc.	Frogs, fish etc.

by man), but for conciseness not all of the possible combinations are shown in the Table.

Multiplication by whole-body fission

The simplest way organisms can multiply is by whole-body subdivision, i.e. 'binary' or 'multiple fission', most evident in the Protista. Binary fission involves cleavage into two parts immediately after mitosis, whereas in multiple fission the nucleus commonly divides several times within the cell body, and the cytoplasm fragments terminally. Many Protozoa maintain continuity and increase for long periods by means of a series of mitotic cell divisions; the method is highly efficient, with every member involved directly in multiplication, but it perpetuates uniformity, unless mutations occur, and the resulting population is deficient in the genetic diversity that allows selection and adaptation to changing circumstances. Multiple fission in Protozoa is well illustrated in the life cycle of the malarial parasite *Plasmodium vivax*, which displays 'sporogony' on the gut wall in the mosquito and 'schizogony' in the liver of the human host; this is in addition to sexual reproduction involving meiosis, with the formation of micro- and macrogametes, within the gut of the mosquito.

Multiplication by fission also occurs in the 'vegetative reproduction' of Metazoa, well illustrated by sea anemones which may detach small portions of the body while moving across rock surfaces, these portions then developing into new adult forms, or the anemones may simply divide themselves into two individuals. Not only coelenterates but also some echinoderms employ this method. Alternatively, multiplication in the Metazoa may take place by budding, as seen in bryozoans, coelenterates, polychaets, cestodes and ascidians; groups of cells assemble and grow rather like a neoplasm in the body of the host, and then become separated to found a new individual. An allied process is that of *Polyembryony*, in which an embryo arising from a single fertilized egg can subdivide, giving rise to two or more embryos. The process is exploited by the liver fluke, *Fasciola hepatica*: fertilized eggs hatch into miracidia which metamorphose into sporocysts in the pond snail. Within the sporocysts develop many rediae by polyembryony and these produce further rediae over several generations, finally becoming cercariae which leave the pond snail and reinfect the sheep. Polyembryony is also to be seen in certain parasitic hymenoptera, where a fertilized egg may divide to produce 100 + progeny. Finally, the process identified as 'identical twinning' is well known in the human subject, where the Dionne quins could still hold the record for the number surviving to adulthood, and also in armadillos: *Dasypus novemcinctus* regularly produces litters of identical quadruplets, while *Dasypus hybridus* can achieve litters of eight to twelve identical young.

A system allowing much greater variation and adaptation than multiple fission is sexual reproduction, in which organisms produce gametes, small aliquots of their genetic information, and new organisms arise from the union of these.

The emergence of gametes in evolution

Gametes are essentially packets of chromosomes, and a basic tenet in the theory of evolution is that chromosomes play the primary role in this process, since they carry the great majority of the genes and these, in turn, specify virtually all somatic characters. Chromosomes, though commonly depicted as stable structures, are in fact moderately fragile, being prone to breakage and random repair, so that genes can become displaced on the same chromosome or exchanged for genes on other chromosomes or lost altogether. Genes have specific molecular configurations but they too are liable to undergo structural changes ('mutations'), with resultant alterations to the specified characters. The great majority of such mutations are deleterious ('non-adaptive') and generally fail to be conserved in the population, their removal depending on the process of natural selection.

A regular feature of populations is genetic polymorphism, the predominant characteristics shown being dependent upon the frequency with which the genes appear. In small populations, gene frequency may change through 'genetic drift', seen as a progressive change in expressed characters throughout the group (Bodmer & Cavalli-Sforza, 1976). The transfer of genes between individuals can occur in several ways, including autogamy, endogamy, transduction, transformation, and syngamy.

Autogamy

Autogamy is seen, for example, in the protozoan *Actinophrys sol*, when after a succession of mitotic cell divisions, it builds a wall around itself thus forming a cyst. In this, it divides into two, and each new cell undergoes *meiotic* divisions, whereby half the chromosomes in each cell are discarded. The two cells then reunite and their nuclei fuse into a single nucleus; the organism emerges from the cyst, apparently refreshed by its experience, and resumes its multiplication by mitosis. The manoeuvre is thought to involve a 'shuffling' of the genes, the new relationships conferring some benefit. Autogamy has also an intriguing feature, namely that when the two *Actinophrys* cells reunite they do not simply fuse, but one cell *actively invades* the other in a manner vaguely prophetic of sperm–egg union. Certain other protozoa have the same suggestive pattern of behaviour, and the participating cells could be regarded as actual forerunners of the gametes, from the evolutionary point of view; the phenomenon is similar to 'hologamy' (discussed later under 'Sexual reproduction').

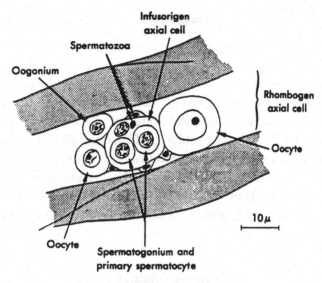

Fig. 1. Gametogenesis and fertilization in the mesozoan *Dicyaema*, which is a self-fertilizing hermaphrodite. (From Austin, 1965.)

Endogamy

Endogamy is exhibited by, for example, another protozoan *Paramecium aurelia*. After only a few mitotic divisions, pairs of cells among the descendants of a single cell may conjugate, undergo meiosis and then take part once more in a series of mitotic divisions. As with autogamy, the benefit is thought to arise from the reassortment of genes. Much the same process is seen in the self-fertilization of higher plants and of mesozoan and metazoan hermaphrodites.

The mesozoan *Dicyaema* (Fig. 1), which is a parasite of cephalopod kidneys, is made up of several cells but has no body cavity; its core consists of a long 'rhombogen axial cell' and this is surrounded by a single layer of ciliated surface cells. Within the rhombogen axial cell is an 'infusorigen axial cell', and within this again a spermatogonium cell produces spermatocytes, which in due course become amoeboid spermatozoa. When mature, these escape from the infusorigen axial cell and fertilize oocytes that have been produced by an oogonium cell resident in the rhombogen axial cell. After the resulting zygote has undergone several divisions, it makes its way out of the mother organism to proceed with independent existence.

Many metazoan species have a bar to self-fertilization, but it does occur in certain cestodes, nematodes and molluscs. Self-fertilization can presumably happen even in some vertebrates, notably teleost fish in the genera *Serranus* and *Sagus*, which shed male and female gametes simultaneously.

Transduction

Transduction takes place through the carriage of genomic DNA by bacterium, virus or plasmid. This is best known as an experimental procedure in genetic engineering, but viruses (bacteriophages) can certainly pass fragments of DNA between their bacterial victims; should the new victim survive, the foreign DNA becomes lodged in the new genome and expressed in the owner. The effect can be produced artificially by adding to cultures of bacteria cell-free extracts of other bacteria possessing distinguishable characteristics, when the recipients come to express heritable features of the donor. This variation is identified as *transformation*, and there is evidence that it can occur naturally, the death and lysis of a bacterium freeing fragments of DNA that are taken up and expressed by other bacteria.

Syngamy (fertilization)

This is distinguished from the other processes just described chiefly by the fact that it involves the orderly union of balanced quanta of DNA from two separate individuals, but otherwise there is no hard and fast line of demarcation.

Gametogenesis in animals

Weismall (1887; see Wilson, 1928) first established that, for gamete production, there would need to be a specific mechanism inducing a reduction in chromosome number, and the reduction had, of course, to be exactly half the original number, a state to be compensated for by union of the gametes. In addition, it came to be appreciated that the chromosomes must exist in homologous pairs, so that union of gametes would restore the chromosome complement appropriately.

In relatively simple organisms like *Parascaris equorum*, the origin of the gametes is demonstrable through a difference in chromosomal material: one of the four cells formed by the second cleavage division of the fertilized egg retains its chromosome complement intact, while in the other three cells a large part of each chromosome passes into the cytoplasm and breaks up (e.g. Wilson, 1928). At the third cleavage division, the first cell divides and one of its daughter cells shows the distinctive 'chromatin diminution' but not the other, nor do the remaining cells; the process is repeated at the fourth cleavage division. Thus one cell stands out alone as having an intact chromosome complement: it is from this cell that the *primordial germ cells* will eventually develop. The factor responsible for preserving the integrity of this cell is identified as the 'germ-cell determinant', and in many eggs its presence can be inferred from the existence of certain deeply-staining granules in the vegetal cytoplasm. Similar events have been described in the eggs of scyphozoans, chaetognaths, rotifers, insects, crustaceans and amphibians. The behaviour of the germ-cell determinant gives support to the 'germ-plasm' theory, which was put forward towards the end of the last century. This held that the germ cells are not really the products of the parent body but share an origin with it from a preceding germ cell, and because a clear distinction between germ cells and somatic cells is generally difficult to draw, emphasis was placed rather on a specifically organized 'germ-plasm' which is transmitted from generation to generation (Wilson, 1928).

In mammals, primordial germ cells first become recognizable in an extra-embryonic location, namely the posterior yolk-sac endoderm of the early embryo (at about the 24th day in the human subject), and they migrate in amoeboid fashion from here through the connective tissue of the hind gut into the gut mesentery, and then, passing close to the developing kidneys, congregate in the genital ridges which represent the gonadal primordia (Byskov, 1982). Observations of germ cells *in vitro* suggest that their migration is guided chemotactically. When first recognizable, the germ cells number rather less than 100, but they multiply rapidly during transit, and after final congregation. (In birds, many more germ cells reach the left gonad than the right, consistently with the left ovary normally being the sole functional entity throughout the life of the bird.) Anomalies too can arise: for some germ cells, migration is faulty and small regions of accessory gonadal tissue may later be found; in certain chromosomal disorders the germ cells may all degenerate, the loss underlying states of sterility. The cells may also migrate into blood vessels and so be carried to anomalous regions, or in the cases where fusion has occurred between the placental blood vessels of non-identical twins, such migration may underlie cases of germ-cell chimaerism.

During fetal life, the germ cells in the embryonic ovaries, now called oogonia, multiply dramatically, reaching a peak in the human subject of around 7 million at about the fifth month of pregnancy (Baker, 1982). Thereafter, the number falls equally dramatically, so that by the time of birth there are generally rather less than 2 million. During the latter part of prenatal life, the oogonia enter upon the prophase of the first meiotic division (thus becoming primary oocytes) and this change ends their capacity for division. After birth, and especially after puberty, the primary oocytes grow in size. In some species (dog, fox), ovulation takes place at this stage and sperm penetration may occur; in others (most mammals), the first meiotic division precedes ovulation, and sperm penetration is thus into the secondary oocyte; fertilization follows with the egg emitting the second polar body and becoming an ootid. Cleavage of the egg at the end of fertilization marks the start of embryonic life. In the first meiotic division, chromosome pairs are formed (maternal and paternal) and portions of some chromosomes are exchanged between pairs; with separation of the two sets of chromosomes, the total number is halved (diploid to haploid), hence the first meiotic division is known as the reduction division. One group of now modified chromosomes passes into the first polar body leaving the egg in a haploid condition, and the other group proceeds to undergo the second meiotic division. This is 'equational', so the ploidy of the egg is unaffected. With fertilization by a similarly haploidized sperm, the normal diploid state is restored. Meiosis like fertilization is a process of great antiquity, and may have been employed by blue-green algae which are thought to have originated about 3000 Myr.

Throughout post-natal life, the number of oocytes steadily decreases through atresia and, after the menarche, through ovulation as well. Their final disappearance marks the time of menopause.

Parthenogenesis

A serious drawback to multiplication by an unbroken series of ameiotic cell divisions (i.e. involving only mitosis and so without gene-shuffling) is the resulting genetic uniformity which is highly prejudicial to the prospects of change by natural selection, and species practising such a method live in serious risk of extinction. This problem is partially remedied by the inclusion of meiosis with its gene-shuffling feature of 'crossing-over' and this addition is seen in diploid parthenogenesis, which has the virtue that all members of the population can take part in maintaining the race (this and other features of parthenogenesis are discussed helpfully by Maynard Smith, 1978). Parthenogenesis is found in rudimentary or fully developed form in many groups of animals, including coelenterates, rotifers, platyhelminths, nematodes, annelids, molluscs, crustaceans, myriapods, insects, arachnids, fishes, amphibians, birds, and mammals. In rotifers, water fleas, aphids and gall wasps, cyclic parthenogenesis is common, a sexual generation being included in a series of parthenogenetic generations. Among the vertebrates, there are about 30 races of lizards that reproduce parthenogenetically (Maslin 1971), also the bony fish *Poecilia* and *Poeciliopsis* and the salamander *Ambystoma* (Cuellar, 1974).

Parthenogenesis is manifest in angiosperms, such as *Alchemilla, Thalictrum, Taraxacum* and *Hieracium*; almost always, it occurs in the 'egg-cells' which differ from the female gamete by being diploid. The process is known as 'apogamy', another form of which involves development from various other cells of the megaspore. Parthenogenesis also occurs in algae that exhibit isogamy or anisogamy.

Development by parthenogenesis may lead to the production of males (arrhenotoky) or females (thelytoky) or both (deuterotoky or amphotoky). *Apis*, and most of the Hymenoptera that have arrhenotoky in addition to the sexual production of females, have the advantage that the species enjoy the long-term evolutionary benefit of sex, with its components of paedogenesis or of obligate, cyclic or facultative parthenogenesis. Paedogenesis is seen in gall flies and midges: under appropriate circumstances, germ cells within *larvae* undergo precocious maturation, without meiosis, and develop into larvae that parasitize and consume the mother larva. While conditions remain favourable, successive generations of paedogenetic larvae are produced, each consuming its mother, but eventually larvae of a new kind are formed and these, after pupating, develop into adult male and female gall flies (White, 1954).

Parthenogenesis (in the form of 'gynogenesis', development from eggs penetrated by sperms but not fertilized) has been successfully induced in trout and salmon (Refstie, 1983). When selected for in the turkey, in which the male is the homogametic sex, diploid parthenogenesis can proceed to the birth of fully viable males (Olsen, 1965). The situation with mammals is quite different. Despite the fact that the early stages of embryonic development appear to be proceeding normally, and that chimaeras between parthenogenetic and fertilized embryos develop to term (Surani, Barton & Kaufman, 1977), there is no certain evidence that far-going mammalian parthenogenesis is possible, despite very many observations and attempts at experimental induction (Barton *et al.*, 1985; Surani, Barton & Norris, 1987). The current conviction is that normal development in mammals requires *both* male and female contributions, but *only one* of each, the controlling mechanism depending upon 'genome imprinting' (Surani *et al.*, 1990). Little is known about the actual change(s) involved in imprinting, but the result is a functional difference in the homologous regions of the maternal and paternal chromosomes. Catternach (1986) has assembled evidence showing that anomalies of development are highly likely to occur if one parent is the sole source of genetic material.

Sexual reproduction

In many single-celled organisms, the gametes differ little in size or structure from the adult form; this state is known as hologamy (which resembles autogamy', discussed earlier under 'The emergence of gametes in evolution'). Other members of the Protista have both macro- and microgametes, a relationship referred to as anisogamy where the differences are small, and heterogamy where they are large. In species, such as *Chlamydomonas*, some strains show isogamy (structurally identical male and female gametes) and others anisogamy. Where heterogamy exists, the microgamete is usually motile; an exception occurs in the gregarine

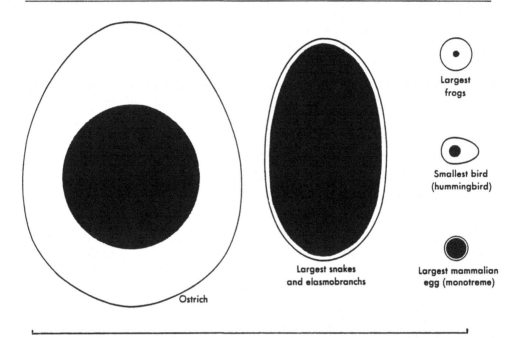

Fig. 2. Relative sizes of the largest eggs, mostly those of non-mammals. The largest known egg (9.5 inches long) was that of the extinct flightless bird *Aepyornis*; its relative length is indicated by the horizontal line. (Based on Fig. 3.11 in Austin, 1965.)

Stylocephalus, which has a motile megagamete, Even with isogamy, there is evidence of functional differences between the cells.

Egg, macrogamete, ovum

In mosses and ferns, the female gametophyte contains an archigonium, a cell in the centre corresponding to the egg. In higher plants, the gametophyte and archigonium are much reduced, and the egg comes to be represented by a single nucleus within the embryo sac; the developing embryos depend upon nutrients stored in endosperm or cotyledons.

Moving to more complex organisms, one encounters an impressive increase in size among the macrogametes (Figs. 2, 3 and 4), though they in no way match the microgametes in complexity of structure and function. The size of macrogamates is due chiefly to the quantity of stored yolk or nutrient material, the relative amount reflecting the duration of nutritionally independent existence of the embryonic organism. Eggs with little or much yolk are referred to, respectively, as microlecithal and megalecithal. Microlecithal eggs yield embryos

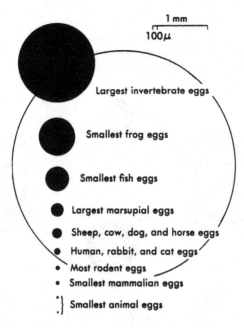

1 mm

100μ

Largest invertebrate eggs

Smallest frog eggs

Smallest fish eggs

Largest marsupial eggs

Sheep, cow, dog, and horse eggs

Human, rabbit, and cat eggs

Most rodent eggs

Smallest mammalian eggs

} Smallest animal eggs

Fig. 3. Relative sizes of the smallest eggs. The outline represents the monotreme egg. (From Austin, 1976.)

that must rapidly develop to an active food-seeking larval stage (insects, tunicates, marine invertebrates, etc.), or become parasitic on the maternal organism, as in mammals and some teleost fish, elasmobranchs, amphibia and coelenterates. In the megalecithal eggs of reptiles, birds and monotremes, a layer of albumen surrounds the yolk, providing protection and additional nutritive material; this layer is small in reptiles and virtually absent in snakes. Species with megalecithal eggs (with the exception of the monotremes) can be said to represent a stock that is evolutionarily separate from that of the mammals. The largest bird eggs known (24 cm in length and found only as fossils), belong to *Aepyornis titan*, a bird that exceeded 4 metres in height, which finally became extinct about 500 years ago.

Animal eggs differ as to the stage of maturation at which fertilization begins (Table 3), and in this there appears to be a complete lack of correlation with systematic status, with mesozoans opting for the same stage (the mature primary oocyte) as the dog and fox, and most of the remaining mammals that have been investigated sharing the second metaphase with *Amphioxus*.

The mammalian egg

As already indicated, the mammalian egg differs in size and form quite strikingly among the three subclasses Prototheira, Metatheria and Eutheria (Figs. 2, 3 and

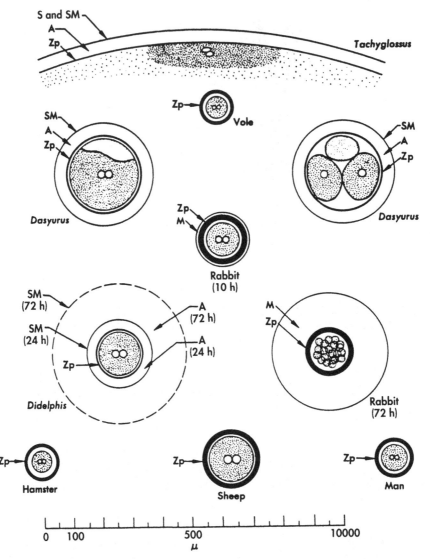

Fig. 4. Major features of mammalian eggs. A, albumin layer; M, mucoid coat; S and Sm, shell and shell membrane; Zp, zona pellucida. The times given represent periods after ovulation. (From Austin & Amoroso, 1959.)

4); background information on this subject can be found in the publications by Austin & Walton (1960), Austin (1961), Blandau (1961), Pincus (1936) and Thibault (1969). The Prototheria (Monotremata) are the most distinctively different among the mammals, and are, in fact, thought to have evolved from a separate reptilian order from that leading to the other two subclasses, the separation occurring about 175 Myr. Certainly, their reproductive method is unique. Both the echidna

Table 3. *Stages of egg maturation at which sperm penetration occurs*

Young primary oocyte	Fully grown primary oocyte	First metaphase	Second metaphase	Female pronucleus
Platyhelminthes *Otomesostoma*	Mesozoa *Dicyema*	Nemertia *Cerebratulus*	Cephalocordata *Amphioxus*	Coelenterata *Actinaria*
Annelida *Dinophilus*	Phasmidia *Ascaris*	Mollusca *Dentallium*	Amphibia *Siredon*	Echinodermata *Echinus Asterias*, etc.
Polychaeta *Histriobdella*	Mollusca *Spisula*	Polychaeta *Chaetopterus*	Mammalia most species	
Onycophera *Peripetopsis*	Polychaeta *Myzostoma*	Polychaeta *Pectinaria*		
Annelida *Saccocirrus*	Polychaeta *Nereis*	Many insects		
	Echiura *Thalassema*			
	Mammalia Dog and fox			

Tachyglossus aculeatus and the platypus *Ornithorhynchus anatinus* lay relatively large 1.7×1.4 cm eggs, with a yolk body around 4 cm in diameter. As in the bird egg, the yolk is surrounded by a broad layer of albumen, limited by a plasma membrane, the whole enclosed by shell membrane and shell. In addition, the yolk body becomes enclosed early in follicular development by a distinctive mammalian membrane, the zona pellucida, which is very thin in the Prototheria and increasingly robust in the Metatheria and Eutheria. The zona has attracted a good deal of research attention, some of which is discussed below. The eggs of Metatheria are similar to those of Eutheria, though of generally larger size, with diameters in the nine species listed by Tyndale-Biscoe & Renfree (1987) ranging from $113–250\,\mu m$; the eutherian range by contrast is roughly $60–180\,\mu m$ (Austin, 1961). The eggs of marsupials, however, resemble those of monotremes by having a mucoid layer and shell membrane deposited in the oviduct; additionally, though, the monotreme egg acquires a leathery shell. Exceptions also occur in the Eutheria with rabbit and hare eggs for they, apparently uniquely, accumulate a broad mucoid layer during their passage through the oviduct.

There are distinctive and unusual features of metatherian and eutherian eggs (and sperms) in relation to fertilization because of the presence of the zona pellucida with its unique properties (see Timmons, Skinner & Dunbar, 1990, Dunbar & Rand, 1991) and because it evidently poses a significant barrier against the entry of the sperm, and so is associated with major new developments in the structure and properties of the eutherian sperm head (Bedford, 1990, 1991). Bedford (1983) points out that the zona pellucida seems to be an unusually resistant membrane, requiring the sperm to have a highly indurated nucleus and a stabilized inner acrosome membrane to enable sperm entry by the characteristic 'slicing' action shown during the process of zona penetration. Toughness of the zona seems to be achieved by the cross-linking of free thiols in its cystine-rich protamine component (Calvin & Bedford, 1971). In order to expose the acrosome, the sperm must undergo capacitation and the acrosome reaction (in common with the sperms of a few non-mammalian species, see companion paper on 'Evolution of human gametes–spermatozoa'), the former process depending on entry of calcium ions from the medium; in invertebrates, by contrast, acrosome exposure is evoked by substances deriving from the egg coatings. Zona penetration apparently requires also the additional force derived from 'hyperactivation' in the mammalian sperm. The unique features of the mammalian sperm head have their consequences, in that the stabilized inner acrosome membrane evidently requires both its separate engulfment by the egg cortex and sperm–egg fusion at a novel site on the sperm head, namely the equatorial segment. Finally, the sperm is taken into the vitellus in a singular manner, with membrane fusion and a phagocytic response by the oocyte. Overall, for sperm entry into the eutherian egg, it would seem that physical forces are more important than in other groups.

The human egg is relatively undistinguished among the primate eggs, except for minor differences in size, and under laboratory conditions exhibits properties similar, in many respects, to those of mouse and hamster eggs.

Is fertilization specificity advantageous through maintaining species integrity?

According to Yanagimachi (1977), neither capacitation nor the acrosome reaction represent truly specific responses to unique stimuli, but the interaction between the sperm and the zona surface does appear to be highly species specific, resembling an antigen–antibody reaction. Penetration of the zona pellucida, which is assisted by the sperm's zona lysin, evidently requires something like a lock-and-key relationship, with appropriate physical and chemical compatibilities. After completion of the 'zona reaction', sperm penetration of the zona is essentially precluded (Braden, Austin & David, 1954). By contrast, fusion between the sperm head and the vitelline surface is a more general kind of reaction, for sperms can fuse with the eggs of some other species, though this capability varies rather

Table 4. *Species of which the sperms were reported to be capable of penetrating the zona-free eggs of other species*

	Zona-free eggs					
Spermatozoa	Golden hamster	Chinese hamster	Mouse	Rat	Guinea pig	Rabbit
Golden hamster	+	–	±	±	+	–
Chinese hamster		+				
Mouse	+		+	+	+	+
Deer mouse	+		–	–		
Rat	+		±	+		+
Guinea pig	+		–	–	+	–
Rabbit	+					+
Dog	–					
Bat, dolphin, pig, bull, goat, horse, marmoset, monkey	+					
Human	+	–	–	–	–	

+ = yes; – = no; ± = opinions divided.
Data from Yanagimachi, 1984.

unpredictably (Table 4) (Yanagimachi, 1984). Even fusion with somatic cells under the appropriate conditions has been observed (Austin, 1959, Austin & Bishop, 1959, Austin & Walton, 1960). A lack of strict specificity is also seen in the transformation of sperm nuclei into male pronuclei and the subsequent events leading to the first cleavage division: zona-free hamster oocytes fertilized by human sperms proceed through the pronuclear phase to the two-cell stage in an apparently normal manner (Yanagimachi, 1984). Investigation into the possibility of further development could incur ethical censure.

The mechanisms that are generally recognized to ensure species integrity include several *in addition to* fertilization specificity, namely:

Geographical location. Species live in different areas separated by sufficiently formidable barriers, such as mountain ranges, wide rivers, and seas.
Ecology. Though potential mates occupy the same geographical area, they frequent different habitats and so generally do not meet.
Season. The periods of sexual activity differ and the times of receptivity do not coincide.

Anatomy. The structure of the sexual organs is such that there are difficulties in performing coitus. In many instances there is an actual aversion between the sexes.

The prospects for hybridization

Hybridization fails because of faults in embryonic or post-natal development. Some investigation of the mechanism of failure of hybridization was made by Chang & Hancock (1967), who found that attempted crosses between rabbit and hare, goat and sheep, and ferret and mink were all sterile. There were some curious differences in the details, depending on which species were chosen as sire or dam. Thus, if rabbits were inseminated with hare semen, all eggs were generally fertilized, but with the reciprocal cross very few eggs were fertilized, and essentially the same kind of result was obtained with attempted crosses between goat and sheep. The points at which embryonic development failed also differed. Thus, with the rabbit and hare cross, development did not proceed past the blastocyst stage. Ferret–mink hybrid embryos did not survive past the 23rd day, and those from the goat–sheep cross not longer than about 6 weeks. Gray (1954) lists a large number of instances in which hybrid pregnancies failed to go to term, or the progeny were born dead, or the young hybrids survived for only a few days or, at most, weeks.

Nevertheless, many hybrids do survive and may even surpass their parents in productivity and vitality, this effect being termed 'hybrid vigour' or 'heterosis', notable examples being the mule (by she-ass out of mare) and hinny (by stallion out of she-ass). Among the survivors, the more remarkable are the products of *intergeneric* crosses. Marshall (1922) mentions as examples of these the hybrids between the cow (*Bos taurus*) and representatives of four other genera, namely the yak (*Bibos grunnicus*), the gaur (*Bibos gaurus*), the gayal (*Bibos frontalis*) and the bison (*Bison americanus*). Much more detail is offered by Gray (1954), who lists records of hybrids, including those between different *genera* of mammals; just in monkeys of the Cercopithecidae and Cebidae, she gave 14 authenticated instances, the progeny surviving from 1–22 months.

Successful hybrids could, of course, serve to initiate new species, but as Bodmer and Cavalli-Svorza (1976) point out, speciation is a long and complex process and depends heavily on isolation between various groups of the original species; speciation can also result from selective adaptation and genetic drift with random accumulation of mutations. In their view, it could take something like a million years for two isolated groups of a species to pass from inter-fertility to inter-sterility. In this connection, the characteristics of the 'naked mole rats' of the genus *Spalacinae* are of interest. Colonies of these animals inhabit complex burrows in the desert regions of the Middle East, each colony being sufficiently isolated to have achieved such genetic uniformity as would require 60 generations of inbreeding (Young, 1990). In some instances, attempted breeding between members of different colonies is sterile, suggesting the start of separate subspecies, Such 'assortive mating' can lead to 'sympatric speciation' (Partridge, 1983).

Summary and conclusions

1. The earliest evidence of life on Earth is believed to be provided by certain microscopic spheres and filaments found in cherts and similar quartz-like minerals dated at 3900–3400 Myr. Undoubted stromatolite remains have persisted from about 3000 Myr. No sign of gametes has yet been reported among these relics, but early forms of multiplication may have been asexual.

2. The earliest evidence of small primate-like species is dated at about 65 Myr, becoming more abundant and ape-like later.

3. Genomic and mitochondrial DNA sequencing, restriction mapping of mitochondrial DNA, DNA hybridization and amino acid sequencing all support the time of separation of human and chimpanzee stocks at between 10 and 5 Myr.

4. An important milestone was *Australopithecus afarensis* which lived about 4 Myr and provided the first evidence of an erect posture and bipedal mode of progression, though the skull and jaw closely resembled those of apes. A more distant forerunner of modern man appears to have been *Homo erectus* at 3.0–1.5 Myr.

5. The simplest way organisms can multiply is by whole-body fission, as practised by the Protista. Rather surprisingly, it also occurs in many Metazoa, including mammals, in the form of polyembryony or identical twinning.

6. Gametes are, in effect, packets of genes arranged on chromosomes, which underlie the process of heredity and thus the progress of evolution. Both chromosomes and genes are prone to structural changes that produce mutations; these are mostly deleterious and commonly removed by natural selection.

7. Genes can be passed from one individual to another in several different ways, but the union of gametes appears to be the most orderly method.

8. Gametes derive from primordial germ cells, which are identifiable early in development, even in the egg in some species, as a region of granular cytoplasm. In mammals, rapid multiplication produces very large numbers of germ cells, but nearly all regress later; those that survive undergo meiosis, halving their chromosome number around the time of fertilization. Final exhaustion of the germ-cell population marks the end of reproductive life. Gametogenesis requiring reduction in chromosome number is widespread in the plant and animal kingdoms, compensatory increase depending on automixis or fertilization.

9. Parthenogenesis occurs in members of most invertebrate and vertebrate orders,

and has the advantages that males do not need to be produced and all members of the group can participate in multiplication. It has the disadvantages that adaptation to changing environments is severely limited and parthenogenetic species are seen to be doomed to extinction relatively early. The situation is somewhat improved by the inclusion of meiosis, with its gene-shuffling feature, which typifies most systems of this kind.

10. Sexual reproduction which includes union of chromosome complements from two individuals as well as meiosis, greatly improves the adaptability and prospects of the offspring.

11. Exhaustive enquiry reveals that fertilization specificity only partially maintains species integrity, viable crosses occurring between species and even between genera in mammals. Other factors working for species integrity include body size and form, genetic compatibility, sexual season and behavioural pattern, and geographical distribution.

12. Hybridization nevertheless readily occurs, such hybrids being sterile, of low fertility or more fertile than the parent stocks, the third state representing the condition of 'hybrid vigour'. Viable hybrids can give rise to new species, provided isolation is adequate, but, according to one estimate, to pass from inter-fertility to inter-sterility might take of the order of a million years. The contrasting procedure of 'inbreeding' can either have no detectable effect on fertility or else lead to 'inbreeding depression', ending in sterility.

References

Austin CR. Entry of spermatozoa into the Fallopian tube mucosa. *Nature, Lond* 1959; **183**: 908–9.

Austin CR. *The Mammalian Egg*. Oxford: Blackwell Scientific Publications, 1961.

Austin CR. *Fertilization*. Englewood Cliffs, New Jersey; Prentice-Hall Inc., 1965.

Austin CR. Specialization of gametes. In: Austin CR, Short RV, eds. *Reproduction in Mammals. Book 6. The Evolution of Reproduction*. Cambridge, London, New York, Melbourne: Cambridge University Press, 1976: 149–82.

Austin CR, Amoroso EC. The mammalian egg. *Endeavour* 1959; **18**: 130.

Austin CR, Bishop MWH. Presence of spermatozoa in the uterine-tube mucosa of bats. *J Endocr*, 1959; **18**: viii–ix.

Austin CR, Walton A. Fertilization. In: Parkes, AS, ed. *Marshall's Physiology of Reproduction*, 3rd ed. London: Longmans, Green & Co., 1960; **1**: 310–416.

Baker TG. Oogenesis and ovulation. In: Austin CR, Short EV, eds. *Reproduction in Mammals*. Cambridge, London, New York, New Rochelle, Melbourne, Sydney: Cambridge University Press, 1982; **1**: 17–45 (Fig. 2.9).

Barton SC, Adams CA, Norris ML, Surani MAH. Development of gynogenetic and parthenogenetic inner cell mass and trophectoderm tissues in reconstituted blastocysts in the mouse. *J Emb Exp Morph* 1985; **90**: 267–85.

Beatty RA. *Parthenogenesis and Polyploidy in Mammalian Development.* Cambridge: University Press, 1957.

Bedford JM. Form and function of eutherian spermatozoa in relation to the nature of egg vestments. In: Beier HM, Lindner HR, eds. *Fertilization of the Human Egg in Vitro.* Berlin, Heidelberg, New York, Tokyo: Springer-Verlag, 1983: 133–46.

Bedford JM. Fertilization mechanisms in animals and man: current concepts. In: Edwards RG, ed. *Establishing a Successful Human Pregnancy.* Serono Symposia Publications from Raven Press. New York: Raven Press, 1990; **65**: 115–31.

Bedford JM. The coevolution of human gametes. In Dumbar BS, O'Rand MG eds. *A Comparative Overview of Mammalian Fertilization,* New York: Plenum Press, 1991: 457.

Blandau RJ. Biology of eggs and implantatation. In: Young WC, ed. *Sex and Internal Secretions.* London: Baillière, Tindall & Cox, Ltd, 1961: 797–882.

Bodmer WF, Cavalli-Sforza LL. *Genetics, Evolution and Man.* San Francisco: W.H. Freeman and Company, 1976.

Braden AWH, Austin CR, David HA. The reaction of the zona pellucida to sperm penetration. *Aust J Biol Sci* 1954; **7**: 391–409.

Byskov AG. Primordial germ cells and regulation of meiosis. In: Austin CR, Short RG, eds. *Reproduction in Mammals,* Second Edition. *Book 1, Germ Cells and Fertilization.* Cambridge, London, New York, New Rochelle, Melbourne, Sydney: Cambridge University Press, 1982: 1–16.

Calvin HI, Bedford JM. Formation of disulphide bonds in the nucleus and accessory structures of mammalian spermatozoa during maturation in the epididymis. *J Reprod Fert* (Suppl) 1971; **13**: 65–75.

Campbell BG. *Humankind Merging,* 2nd edn. Boston, Toronto: Little, Brown and Company, 1979.

Cann RL, Stoneking M, Wilson AC. Mitochondrial DNA and human evolution, *Nature, Lond* 1987; **325**: 31–6.

Catternach BM. Parental origin effects in mice. *J Exp Morph* 1986; 97 (Suppl): 137–50.

Chang MC, Hancock JL. Experimental hybridization. In: Benirschke K, ed. *Comparative Aspects of Reproductive Failure.* New York: Springer-Verlag, 1967: 206–17.

Cuellar O. The origin of parthenogenesis in vertebrates: the cytogenetic factors. *Am Natur* 1974; **108**: 625–48.

de Duve C. *Blueprint for a Cell; the Nature and Origin of Life.* Burlington, North Carolina: Neil Patterson Publishers, Carolina Biological Supply Company, 1991.

Dunbar BS, O'Rand MG. *A Comparative Overview of Mammalian Fertilization.* New York: Plenum Press, 1991: 452.

Gray AP. *Mammalian Hybrids.* Farnham Royal, England; Commonwealth Agricultural Bureaux, 1954.

Marshall FHA. *The Physiology of Reproduction.* London, New York, Toronto, Bombay, Calcutta, Madras: Longmans, Green & Co., 1922.

Maslin PT. Parthenogenesis in reptiles. *Am Zool* 1971; **11**: 361–80.

Maynard Smith J. *The Evolution of Sex.* Cambridge, London, New York, Melbourne: Cambridge University Press, 1978.

Ohno S. Genes, evolution, and the immortality of the monophyletic germ line. In: Metz CB, Monroy A, eds. *Biology of Fertilization, volume 1, Model Systems and Oogenesis.* Orlando, Sand Diego, New York, London, Toronto, Montreal, Sydney, Tokyo; Adacemic Press Inc., 1985: 3–21.

Olsen MW. Twelve year summary of selection for parthenogenesis in the Beltsville small white turkey. *Br Poultry Sci* 1965; **103**: 1–6.

Partridge L. Non-random mating and offspring fitness. In: Bateson P, ed. *Mate Choice.* Cambridge, London, New York, New Rochelle, Melbourne, Sydney: Cambrige University Press, 1983: 227–55.

Pincus G. *The Eggs of Mammals.* New York; Macmillan, 1936.

Refstie T. Induction of diploid gynogenesis in Atlantic salmon and rainbow trout using irradiated sperm and heat shock. *Can J Zool* 1983; **61**: 2411–6.

Strother PK. Pre-metazoan life. In: Allen KC, Briggs DEG, eds. *Evolution and the Fossil Record,* London: Belhaven Press, 1989: Chap. 3, 51–72.

Surani MA. Influence of genome imprinting on gene expression, phenotypic variations and development. *Hum Reprod* 1991; **6**: 45–51.

Surani MAH, Allen ND, Barton SC, Fundele R, Howlett SK, Norris ML, Reik W. Developmental consequences of imprinting of parental chromosomes by DNA methylation. *Phil Trans R Soc, Lond* 1990; **B326**: 313–27.

Surani MAH, Barton SC, Kaufman MH. Development to term of chimaeras between diploid parthenogenetic and fertilized embryos. *Nature, Lond* 1977; **270**: 601–2.

Surani MAH, Barton SC, Norris ML. Experimental reconstruction of mouse eggs and embryos: an analysis of development. *Biol Reprod* 1987; **36**: 1–16.

Thibault C. Formation et maturation des gametes. In: Grasse P-P, ed, *Traité de Zoolgie: Anatomie, Systematique, Biologie.* Paris: Masson et Cie, 1969; **16**: 799–853.

Timmons TM, Skinner SM, Dunbar BS. Glycosylation and maturation of the mammalian zona pellucida. In: Alexander NJ, Griffin D, Spieler JM, Waites GMH, eds. *Gamete Interaction; Prospects for Immunocontraception.* New York, Chichester, Brisbane, Toronto, Singapore: John Wiley & Sons Inc., 1990: 277–92.

Tyndale-Biscoe H, Renfree M. *Reproductive Physiology of Marsupials.* Cambridge, London, New York, New Rochelle, Melbourne, Sydney: Cambridge University Press, 1987.

Valentine JW, Erwin DH. Interpreting great developmental experiments: the fossil record. In: Raff RA, Raff EC, eds. *Development as an Evolutionary Process.* New York: Alan R. Liss, Inc., 1987: 71–107.

White MJD. *Animal Cytology and Evolution.* Cambridge: Cambridge University Press, 1954.

Wilson EB. *The Cell in Development and Heredity.* New York: The Macmillan Company, 1928.

Yanagimachi R. Specificity of sperm–egg interaction. In: Edidin M, Johnson MH, eds., *Immunobiology of Gametes.* Cambridge, London, New York, Melbourne: Cambridge University Press, 1977: 255–95.

Yanagimachi R. Zona-free hamster eggs: their use in assessing fertilizing capacity and examining chromosomes of human spermatozoa. *Gam Res* 1984; **10**: 187–232.

Young S. Naked mole rats keep it in the family. *New Sci* 1990; vol. 126, no. 1716: 16.

2

Molecular and cellular aspects of oocyte development

R. G. GOSDEN AND M. BOWNES

The frontispiece to William Harvey's book, *De Generatione Animalium* (1651), depicting Jove holding up an egg, carries an inscription, 'ex ovo omnia'. The pivotal role of eggs in the life histories of all vetebrate animals has stimulated scientific attention since the era of Aristotle, and has been responsible for as much speculative philosophy as experimentation in the past. Both ancient and modern scientists alike have been fascinated by the apparently paradoxical capacity of the egg to be highly specialized yet totipotent at the same time. It is uniquely able to give rise to every cell type in a new organism and, through the production of germ cells, to an indefinite number of descendants besides. Interest in oogenesis is, however, driven as much by practical objectives as sheer intellectual curiosity. Revolutionary progress in human and animal reproductive technology and astonishing advances now being made in developmental biology provide impetus for investigating oogenesis.

Experimental studies of mammalian oocytes have, mainly for practical reasons, lagged behind those of oviparous species. The eggs of species such as the fruit fly (*Drosophila*), sea urchins and amphibia (especially *Xenopus*) are relatively large and produced in far greater numbers than in mammals. With the notable, but rare, exception of Australian monotremes, mammalian eggs are small, shed singly or in small numbers from the ovary and retained within the body. Until relatively recently, few clinicians or biologists had ever observed living human oocytes and the prospects for studying them seemed bleak. That situation has abruptly changed, and research on mammalian, including human, eggs will in due course reward the investment with a better knowledge of oogenesis and the possibility of controlling the quality and fertility of oocytes.

Rapid progress is being made in early human embryology, and in technologies for monitoring and even treating unborn children, but we still have comparatively little understanding or control of the quantity and quality of gametes produced by the gonads. The processes of gametogenesis are, compared with pre-

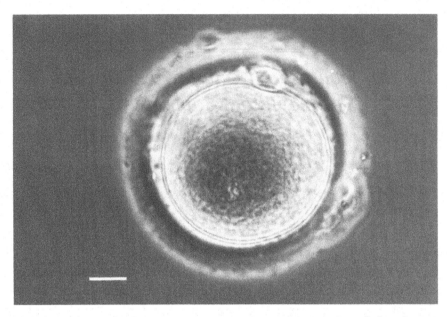

Fig. 1. A human oocyte undergoing fertilization *in vitro*. Cumulus cells have been removed to show the first polar body under a zona pellucida which is being penetrated by spermatozoa. (By courtesy of Dr Ros Evans, MRC, Edinburgh.) (Magnification bar = 30 μm.)

implantation embryo development, more difficult to study and experimentally manipulate, yet they crucially determine whether reproduction will be possible and the potential degree of success. According to Trounson (1989), 'Determination of egg quality is the single most difficult task in human IVF'. Better criteria of quality are required than the mere appearance of an oocyte (Fig. 1). We also need a sound knowledge of the physiological requirements for making 'good eggs' to improve the quality of those harvested during controlled cycles and to assess the prospects of growing large numbers of oocytes to maturity entirely *in vitro* for clinical treatment and investigation.

In this chapter we describe the development of follicular oocytes from the primordial stage to the emergence of a mature cell in a Graafian follicle. Although excellent reviews have been published in recent years (Bachvarova, 1985; Schultz, 1986; Wassarman, 1988a), it is timely to update this advancing field. This chapter presents a cytological profile of the oocyte before reviewing current knowledge of the molecular biology of oogenesis and physiological interdependence between oocytes and follicle cells. Since human oocytes are rare and precious cells, experimental studies will rely for the foreseeable future on animal models, particularly the laboratory mouse. Such heavy dependence on one model species raises the question of the validity of extrapolating to others. Nevertheless, we bear in mind that the comparative biology approach has already been very fruitful for oogenesis research in lower organisms. The production of fertile eggs is vital for survival of the species and, despite superficial differences in size and yolkiness, we might expect to find some phylogenetically ancient developmental mechanisms conserved because evolutionary 'tinkering' at this critical stage of life history is risky. The following account will therefore also compare and contrast oogenesis in humans and a number of animal species, indicating the potential value of these models for understanding this stage of development.

Oocyte growth

Eggs are impressively large by comparison with most somatic cells. Although this is most obviously true of the yolky eggs of oviparous species, the eggs of humans and domesticated mammals are still among the largest cells in the body. For instance, the maximum diameters of mature, fresh oocytes in mice and humans are approximately 80 and 120 μm, respectively. Such differences (three-fold in volume) are not so easily explained, however, and probably do not simply reflect scaling to follicle or body size since no simple relationship was found across a wide spectrum of mammalian species (Gosden & Telfer, 1987). The range of egg sizes is narrow compared with many other classes of animals. The size and character of eggs reflect the requirements for survival as embryos. Mammalian embryos by and large have similar requirements for preimplantation development which takes place in the protected environment of the genital tract and generally lasts for only about a week.

The vast majority of ovarian oocytes are immature and rest in primordial follicles in the ovarian cortex (see Chapter by Gosden). These small oocytes measure approximately 15 and 35 μm in diameter in mice and humans, respectively, and must therefore expand in volume 150- and 40-fold to reach full size. Besides accumulating water, ions and lipids, the rate of protein synthesis and total cellular protein rise in parallel with expanding cell volume (Fig. 2). At full size, the mouse egg contains 25 ng protein, excluding the 3 ng of the zona pellucida.

Oocytes are able to undergo a remarkable enlargement because their growth is not interrupted by mitosis and cleavage of the cytoplasm. This peculiarity, all the more striking by contrast with the economical size of spermatozoa, has stimulated much experimental interest over the years. For more than 50 years it has been known that oocytes arrested at diplotene of meiosis become competent to resume nuclear maturation towards the end of the growth phase, but actual progression is restrained by the inhibitory influence of the follicular environment.

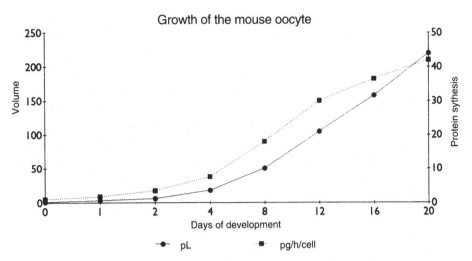

Fig. 2. During the full growth-span of mouse oocytes, which lasts approximately 2 weeks, increases in cell volume closely parallel the rate of protein synthesis.

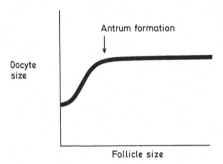

Fig. 3. Diagrammatic representation of the correlation between oocyte and follicular diameters during the early stages of follicle development. Attainment of full size by the oocyte and early stages of follicular antrum formation approximately coincide.

Whilst it is well established that this inhibition is relieved by the mid-cycle surge of gonadotropic hormones, the mechanism of signal transduction to the oocyte via somatic cells remains unclear. Much attention has been paid to the potential role of cyclic AMP and, more recently, to the interacting effects of cytostatic factor (the proto-oncogene *c-mos*) and maturation promoting factor with the cytoskeleton. These aspects are discussed in detail in the chapter by Downs (p. 150).

Enlargement of the oocyte is one of the early signs of follicle recruitment and is well advanced when the second layer of granulosa cells is forming. The diameters of oocytes correlate with those of their follicles during preantral stages and they approach full size when antrum formation is incipient (Fig. 3). At this time, the cells first become competent to undergo germinal vesicle breakdown and resume meiosis. The mouse oocyte normally takes approximately 2 weeks to reach full size and a further week to reach preovulatory ripeness.

Dimensions are useful indicators of developmental stage, but full-size does not necessarily imply full maturity. During the growth phase oocytes become competent to resume meiosis and cleave but the cytoplasmic mechanisms required for sperm head penetration, decondensation of chromatin and the polyspermy block are progressively acquired during the final days of maturation before ovulation. They acquire meiotic competence and fertile potential in a stepwise manner during Graafian stages: first, the capacity of the nuclear membrane to breakdown and for progression to Metaphase I and, secondly, the ability to reach Metaphase II and to decondense the chromatin of penetrating spermatozoa (Sorensen & Wassarman, 1976; Crosby & Moor, 1984). The principal aim of oogenesis research is to discover the cellular and molecular bases of this fertility.

Cytological changes

Compared with primordial follicles, mature oocytes have a much more complex cytoplasmic organization, are competent to resume meiosis and are able to undergo fertilization and cleavage divisions (Fig. 4). These changes are dependent on the production of new gene products and organelles during oogenesis, as well as involving modification and redistribution of existing ones. The cytological features of developing oocytes described below refer to the mouse unless stated otherwise.

The appearance of the oocyte nucleus is unlike that of any interphase somatic cell, and is reflected in the special term, *germinal vesicle*. The large size and absence of much heterochromatic material are the chief characteristics of this nucleus which is suspended at diplotene (Fig. 5). It increases in diameter from about 10–20 μm during oocyte growth, but this represents a shrinking proportion of cell volume as the cytoplasm enlarges faster. The nuclear membrane becomes undulated with more pores, presumably reflecting greater nucleo-cytoplasmic traffic of substrate and informational molecules during oocyte growth. Finally, it becomes more deeply folded shortly before germinal vesicle breakdown.

Primordial follicle oocytes are commonly, and misleadingly, described as 'quiescent'. It is only the state of the nucleus that is resting, and this is the G_0 equivalent of G_2 in an interphase somatic cell. The presence of one or more nucleoli, RNA polymerase activity and the continuous uptake of amino acids and ribonucleosides into small oocytes demonstrate their active state. Since these cells may survive for 50 years or more in human ovaries, it is not surprising that they continuously repair and replace damaged organelles and macromolecules in order to maintain the *status quo*.

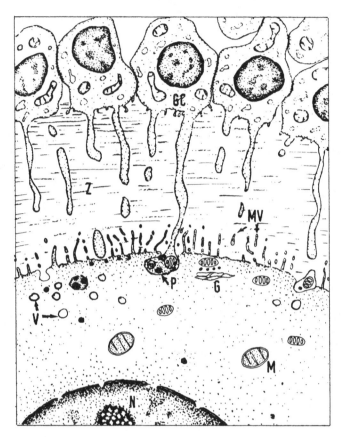

Fig. 4. Diagrammatic representation of the fine structure of an oocyte and adjacent granulosa cells (GC) (corona radiata). The following structures are depicted: zona pellucida (Z), germinal vesicle nucleus (N), mitochondria (M), microvilli (MV), Golgi apparatus (G), vesicles (V) in the cortical ooplasm and processes (P) extending from granulosa cells to the oocyte surface. (Adapted from, and published by permission of Baker & O, 1976.)

The germinal vesicle nucleus in rodents is particularly pale and featureless, giving rise to the term 'dictyotene' to describe the unusual character of diplotene in these animals. Distinct chromosomes are no longer visible either by light or electron microscopy because the chromosomal axes become unravelled and extensive lateral loops form. In primate oocytes, the chromatin is more condensed and chromosomal threads are recognizable through diplotene.

The lateral loops of these chromosomes, like those of pachytene-diplotene cells in fetal ovaries (see p. 119), have sometimes been compared with the 'lampbrush chromosomes' of growing oocytes in amphibians, fish and some non-vertebrates. In those species, thousands of loops measuring as much as several microns in

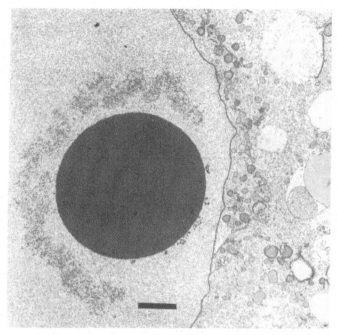

Fig. 5. The germinal vesicle nucleus of a human oocyte with a characteristic ring
of chromatin around the nucleolus. (Bar = 1.25 μm.)

length extend laterally from the axis and are sites of intense transcriptional activity
(Davidson, 1986). But, it is a matter of definition and degree whether the
chromosomes of mammalian oocytes should be regarded as being in a strictly
comparable state. Oocytes at the mid-growth stage produce more than ten times
as much RNA (particularly ribosomal RNA) than most somatic cells and the
nucleoli become large and dense (from 2 or 3 to 10 μm diameter) with
extranucleolar satellite material at specific stages, also representing sites of
transcription (Chouinard, 1973). Because the loops in mouse oocytes are far
smaller and the overall rate of transcription is much lower than in oviparous
species, some authorities have concluded that 'True lampbrush chromosomes do
not exist at any point in development of mouse oocytes' (Bachvarova, 1985).

Although we might expect oocytes to be endowed with the normal household
inventory of cytoplasmic organelles, there is one notable absence. They lack the
centrioles which, except in plants and a few rare exceptions in mitotic animal
cells, are responsible for assembling the spindle apparatus which segregates
chromosomes during cell division. While present in primordial oocytes, centrioles
have disappeared by the mid-growth stage and do not reappear until an embryo
has completed several cleavage divisions (Szollosi, Calarco & Donahue, 1972).
This is generally true in mammals and, even when sperm centrioles are introduced

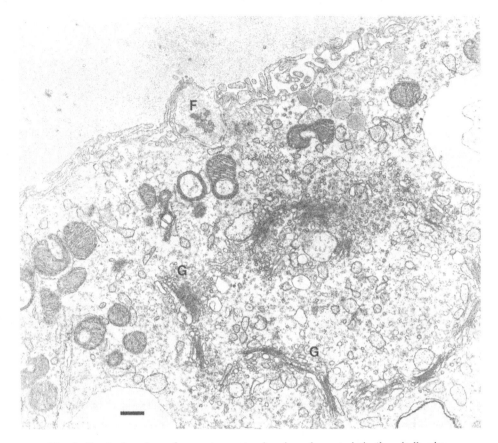

Fig. 6. Cortical region of a goat oocyte showing characteristic 'hooded' mitochondria. Golgi apparatus (G) is abundant and a foot process (F) from a corona
cell can be seen embedded in a pit in the oocyte surface. (Bar = 0.45 μm.)

into oocytes, they do not appear to contribute to the formation or polarity of
the spindle, although there may be exceptions.

Small oocytes have a scanty population of cytoplasmic organelles which, in
primates, are mainly clustered around the nucleus. Under the light microscope
these can be observed as a definite perinuclear structure, the so-called Balbiani
vitelline body ('yolk nucleus'), consisting of various membranous organelles
including the Golgi apparatus, mitochondria and lipid droplets.

Once the oocyte begins to grow, these organelles migrate closer to the periphery
without any hint of polarizing the cell. The *Golgi apparatus* breaks up into
separate units in the cortical region, which is appropriate for its role in the
production of glycoproteins for export (Fig. 6). The stacks of parallel lamellae
become vacuolated and accumulate granules, some of which are likely to include
zona glycoproteins and zymogen-like cortical granules. A large proportion of

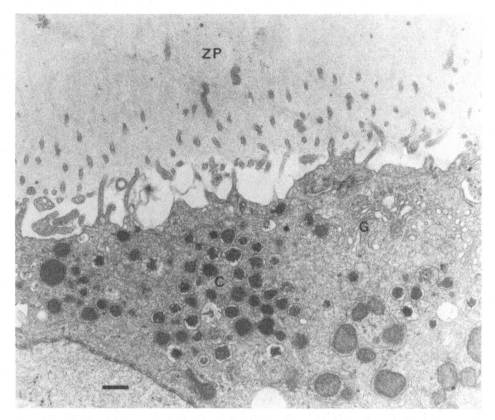

Fig. 7. The surface of this growing oocyte from a sheep is covered by many microvilli which project a short way into the zona pellucida (ZP). Beneath the oolemma there are layers of cortical granules (C) in the neighbourhood of the Golgi apparatus (G). (Bar = 0.45 μm.)

total protein synthesis is accounted for by these two activities but, once they are complete and the oocyte is approaching maturity, Golgi activity wanes.

Cortical granules were first discovered in sea urchin eggs and are now assumed to be of general importance. In mammalian eggs, they are refractile, spherical bodies measuring 300-500 nm in diameter and consisting of an electron-dense core bounded by a unit membrane (Fig. 7). Granule production commences soon after the onset of oocyte growth in rodents, later in some other species, and may continue into the post-ovulatory phase until some 5000 are present *in toto*. At maturity, they are found just beneath the cell membrane to which they become firmly attached in some species in readiness for discharge into the perivitelline space in response to fertilization or other activating stimuli. Exocytosis can be prematurely induced and sometimes occurs spontaneously, with potentially deleterious effects on sperm penetration. Although still poorly biochemically

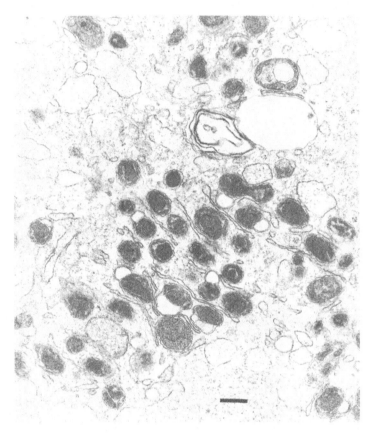

Fig. 8. Rows of mitochondria lie between flattened sacs of smooth endoplasmic
reticulum in this immature human oocyte. (Bar = 0.23 μm.)

characterized, their proper role in preventing polyspermic fertilization is not in
doubt, and assumes greater importance in our species in which a 'vitelline block'
is comparatively unimportant.

Mitchondria in the oocyte have a number of special features of interest. Apart
from a very small paternal 'leak', the great majority of mitochondrial DNA that
is inherited by the embryo is of maternal origin, and so the fidelity of replication
during oogenesis is crucial (Gyllensten *et al.*, 1991). Secondly, the phenotype of
the mitochondria is peculiar and possibly reflects attentuation of oxidative
phosphorylation as a source of energy in these cells. In small- and medium-sized
human oocytes, where they are often found in the neighbourhood of the
endoplasmic reticulum, mitochondria possess numerous transverse cristae and
are either elongated (1–2 μm) or transform to dumb-bell shapes as a prelude to
undergoing fission (Figs. 8 and 9). The numbers of small, oval or round
mitochondria progressively increase to 10^5 in preovulatory oocytes and the cristae

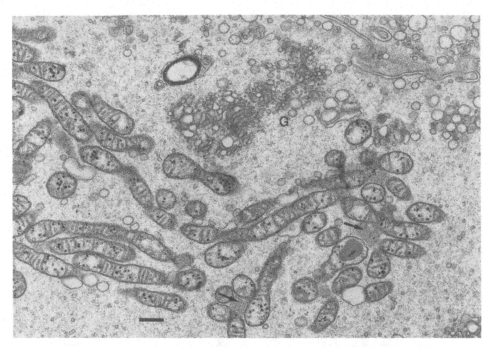

Fig. 9. Oocyte of a spider monkey showing a cluster of mitochondria at various stages of fission and containing dense bodies. Golgi apparatus (G) and homogeneous material of unknown significance, 'nuage' (arrow) are visible. (Bar = 0.17 μm.)

become more columnar and eventually arranged in concentric arches (Szollosi, 1972; Wassarman & Josefowicz, 1978).

In many cases, the fine structure of oocytes is so characteristic that the stage of development and even the species of origin can be identified. Differences in the nucleus have already been mentioned, but they also extend to cytoplasmic organelles and storage materials. For example, the mitochondria of ruminant oocytes have a curved appendage consisting of both inner and outer membranes forming a hood-like structure of uncertain significant (Fig. 6). Human oocytes possess curious structures of unknown significance called annulate lamellae consisting of stacks of up to 100 parallel, paired membranes fused at intervals. They characterize the cytoplasm, and sometimes the nucleus, of small oocytes but similar, if smaller structures have been found in the oocytes of other species as well as in other rapidly growing cells in embryos and neoplasms. Growing oocytes from different species of rodents can be distinguished simply on the basis of the morphology of fibrous lattices (see below).

Both rough and smooth *endoplasmic reticulum* (ER) are present throughout oogenesis, but the former is sparse and the latter becomes less prominent in mature eggs, perhaps as they are recycled for assembly into other structures. The

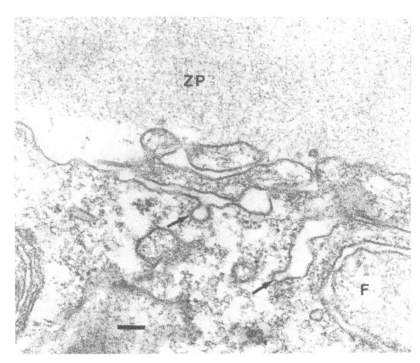

Fig. 10. Detail of the cortical region of a sheep oocyte showing goblet-shaped invaginations of the oolemma characteristic of coated pit endocytosis (arrows). A foot process associated with adhesive-type junctions is embedded in the oolemma (F) beneath the zona pellucida (ZP). (Bar = 0.12 μm.)

ER may be very close to and fuse with the Golgi apparatus where proteins and polysaccharides, respectively, are being processed. The cisterns of the ER are also sites at which heritable retrovirus-like particles have been observed. These RNA-containing viruses are universally present in mouse oocytes and preimplantation embryos and have also been observed in a number of other species, including humans (Yotsuyanagi & Szollosi, 1984). Several types have been recorded although it is the A-type particles, measuring about 50 nm diameter and consisting of two concentric shells around a clear centre, that dominate the mouse oocyte. Like the transposons of *Drosophila,* the significance of these potentially harmful agents is unknown and it is unclear why they have not been eliminated by natural selection.

Many membrane-bound *vesicles* as well as multivesicular bodies exist in the cytoplasm of growing oocytes and are probably involved in moving materials across the cell membrane. The vesicles in the cortex belong to a heterogeneous population, some being products for export while others contain material taken up from granulosa cell secretions and serum transudation into the follicular fluid.

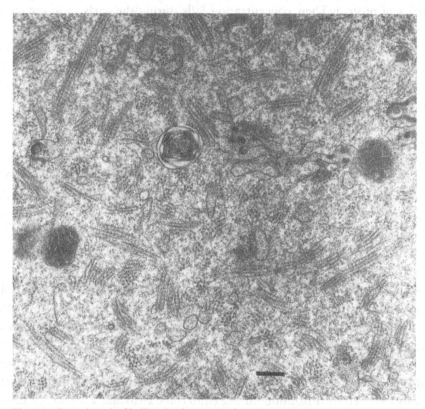

Fig. 11. Cytoplasmic fibrillar lattices, seen here in transverse and cross-section, are the most striking storage material of rodent oocytes and reach peak abundance near the time of ovulation. (Bar = 0.16 μm.)

That endocytosis takes place at the surface of oocytes of all sizes and stages is indicated by the presence of coated vesicles and pits and scattered heterolysosomes from the earliest stages of development (Fig. 10).

Large numbers of *ribosomes* accumulate in the mature egg (10^8), though polyribosomes are scarce. The total number rises four-fold during mouse oogenesis but, because of proportionately greater expansion of the ooplasm, their density actually falls considerably. While these changes are consistent with the trends in protein and rRNA synthesis to be described in the next section, the question of ribosomal storage still remains to be settled.

Paracrystalline *fibrous lattices* are one of the dominant features of the cytoplasm of the growing and mature oocyte in rodents (Weakley, 1968). They are absent from primordial oocytes but rapidly accumulate throughout the cytoplasm in growing oocytes and reach peak abundance at maturity when they occupy > 10% of the volume (Fig. 11). The lattices have a periodic structure and the staining properties of protein. Their concentration falls during the early cleavage stages of embryos and completely disappears from diapausing blastocysts.

Such abundant material is likely to be important, but until it can be isolated for biochemical characterization its significance will remain largely a matter of conjecture. Some investigators have proposed that the lattices represent ribosomal storage for early embryogenesis (Burkholder, Comings & Okada, 1971; Bachvarova, De Leon & Spiegelman, 1981) while others suggest they may be a form of mammalian 'yolk' (Szollosi, 1972; Piko & Clegg, 1982). In our view, the balance of experimental evidence currently favours the second hypothesis because the material is resistant to alkaline hydrolysis which would degrade RNA, ribosomes have never been observed budding off from the narrower fibres during embryogenesis and the number of conventional ribosomes can account for the ribosomal RNA content of the oocyte. These contrasting hypotheses are in agreement, however, in so far as they point to some sort of storage function, at least in rodents.

Although lattices are absent from primate and ruminant oocytes, other storage materials may exist. Flocculent proteinaceous materials occur in ribosomal-studded cisternae of ER or freely in the cytoplasm of primate and farm animal oocytes (Fig. 12), and small electron-dense granules are frequent in monkey mitochondria (Fig. 9) as well as in pig and rabbit ooplasm. To be properly regarded as protein stores we should expect to find gradual accumulation during oogenesis followed by utilization during embryonic cleavage. Further studies are needed to verify this theory, though the electron dense 'nuage' (Fr. cloud) material found near mitochondria presumably has a different significance since it characterizes oocytes of primordial follicles. While the question of protein storage in mammalian oocytes requires attention, there is no doubt that the scattered glycogen granules and lipid droplets which accummulate to varying extents in the eggs of all species probably provide energy and substrates for the synthesis of new membranes after fertilization. On these grounds alone, it would seem that mammalian oocytes contain material fulfilling the conventional criteria for 'yolk'. Those denying the existence of mammalian yolk are influenced by the obvious differences between the comparatively small size and nourishing medium of tubal fluid for mammalian eggs compared with the large yolky eggs of species that are shed into the external environment where they require a 'survival package' until the embryos can feed for themselves. Since pre-implantation embryos can develop *in vitro* in a simple medium consisting of only salts, albumen and pyruvate, it would appear that they either have very efficient molecular recycling processes and/or depend on stored materials. Much more experimental attention needs to be paid to the question of storage of non-informational molecules which may contribute importantly to embryonic viability.

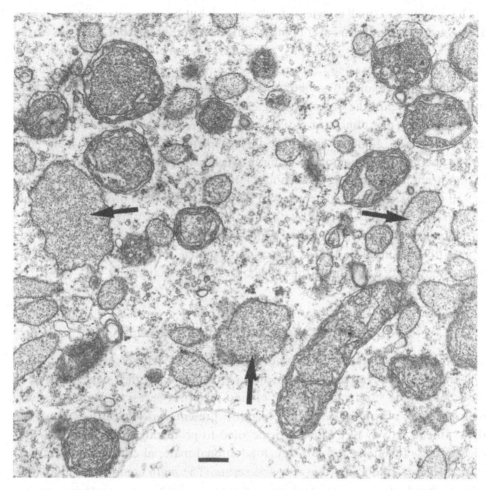

Fig. 12. Oocytes from humans and some farm species contain proteinaceous material accumulating in dilated sacs of endoplasmic reticulum (arrows). (Bar = 0.10 μm.)

One of the most conspicuous changes occurring during oogenesis is secretion of a glycoprotein coat, the *zona pellucida* (ZP), which is a general feature among mammals. The functions of the zona include presentation of species-specific receptors to sperm and induction of the acrosome reaction before fertilization and a polyspermy block and physical protection of the embryo afterwards. Once the eggs is fertilized, the zona becomes harder, more insoluble and perhaps less permeable as a result of steric changes in glycoproteins. It progressively separates the oocyte from the bulk of its enveloping follicle cells, although remaining porous to large molecules and permitting somatic cell processes continuing contact with the oolemma (Fig. 7).

The oolemma of small oocytes is fairly smooth but becomes increasingly folded during growth. A uniform cover of microvilli with cores of microfilamentous actin extend a short way into the zona pellucida and sometimes makes junctional contact with granulosa cell processes traversing in the opposite direction. These processes terminate in button-like swellings containing few organelles on the cell surface or in pits in the oolemma (Figs. 4 and 6). The surface properties of the oolemma are of the utmost importance for further development and one of the most crucial is the ability to bind the fertilizing spermatozoon. A protein identified on the spermatozoal membrane using monoclonal antibody PH-30 appears to be important for sperm–egg fusion and is homologous to snake venom disintegrin as well as related to a highly conserved family of viral fusion proteins (Blobel *et al.*, 1992). Evidence that peptides with affinities for fibronectin-like molecules bind to the oolemma suggests that the ligand on this membrane is an integrin (Fusi *et al.*, 1993). Attention to the molecular aspects of oogenesis is becoming increasingly successful, and is the subject of the next section.

Biosynthesis and uptake of macromolecules

The synthesis and uptake of macromolecules into the oocyte serves two purposes. The first is for the growth, development and maturation of the oocyte itself, and the second is the storage of information and materials necessary for the first 24 hours or more of embryonic development. At present, it is unclear how much of the synthetic activity of the oocyte is devoted to producing macromolecules for each of these functions and how much additional material comes from external sources such as the granulosa cells and serum. The main components that will be considered below are the synthesis and storage of RNA and proteins because they provide much of the informational and structural requirements for development. We have already noted the increased mitochondrial population which is active in transcription throughout oogenesis.

Ribonucleic acids

The oocyte synthesizes large amounts of RNA and the mature mouse egg contains 0.3–0.55 ng of RNA *in toto*. This is a minute amount compared with the 4000 ng present in the oocyte of *Xenopus* but, when adjusted for the 4000-fold difference in cell volume, the concentrations are roughly comparable. Approximately 65% is ribosomal RNA, 20% is 5S RNA and tRNA and 15% is heterogeneous RNA (Fig. 13); these RNAs steadily accumulate until meiosis is resumed when their levels begin to fall. Poly(A)+RNA in the latter fraction is potentially available

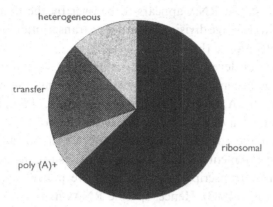

Fig. 13. Fractional amounts of different classes of RNA in fully grown mouse oocytes. (Data adapted from Piko & Clegg, 1982.)

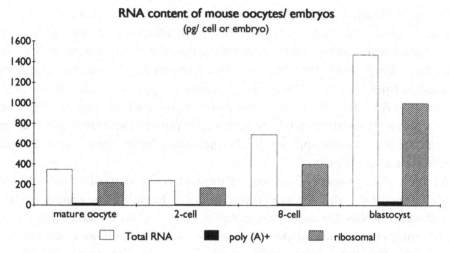

Fig. 14. Changes in the amounts of total, poly (A)$^+$ and ribosomal RNA from the mature oocyte to the blastocyst stage in the mouse. The amounts notably decline after the onset of oocyte maturation and rise after the embryonic genome has been activated. (Data adapted from Piko & Clegg, 1982.)

for translation into protein and amounts to about 8%, which is large by the standards of most somatic cells and four-fold greater than *Xenopus* eggs. Amplification of ribosomal genes is evidently unnecessary because the embryonic genome is activated early, which is another contrast with *Xenopus* in which a 1000-fold increase is needed to produce the ribosomes to last until the tadpole stage. When the two-cell embryonic stage has been reached, most of the stored ribosomal RNA has been degraded and 70% of the poly(A)+ has been removed (Fig. 14). Thus, although the stability of RNAs in the oocyte is high, the functional role of much of the stored RNA appears to be over by the time that embryos undergo their second cleavage division when active transcription of the embryonic genome begins in the mouse (Flach *et al.*, 1982).

The first 24 hours of development after fertilization depend critically on the information that has accumulated during oogenesis. A mature oocyte contains about 1 pg poly(A) + RNA, though this drops to about 0.7 pg in the unfertilized egg, either by degradation of RNA or by the loss of the poly(A) + tails. However, the poly(A) + RNA in the oocyte is not the only RNA of importance in regulating early embryonic development because the amount rises rapidly after fertilization in the absence of new transcription by the selective polyadenylation of stored mRNAs (Clegg & Piko, 1983). Hence, specific RNAs may be selected from the stored pool for conversion into translatable forms. How specific mRNAs are stored and selectively recruited is not known, but the mechanisms involved must be unravelled if we are to understand the first day or two of mammalian development which depend upon the activity of the maternal genome.

Since very few specific transcripts have been identified or assayed during oogenesis and early embryogenesis, our knowledge of their storage and utilization is limited. We presume that because there are changing patterns of protein synthesis during the one-cell stage in the absence of synthesis of new mRNAs (Magnusson & Epstein, 1981), mechanisms must exist for distinguishing between transcripts and translating and degrading specific populations of molecules rather than global mechanisms applying to all transcripts. Nevertheless, some general mechanisms seem to exist.

We have already noted that most of the maternally derived transcripts are degraded at the two-cell stage when transcription of the embryonic genome begins. The stored mRNAs for actins are notable examples. Actin molecules, being fundamental constituents of the cytoskeleton, are abundant and account for almost 1% of the total protein synthesis in the growing mouse oocyte, though less at maturity (Taylor & Piko, 1990). The 2×10^4 β actin mRNA molecules in the full-grown oocyte have fallen 50% by the one-cell stage and only 10% of the original store remains in the two-cell embryo (Fig. 15). The profiles for gamma actin and several other gene products are known to be broadly similar. Thus, most of the actin mRNA synthesis in the oocyte is probably for utilization by the oocyte rather than after fertilization, which is consistent with most of the actin mRNA being found on polysomes.

Three ribosomal protein genes have been analysed which encode protein components of the 60S and 40S subunits. The large numbers of their transcripts in the oocyte also degrade fairly rapidly at maturity and the genes are not switched on again until embryonic cleavage has commenced. The reported rates of synthesis of ribosomal proteins in mature oocytes are low compared to the numbers of

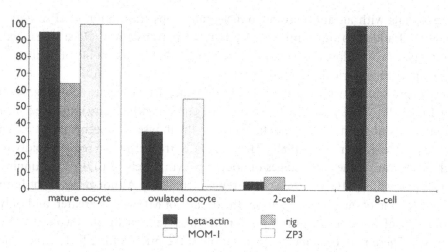

Fig. 15. Relative abundance of transcripts of β-actin (Taylor & Piko, 1990), *rig* (Taylor & Piko, 1991) and MOM-1 and ZP3 (Roller *et al.*, 1989) during oogenesis and early embryonic development in mice. Maternal transcripts of these genes decrease at different rates and the former two are re-expressed by the embryonic genome after the two-cell stage.

transcripts which are present suggesting that utilization of the RNA is being controlled and that storage forms are being used.

The *rig* gene (rat insulinoma gene) of the mouse has been isolated from an embryonic cDNA library and investigated in some detail (Taylor & Piko, 1991). It encodes a 145 amino acid protein with a nuclear localization signal and a DNA binding domain, and probably performs a housekeeping role in cell growth and replication, though it is unclear whether the *rig* gene product is being made during oogenesis, of if the transcript is stored entirely for embryogenesis. A relatively abundant store of transcripts in the mature oocyte declines abruptly to 10% in the ovulated egg, only to rise again during cleavage. The signal for degradation of the *rig* transcripts is probably encoded in the 3′ untranslated region of the mRNA. Interestingly, the *rig* RNA is lost earlier than the bulk of stored maternal mRNAs which largely degrade at the two-cell stage. Another transcript which is degraded during the one-cell stage is that encoding tissue-type plasminogen activator (tPA).

The mRNA encoding tPA is degraded more rapidly than the bulk of stored mRNA and provides an excellent example of how stored transcripts are selectively polyadenylated and translated. Using chimaeric mRNAs, it has been possible to show that both polyadenylation and translation after meiosis require specific sequences within the 3′ untranslated region, where selective polyadenylation signals lie, and a 3′ processing signal (AAUAAA) (Vassalli *et al.*, 1989). Blocking these signals with an antisense oligonucleotide stops translation of tPA, and a similar tail added to other mRNAs leads to their translation. Once translated, the mRNA rapidly loses its stability and is degraded to the point of extinction in fertilized eggs (Strickland *et al.*, 1988).

The expression of two genes encoding LDH-β (heart-type lactate dehydrogenase) and MON-1(a 76 kD protein of unknown function), which are expressed in a variety of tissues and developmental stages in the mouse, has been studied in the mouse oocyte (Roller *et al.*, 1989). The number of transcripts increases rapidly to high levels during the early stages of oocyte growth, levels of LDH-β continuing to increase whilst MON-1 transcripts remain constant. Although levels of both fall at the time of meiotic maturation, the decline of MOM-1 is greater, and only about 1% of the oocyte transcripts for MOM-1 remain by the two-cell stage (Fig. 15). There may be some de-adenylation of the mRNA for LDH at the time of meiotic maturation since synthesis of the protein LDH falls faster than the observed drop in level of transcripts encoding it and there is a corresponding decline in size from 1.4 to 1.3 kb. Similar findings have been reported for actin (Bachvarova *et al.*, 1985).

Expression of the zona pellucida gene, ZP3, has been studied in detail because it is abundant and has a key role in fertilization. A cDNA encoding murine ZP3 has been isolated and found to be approximately 10 kb in length with a number of exons. The regulation of transcription and translation of the gene has been described above. Once a cDNA was identified, it was possible to characterize the behaviour of the ZP3 gene in the oocyte and its unique site of expression. Transcript levels rise continuously during early oocyte growth to 3×10^5 copies per cell or more, drop somewhat in the final stages of oocyte growth and fall precipitously to undetectable levels at the time of meiotic maturation and ovulation (Fig. 16). The sudden loss of ZP3 transcripts suggests that a sequence-specific degradation mechanism may be involved. Unlike some of the more complex examples mentioned above, changes in the translation of ZP3 simply reflect changes in transcript levels (Wassarman, 1988*b*).

From this survey of the molecular biology of mammalian oogenesis, we have seen that most attention has been paid to expression of some of the genes encoding housekeeping and abundant proteins, such as histones, actin, some ribosomal proteins, ZP3 and LDH. Even though so few have been studied, we can see that several patterns of transcript synthesis, storage, activation for translation and degradation have emerged. We know nothing of the transcripts which are much less abundant, and which may be critically important for the development of the oocyte and the embryo. Some of these are likely to be as yet uncharacterized genes which are uniquely expressed in the germ cells of both sexes or even more specifically in the oocyte. Isolation and analysis of these genes is a major challenge for future research and will require cDNA libraries from ovaries and oocytes.

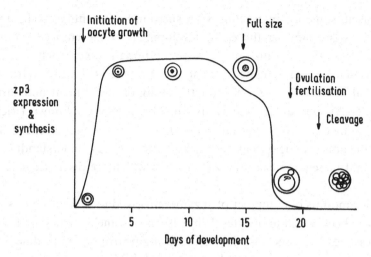

Fig. 16. Covariation of gene expression and translation of ZP3, a component of the murine zona pellucida produced only by the oocyte and involved in sperm binding and the acrosome reaction. This is confined to oogenesis from the initiation of follicle growth to formation of the mature oocyte.

Although the small amounts of material which can be collected have in the past prevented such experiments, recent advances in cloning technology, especially the use of the polymerase chain reaction (PCR) to amplify sequences, means that such experiments are now feasible.

As well as the RNAs which encode proteins needed by the embryo, there are some interesting RNA species which may have regulatory functions. In the mouse there are repeat sequences of 130 bp and 180 bp in length related to the human 300 bp Alu repeat sequences and called B1 and B2 repeats, respectively (Taylor & Piko, 1987) which are transcribed by RNA polymerase III. B1 and B2 make up some 2% of the mRNA and can be found interspersed in the 3' untranslated regions of cytoplasmic RNAs and as small poly(A)+RNAs. Both B1 and B2 transcripts are found in mature oocytes, but their levels differ from each other during early development suggesting independent recruitment and possibly different functions. Unfortunately, it is not yet clear what these transcripts do, but they may be involved in utilization of RNAs or they may affect the stability of specific subclasses of mRNAs. Their presence in the stored RNA may be an important part of the regulated recruitment of specific RNAs for translation. Clearly, there is a great deal of uncharted territory to explore in this field.

Cellular proteins

The growing oocyte is very active in the synthesis of proteins from nuclear and mitochondrial transcripts. Some of these are required for the differentiation of the oocyte itself, some for interacting with surrounding granulosa cells and yet others will be significant for the early development of the embryo. Many are important for growth in a range of cell types, although some which are specific to the oocyte have been investigated. One specific protein, D14, which is translated from maternal mRNA will be useful for the study of recruitment and turnover of stored mRNAs, but unfortunately its function is not yet known (Richoux, Renard & Babinet, 1991). Rapid advances in the study of genes encoding the proteins of the zona pellucida have contributed to a better understanding of its production and the character of the ZP proteins which are discussed separately below.

Detectable amounts of a number of enzymes involved in cellular housekeeping functions have been found in oocytes. While levels of some enzymes are low until embryogenesis (e.g. α- and β-galactosidase, β-glucuronidase, uridine kinase, hypoxanthine guanine phosphoribosyl transferase (HPRT), adenine phosphoribosyl transferase), others are present in greater concentrations in mouse eggs and remain stable or rise even higher after fertilization (e.g. glucose-6-phosphate dehydrogenase, glucose phosphate isomerase (GPI), phosphoglycerate kinase, creatine kinase, lactate dehydrogenase (LHD)). Some of these enzymes can be remarkably abundant. For instance, 200–400 pg LDH is present in the full-grown mouse oocyte and is responsible for 2–5% of total protein synthesis at some stages. For the purposes of diagnosing genetic defects by enzymic assay of embryonic biopsies, it is important to know how much of the maternally encoded enzyme remains compared to that being expressed by the human embryo, which expresses its genome after the 4- to 8-cell stage (Braude, Bolton & Moore, 1988). Significant amounts of maternally-derived key enzymes such as HPRT and GPI may remain as late as the eight-cell stage in the mouse. We have comparatively little information about enzymes in human eggs, but it is clear that simple extrapolations from the mouse may be unreliable. For example, there is six times as much GPI in human, compared with mouse, oocytes whereas the difference in cell volume is only three-fold (West *et al.*, 1989).

With the exception of actin, comparatively little is known about the role of maternal transcripts in the synthesis of structural proteins in embryos. In the case of protein components of gap junctions, which are established at the eight-cell stage, no corresponding mRNA was detected until the 4-cell stage denying an earlier claim that the protein was inherited as an oogenetic product (Nishi, Kumar & Gilula, 1991).

Some of the proteins which are found in the oocyte may not be synthesized there but taken up from the follicular fluid. In developing oocytes of most species, there is a macromolecular component which is endocytosed by specific mechanisms from the surrounding body fluids or blood, and the evidence of certain serum proteins in ooplasm suggested that the mammalian oocyte is no exception (Glass, 1971). Despite the ultrastructural and cytological evidence of endocytosis in oocytes, we have few clues about the identity of molecules being transported.

Some proteins taken up into oocytes, such as albumen-like molecules, may carry other molecules into the oocyte for metabolism or regulatory functions in the nucleus and elsewhere. There have been suggestions that they may be involved in masking stored RNA, but this hypothesis seems unlikely to us. In oviparious species, the major storage proteins for vitellogenesis are produced in other organs, such as liver, and transported in the blood to the oocyte for endocytosis after binding to specific receptors on the cell surface (Byrne, Gruber & Ab 1989). Thus, we might expect that, if such a mechanism exists in mammals, we might look first at the more abundant proteins with a possible storage function, such as the protein lattices of rodent oocytes.

Zona pellucida proteins

The ZP is a fibrillar coat of glycoproteins up to 7 μm thick secreted by the oocyte into the perivitelline space. The composition of the glycoproteins which make up the ZP is quite variable as a result of carbohydrate moieties added to a small number of polypeptides. The ZP proteins have been isolated and characterized from a number of mammalian species and consist of just three glycoproteins in the mouse (two to four in the pig, rabbit, monkey and human) (Wassarman, 1988b). The three glycoproteins are ZP1 (average size 200 kD), ZP2 (120 kD), and ZP3 (83 kD). ZP2 and 3 are present in equimolar amounts whilst ZP1 is much less abundant. Much of their molecular weight is from the post-translational modifications, the native polypeptides having been estimated to be 81 kD, 44 kD, and 75 kD for ZP1, 2 and 3, respectively. They are not only different molecular species, but also have different biological functions and variable patterns of glycosylation, the murine ZPs having N-linked oligosaccharides and ZP2 and 3 also have sites for O-linked glycosylation. The porcine zona pellucida, which has also been characterized in some detail, has a small number of basic polypeptide chains which are differentially glycosylated to give a variety of different molecular species.

The ZP proteins belong to a unique class of macromolecules which is not related to components normally found in the extracellular matrix, such as collagen or fibronectin. In mice, it has been clearly established that they are secreted by the oocyte, and this is likely to be the case for other mammals, although the experimental evidence is less complete. The ZPs are evidently representatives of

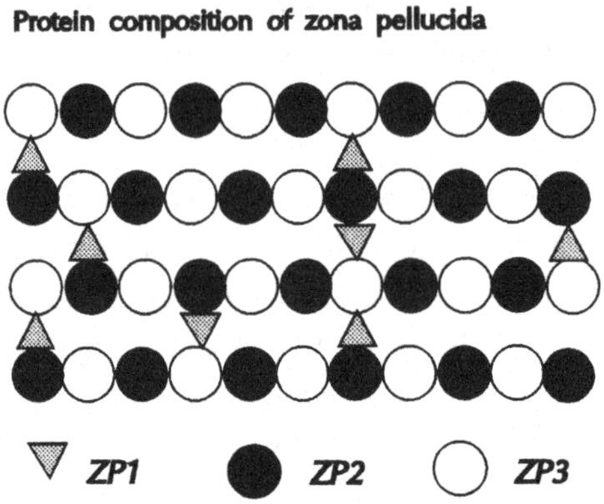

Protein composition of zona pellucida

Fig. 17. Diagrammatic representation of the murine zona pellucida showing chains of ZP2 and ZP3 glycoproteins joined by ZP1 heterodimers.

a family of highly conserved genes since 60% of the amino acid sequence of human and murine ZP3 is similar.

The molecular structure of the ZP helps to clarify how it functions as a protective and sperm-binding membrane. Chains of ZP2 and 3 are joined by heterodimeric ZP1 to produce a mesh of fibrils (Fig. 17). ZP3 is the primary sperm receptor which binds specifically to the sperm head and induces the acrosome reaction. Receptor recognition lies not, however, within the polypeptide chain but with a specific class of O-linked (serine/threonine) oligosaccharide, and the great diversity of these allows the generation of species-specific sperm recognition. The complementary part of this system is the enzyme β-1,4-galactosyltransferase located on the surface of the sperm head which specifically recognises the N-acetylglucosamine on ZP3 (Miller, Macek & Shur, 1992). If the binding site for Gal-transferase is blocked on the ZP3, sperm are no longer able to bind or penetrate the zona. ZP2 is a secondary sperm receptor which binds acrosome-induced sperm and facilitates penetration of the coat. Thus, dimers of ZP2 and 3 have key roles in fertilization: first in sperm activation and penetration and second in excluding supernumerary sperm as a result of the actions on the ZP of enzymes released from cortical granules.

Interactions with follicle cells

Oocytes and granulosa cells are mutually interdependent for survival and normal development, which has practical implications for strategies aimed at growing them in culture (Gosden & Boland, 1992). On the one hand, follicular integrity depends on the presence of the oocyte and, on the other, oocytes require granulosa cells to survive and for controlling development. There are some experimental conditions *in vivo* and in organ culture that permit oocyte growth to occur independently of follicle growth, but it is far from clear whether the cells become fully mature and fertile. Small oocytes completely denuded of follicle cells fail to thrive and grow in follicle-conditioned culture medium, but limited development is possible when contact is maintained *in vitro* on a lawn of granulosa cells. Interestingly, the period required for reaching the same degree of development *in vivo* and *in vitro* is similar, implying that oocytes possess an autonomous programme which requires a fixed time for its expression (Canipari *et al., 1984*).

Although lying within a zona pellucida near the centre of an avascular follicle, the oocyte is not cut off from influences in the external environment. The porous zona permits exchange of molecules with follicular fluid and the foot processes of cells in the corona radiata extend for about $10\,\mu$m through the zona and terminate as buttons on the oolemma with adhesive (intermediate)-type junctions as well as gap junctions (Anderson & Albertini, 1976) (Fig. 4). During the later stages of follicular growth, granulosa cells become joined to each other by gap junctions which are much larger and reveal more particles by freeze–fracture techniques than the heterologous junctions. The physiological significance of these junctions is that they provide low resistance electrical pathways and pores with a calibre sufficient to permit exchange of ions and molecules of up to about 1000 D. The union is broken within a few hours of the ovulatory gonadotrophin surge when the processes are withdrawn and the vitellus shrinks.

The significance of gap junctions between cells has been well illustrated by experimental studies performed *in vitro* (Lawrence, Beers & Gilula, 1978). Mouse myocardial cells respond to noradrenaline electrophysiologically and by an increasing frequency of contractions mediated by cyclic AMP: they are unresponsive to FSH. Ovarian granulosa cells, on the other hand, respond to FSH by stimulating adenylate cyclase and, hence, the production of plasminogen activator: they do not respond to noradrenaline. When these cell types are in contact *in vitro*, intercellular junctions form and enable noradrenaline to promote PA production from granulosa cells while FSH increases the amplitude of action potentials and beat frequency of heart cells.

The granulosa–oocyte complex is a metabolically coupled unit in which ions, amino acids, nucleotides and other small molecules can equilibrate between the compartments without affecting the distinctive macromolecular phenotype of either cell type. Furthermore, granulosa cells liberate the oocyte from responsibility for some of its nutritional requirements, as demonstrated *in vitro* by incubating growing oocytes in radioisotopically labelled metabolites or their analogues. Granulosa-enclosed oocytes incorporate significantly less uridine, choline, 2-deoxyglucose and some amino acids than naked ones according to the

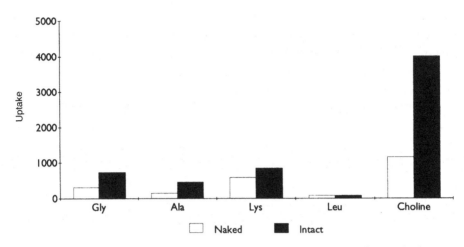

Fig. 18. Incorporation of tritiated choline and amino acids (glycine, L-alanine, L-lysine, L-leucine) by mouse oocytes cultured at mid-growth stages. With the exception of L-leucine, significantly more metabolite was taken up by oocytes enclosed in granulosa complexes than by denuded ones. (Data extracted from Haghighat & van Winkle, 1990) and reproduced by permission from *J Exp Zool* 253: 71–82.)

number of cells attached (Fig. 18) (Heller & Schultz, 1980; Moor, Smith & Dawson, 1980; Haghighat & van Winkle, 1990). The diminished ability of naked oocytes to take up amino acids directly from the medium is a result of a deficiency of the energy-dependent A-transport system which is normally compensated for by supplies from the granulosa cells via gap junctions.

Nucleotides may also pass between cells either as signalling molecules influencing phosphorylation states or as ATP to fuel the intense biosynthetic activities of oogenesis. Surprisingly little is known about the normal sources of energy though it appears that the mature isolated oocyte, like embryos up to the eight-cell stage, requires pyruvate and cannot oxidize either glucose or lactate (Biggers, Whittingham & Donohue, 1967). The very high concentrations of lactate dehydrogenase in oocytes are puzzling in view of the inability to metabolize lactate. One plausible explanation is that the large amounts of lactate produced glycolytically by granulosa cells might shift the equilibrium between lactate and pyruvate in favour of formation of the latter which, in the presence of sufficient NAD+, could contribute to energy production (Boland *et al.*, 1993).

The relationship between granulosa cells and oocytes is, however, one of reciprocal influences rather than unbalanced dependence (Fig. 19). Proliferation, morphogenesis and differentiation of the cumulus cells are all influenced by local factors released by the oocyte (Buccione, Schroeder & Eppig, 1990). The secretory activity of oocytes therefore amounts to much more than the production of a

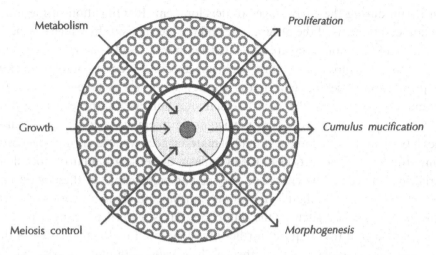

Fig. 19. Interactive character of relationships between the central germinal vesicle oocyte and its surrounding somatic cells.

zona pellucida and cortical granule exocytosis, and another major goal for future research is elucidation of the signalling molecules passing between oocytes and granulosa cells which regulate development of the follicle as a unit.

Prospect

Mammalian oogenesis is still an infant science and it is risky to make generalizations while knowledge remains so heavily weighted on the study of one model species. Nevertheless, some bold predictions can be offered on the basis of comparative biology, on the strength of striking findings in recent years, that some fundamental developmental mechanisms have been well-conserved during evolution. The homology of *hox* sequences involved in laying down the body plan in organisms as diverse as *Drosophila* and mammals is perhaps the most notable example. It would be serendipitous if genes recently shown to be involved in *Drosophila* oogenesis were found to have homologues in mammals. This would offer an additional and faster route for identifying important genes and their products than the conventional ones requiring the production of cDNA libraries and monoclonal antibodies. Genes with a specific role in determining the insect germ line and anchoring stored mRNAs, such as *vasa* and *staufen*, are more likely to be widely important than those responsible for embryonic polarity which has no obvious parallel in most mammalian eggs (Lasko, 1992).

Many other important issues arise from the cell biology of oogenesis, as we have shown. Clearly, the egg acquires during development a stored programme which is run during the early stages of development. Identification of the most important components of the programme and the mechanisms by which synthesis and actions of the molecules are regulated temporally and spatially within the cell are among the most challenging problems ahead. A second notable question is the proportion of cell protein that is synthesized *in situ* or taken up from the environment. This raises the controversial question about the existence and character of mammalian 'yolk' and particularly protein storage. Ultrastructural studies have demonstrated that a variety of material accumulates during oogenesis, ranging from crystalline lattices in the cytoplasm to dense granular or flocculent material in organelles. The character, origins and significance of these materials require clarification. The significance of the unusual and changing forms of some cytoplasmic organelles, such as the mitochondria, is a third puzzling aspect of oocyte development that requires further investigation. Finally, the nature of the association between oocytes and their follicle cells, although clearly one of interdependence, is far from being exhaustively investigated. We need to identify the signalling molecules passing between them and so acquire a better understanding of how the oocyte obtains all the metabolites it requires before we can say whether it will ever be possible to grow naked oocytes to full maturity.

Acknowledgements

We are indebted to Dr Daniel Szollosi (INRA, Jouy-en-Josas, France) for commenting on the manuscript and for permission to use his unpublished electron micrographs. We thank The Wellcome Trust and Medical Research Council for supporting our research on oogenesis.

References

Anderson E, Albertini DF. Gap junctions between the oocyte and companion follicle cells in the mammalian ovary. *J Cell Biol.* 1976; **71**: 680–6.

Bachvarova R. Gene expression during oogenesis and oocyte development in mammals. In: Browder LW, ed. *Developmental Biology. A Comprehensive Synthesis. Volume 1, Oogenesis.* New York: Plenum, 1985: 453–524

Bachvarova R, De Leon V, Spiegelman I. Mouse egg ribosomes: evidence for storage in lattices. *J Embryol Exp Morph* 1981; **62**: 153–64.

Bachvarova R, De Leon V, Johnson A, Kaplan G, Paynton BV. Changes in total RNA, polyadenylated RNA and actin RNA during meiotic maturation of mouse oocytes. *Dev Biol* 1985; **108**: 325–31.

Baker TG, O WS. Development of the ovary and oogenesis. *Clinics Obst Gyn* 1976; **3**: 3–26.

Biggers JD, Whittingham DG, Donahue RP. The pattern of energy metabolism in the mouse oocyte and zygote. *Proc Natl Acad Sci USA* 1967; **58**: 560–7.

Blobel CP, Wolfsberg TG, Turck CW, Myles DG, Primakoff P, White JM. A potential fusion peptide and an integrin ligand domain in a protein active in sperm–egg fusion. *Nature, Lond* 1992; **356**: 248–52.

Boland NI, Humpherson PG, Leese HJ, Gosden RG. The pattern of lactate production and steroidogenesis during growth and maturation of mouse ovarian follicles *in vitro*. *Biol Reprod* 1993; **48**: 798–806.

Braude P, Bolton V, Moore S. Human gene expression first occurs between the four- and eight-cell stages of preimplantation development. *Nature, Lond* 1988; **332**: 459–62.

Buccione R, Schroeder AC, Eppig JJ. Interactions between somatic cells and germ cells throughout mammalian oogenesis. *Biol Reprod* 1990; **43**: 543–7.

Burkholder GD, Comings DE, Okada TA. A storage form of ribosomes in mouse oocytes. *Exp Cell Res* 1971; **69**: 361–71.

Byrne BM, Gruber M, Ab G. The evolution of egg yolk proteins. *Biophys Mol Biol* 1989; **53**: 33–69.

Canipari R, Palombi F, Riminucci M, Mangia F. Early programming of maturation competence in mouse oogenesis. *Dev Biol* 1984; **102**: 519–24.

Chouinard LA. An electron-microscope study of the extranucleolar bodies during growth of the oocyte in the prepubertal mouse. *J Cell Sci* 1973; **12**: 55–69.

Clegg KB, Piko L. Quantitative aspects of RNA synthesis and polyadenylation in 1-cell and 2-cell mouse embryos. *J Embryol Exp Morph* 1983; **74**: 169–82.

Crosby IM, Moor RM. Oocyte maturation. In: Trounson A, Wood C, eds. *In Vitro Fertilization and Embryo Transfer*. Edinburgh: Churchill-Livingstone, 1984: 19–31.

Davidson EH. *Gene Activity in Early Development*. Orlando: Academic Press, 3rd ed., 1986: 328–75.

Flach G, Johnson MH, Braude PR, Taylor RAS, Bolton VN. The transition from maternal to embryonic control in the 2-cell mouse embryo. *EMBO J* 1982; **1**: 681–6.

Fusi FM, Vignali M, Gailit J, Bronson RA. Mammalian oocytes exhibit specific recognition of the RGD (Arg–Gly–Asp) tripeptide and express oolemmal integrins. *Mol Reprod Dev* 1993; **36**: 212–19.

Glass LE. Transmission of maternal proteins into oocytes. *Adv Biosci* 1971; **6**: 29–58.

Gosden RG, Boland NI. Extracorporeal development of mammalian oocytes. In: Templeton AA, Drife JO, eds. *Infertility*. London: Springer-Verlag, 1992: 263–75.

Gosden RG, Telfer E. Scaling of follicular sizes in mammalian ovaries. *J Zool (A)* 1987; **211**: 157–68.

Gyllensten U, Wharton D, Josefsson A, Wilson AC. Paternal inheritance of mitochondrial DNA in mice. *Nature, Lond* 1991; **352**: 255–7.

Haghighat N, van Winkle LJ (1990) Developmental change in follicular cell-enhanced amino acid uptake into mouse oocytes that depends on intact gap junctions and transport system Gly. *J Exp Zool* 1990; **253**: 71–82.

Heller DT, Schultz RM. Ribonucleoside metabolism by mouse oocytes: metabolic cooperativity between the fully grown oocyte and cumulus cells. *J Exp Zool* 1980; **214**: 355–64.

Lasko PF. Molecular movements in oocyte patterning and pole cell differentiation. *Bioessays* 1992; **14**: 507–12.

Lawrence TS, Beers WH, Gilula NB. Transmission of hormonal stimulation by cell–cell communication. *Nature, Lond* 1978; **272**: 501-6.

Magnusson T, Epstein CJ. Genetic control of very early mammalian development. *Biol Rev* 1981; **56**: 369–408.

Miller DJ, Macek MB, Shur BD. Complementarity between sperm surface
β-1,4-galactosyl-transferase and egg-coat ZP3 mediates sperm–egg binding. *Nature, Lond* 1992; **357**: 589–93.

Moor RM, Smith MW, Dawson RMC. Measurement of intercellular coupling between oocytes and cumulus cells using intracellular markers. *Exp Cell Res* 1980; **126**: 15–29.

Nishi M, Kumar NM, Gilula NB. Developmental regulation of gap junction gene expression during mouse embryonic development. *Dev Biol* 1991; **146**: 117–30.

Piko L, Clegg KB. Quantitative changes in total RNA, total poly(A), and ribosomes in early mouse embryos. *Dev Biol* 1982; **89**: 362–78.

Richoux V, Renard J-P, Babinet C. Synthesis and developmental regulation of an egg specific mouse protein translated from maternal mRNA. *Mol Reprod Dev* 1991; **28**: 218–29.

Roller RJ, Kinloch RA, Hiraoka BY, Li SS-L, Wassarman PM. Gene expression during mammalian oogenesis and early embryogenesis: quantification of three messenger RNAs abundant in fully grown mouse oocytes. *Development* 1989; **106**: 251–61.

Schultz RM. Molecular aspects of mammalian oocyte growth and maturation. In: Rossant J, Petersen RA, eds. *Experimental Approaches to Mammalian Embryonic Development* Cambridge: C.U.P., 1986: 195–237.

Sorensen RA, Wassarman PM. Relationship between growth and meiotic maturation of the mouse oocyte. *Dev Biol* 1976; **50**: 531–6.

Strickland S, Huarte J, Belin D, Vassalli A, Rickles RJ, Vassalli J-D. Antisense RNA directed against the 3' noncoding region prevents dormant mRNA activation in mouse oocytes. *Science* 1988; **241**: 680–4.

Szollosi D. Changes of some cell organelles during oogenesis in mammals. In: Biggers JD, Schuetz, AW, eds. *Oogenesis*. Baltimore: University Park Press, 1972: 47–64.

Szollosi D, Calarco P, Donahue RP. Absence of centrioles in the first and second meiotic spindles of mouse oocytes. *J Cell Sci* 1972; **11**: 521–41.

Taylor KD, Piko L. Patterns of mRNA prevalence and expression of B1 and B2 transcripts in early mouse embryos. *Development* 1987; **101**: 877–92.

Taylor KD, Piko L. Quantitative changes in cytoskeletal β- and alpha-actin mRNAs and apparent absence of sarcomeric actin gene transcripts in early mouse embryos. *Mol Reprod Dev* 1990; **26**: 111–21.

Taylor KD, Piko L. Expression of the *rig* gene in mouse oocytes and early embryos. *Mol Reprod Dev* 1991; **28**: 319–24.

Trounson A. Fertilization and embryo culture. In: Wood C, Trounson A, eds. *Clinical In Vitro Fertilization,* 2nd edn. Berlin, Heidelberg: Springer-Verlag 1989, 41.

Vassalli J-D, Huarte J, Belin D, Gubler P, Vassalli A, O'Connell ML, Parton LA, Rickles RJ, Strickland S. Regulated polyadenylation controls mRNA translation during meiotic maturation of mouse oocytes. *Genes & Dev* 1989; **3**: 2163–71.

Wassarman PM. The mammalian ovum. In: Knobil E, Neill JD, eds. *The Physiology of Reproduction,* vol 1. New York, Raven Press, 1988*a*: 69–102.

Wassarman PM. Zona pellucida glycoproteins. *Ann Rev Biochem* 1988*b*; **57**: 415–42.

Wassarman PM, Josefowicz WJ. Oocytes development in the mouse: an ultrastructural comparison of oocytes isolated at various stages of growth and meiotic competence. *J Morph* 1978; **156**: 209–36.

Weakley BS. Comparison of cytoplasmic lamellae and membranous elements in the oocytes of five mammalian species. *Z Zellforsch* 1968; **85**: 109-23.

West JD, Flockhart JH, Angell RR, Hillier SG, Thatcher SS, Glasier AF, Rodger MW, Baird DT. Glucose phosphate isomerase activity in mouse and human eggs and pre-embryos. *Hum Reprod* 1989; **4**: 82–5.

Yotsuyanagi Y, Szollosi D. Virus-like particles and related expressions in mammalian oocytes and preimplantation stage embryos. In: Van Blerkom J, Motta PM, eds. *Ultrastructure of Reproduction*. Boston: Martinus Nijhoff, 1984: 218–34.

3

Cytoskeletal organization and dynamics in mammalian oocytes during maturation and fertilization

C. SIMERLY, C. NAVARA, G.-J. WU AND G. SCHATTEN

Investigations on the organization of the human oocyte

The human oocyte exhibits two remarkable phenomena: the reductional divisions necessary to create the haploid gamete during meiotic maturation and the restoration of the diploid condition when the sperm unites with the mature oocyte during fertilization. Fertilization leads to the extraordinary cascade of events involving metabolic activation, motility, the initiation of the cell cyclical events of DNA replication and chromosome separation at mitosis, and cell surface alterations to effect the block to polyspermy. Ultimately, these divisions lead to the formation of the human embryo and developing fetus.

While information on human oocytes and human fertilization is of tremendous importance for generating a full understanding of the origins of human life, the availability of human oocytes for experimentation is, of course, limited, and most countries have restrictions on the investigation of human fertilization. Consequently, this field has progressed due to the sensible approach of developing methods and learning details about cytoskeletal activity during fertilization in lower animals, lower mammals (such as rodents and domestic species), and then making predictions about the situation in the primate egg. These hypotheses can be tested in non-human primates (such as the Rhesus monkey) where fertilization can be explored without the same sort of ethical and moral dilemmas associated with human fertilization. In addition, surplus unfertilized human oocytes can be obtained from IVF or GIFT clinics.

This chapter will review the state of knowledge regarding the human oocyte structure by considering the organization of the cytoskeleton (in particular microtubules and microfilaments), and the dynamic behaviour and regulation these structures exhibit during maturation and fertilization. Information will be presented from studies on various mammals, including humans, and the gaps in our knowledge on the human oocyte will be highlighted.

Intracellular events

The mammalian oocyte exhibits several motility events mediated by the rearrangement of the egg cytoskeleton which successfully conclude the chromosomal reductional divisions during meiotic maturation, and ensure the correct union of the parental genomes during fertilization. The milestones crucial to achieving mammalian fertilization are depicted in the living mouse oocyte and egg by time-lapse differential interference contrast (DIC) imaging (Fig.1).

Immature primary oocytes released from ovarian follicles are arrested at the dictyate stage, and contain a germinal vesicle (GV) with a prominent nucleolus (Fig.1A), seen here without the accompanying follicular and cumulus cells. Mouse GV-oocytes will resume meiotic maturation spontaneously when placed in the proper culture conditions (Donahue, 1968). Within three hours of culturing *in vitro*, the germinal vesicle disappears (Fig.1B) and the chromosomes condense into circular bivalents (Wassarman, Josefowicz & Letourneau, 1976). Microtubules organize the first meiotic spindle (MetI) at the cell centre within 9 hours of culturing (Fig.1C), and the bivalents align at the metaphase equator. The MetI spindle migrates peripherally to the cell cortex over the next few hours, a process which has been shown to require oocyte-mediated microfilaments (Longo & Chen, 1985). By 12–14 hours post-culturing, the murine oocyte will complete a reductional division and elicit the first polar body (Fig.1D). Since no interphase stage occurs between first and second meiosis, the chromosomes immediately align at the equator of the second metaphase (MetII) spindle, where the oocyte remains arrested until fertilization or activation. MetII arrest is generally achieved *in vivo* shortly before ovulation.

Not all mammalian species will undergo spontaneous meiotic maturation *in vitro* as readily as the mouse oocyte. Other species such as primates and domestic species require the presence of follicular cells and/or exogenous hormones added to the maturation medium to complete meiosis I (for review see Thibault, Szöllosi & Gerard, 1987). Other significant deviations from the murine model include the peripheral positioning of the germinal vesicle next to the egg cortex prior to GVBD and the extended timing of meiotic maturation in these species (24–48 hours post-culturing). A few mammalian species (e.g. dog) are ovulated at the germinal vesicle stage and do not complete first meiosis until 48 hours later (Yamada *et al.*, 1992) but the vast majority of eutherian mammals arrest at metaphase of second meiosis around the time of ovulation (for review see Thibault *et al.*, 1987).

Sperm penetration occurs in the oviduct following ovulation *in vivo* or it can be achieved using *in vitro* fertilization (IVF) technology for many species, including the human (Steptoe & Edwards, 1978). In species with relatively transparent

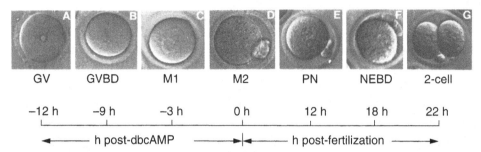

Fig. 1. Time line of development stages of mouse oocytes and zygotes. Differential interference contrast (DIC) microscopy of living oocytes. Stages include: A germinal vesicle (GV); B germinal vesicle breakdown (GVBD); C first meiotic spindle (M1); D first polar body (M2) and second meiotic spindle (invisible); E fertilized egg with male and female pronucleus and second polar body (PN); F pronuclear envelope breakdown (NEBD); G first cleavage (two-cell). Since maturing oocytes naturally arrest at M2, we set that time to 0; events before then are those after dbcAMP removal, but are assigned negative values from M2, while events afterwards have positive values, starting with hours after estimated fertilization. Times represent when 50% of the population reached the indicated stage. For parthenogenetic activation studies, haploid female pronuclear formation occurred 5 h after artificial stimulation; all other times are similarly adjusted by 7 h less. (Reprinted, with permission, from Tombes *et al.*, 1992.)

oocytes such as the mouse and human, the morphological signs of insemination can be confirmed with the appearance of two pronuclei, the second polar body, and the presence of the incorporated sperm axoneme in the cytoplasm beginning 8–12 hours post-insemination (Fig.1E). The first cell cycle is some 12–24 hours long in mammals (Thibault, 1971) and, with confirmation of pronuclear envelope breakdown (Fig.1E) and the alignment of the parental genomes on the first metaphase equator, the fertilization stage is concluded. Cytokinesis signifies the completion of the first cell cycle and occurs some 22–36 hours post-insemination (Fig.1G; Thibault, 1971).

Mammalian fertilization, therefore, encompasses the period between the resumption of meiotic maturation and mid-mitosis, being formally completed when the parental genomes intermix at metaphase of first mitosis. Essential to the successful completion of mammalian meiotic maturation and fertilization are the architectural rearrangements in the oocyte cytoskeleton which are crucial to ensure the successful union of the parental genomes. These events will be highlighted in the following sections for the various mammalian species which have thus far been investigated. Changes in nuclear organization during fertilization have been reviewed by Schatten and Schatten (1987).

Microtubule organization

Microtubules, 25 nm cytoskeletal elements, are essential for chromosome movements as well as other aspects of motility and cytoplasmic architecture (for review see Longo, 1989; Yanagimachi, 1988). In the mammalian oocyte, microtubules are essential for first and second meiosis, and for the swimming of the sperm as well as the union of the male and female pronuclei (sperm and egg nuclei, respectively) during fertilization. This section will consider our knowledge regarding microtubules and related structures in the mammalian oocyte and egg. Since the majority of information is derived from murine oocytes that system will be considered first, next domestic species (e.g. cows) will be discussed and finally primate oocytes (human and rhesus) will be described.

Microtubule organization in mouse oocytes during maturation and fertilization

The dominant microtubule-containing structure in the unfertilized mouse oocyte arrested at metaphase of second meiosis is the meiotic spindle; it is anastral, barrel shaped with broad poles, and anchored to the cell cortex tangentially as depicted in Fig. 2 (Schatten *et al.*, 1986*a*). Curiously, around a dozen cytoplasmic microtubules (cytasters) are also detected in the mouse oocyte cytoplasm. Microtubules in the meiotic spindle are crucial for the proper alignment and separation of the maternal chromosomes during progressive maturation while the cytoplasmic microtubules are responsible for the motions necessary for pronuclear apposition following sperm insemination (Szöllosi, Calarco & Donahue, 1972; Wassarman & Fujiwara, 1978; Messing & Albertini, 1991; Schatten *et al.*, 1986 *a*).

In most animals, the sperm is thought to introduce the dominant microtubule organizing entity at fertilization, the centrosome. This organelle creates the sperm aster, the microtubule-based structure responsible for male and female pronuclear movement and ultimately their apposition (Boveri, 1901; Mazia, 1987). Surprisingly, however, the incorporated mouse sperm does not organize microtubules in the cytoplasm of the oocyte. As shown in Fig. 2, the microtubule-containing cytasters derived from the oocyte increase in size during pronuclear development to fill the egg cytoplasm with a dense matrix of assembled tubulin protein which ultimately moves the pronuclei into close apposition at the cell center. Pronuclear fusion does not occur in the mouse and, by the end of first interphase, the matrix array disassembles, ensheathing the apposed, centered pronuclei in a perinuclear shell of microtubules.

Microtubule configurations during first division in the mouse are shown in Fig. 3. As prophase commences, the paternal and maternal chromosomes, still

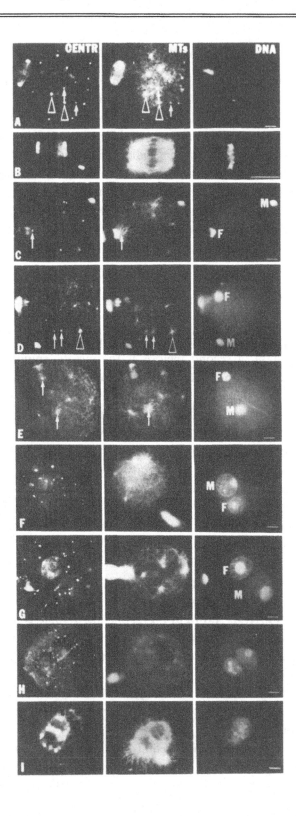

separated by the perinuclear microtubules, condense separately within the monaster array. As mitosis ensues, the chromosomes intermix at the equator of the barrel-shaped, anastral metaphase spindle and successfully conclude the fertilization stage. The mouse mitotic spindle has an atypical shape compared to most animal cells and more closely resembles the spindles of plant cells: only sparse microtubules appear at the spindle poles in anaphase and few non-spindle microtubules are found in the cytoplasm. By telophase, interzonal microtubules form and aggregate into a midbody structure during cell division as a new cytoplasmic array of microtubules develops in the daughter blastomeres.

The dramatic alterations in the patterns of microtubules during mouse fertilization resemble the configurations noted for other animal systems for the segregation of the chromosomes in meiosis and mitosis as well as for the migrations leading to the union of the parental genomes (for review see Schatten, 1982). In contrast to other systems, however, spindle poles in both meiosis and first mitosis are organized without the presence of centrioles (Szöllosi *et al.*, 1972) and microtubules are nucleated by maternal centrosomes rather than the incorporated sperm centriole/centrosome complex (Maro, Howlett & Houliston, 1986*b*; Schatten *et al.*, 1986*a*). These observations raise interesting questions about the inheritance of microtubule-organizing centres, and will be considered in more detail in the section on patterns of centrosomal inheritance in mammals.

Microtubules are dynamic structures and fluorescent tubulin protein micro-injected into interphase or mitotic cells turnover subunits within the polymerized arrays with differing rates, as measured by fluorescent recovery after photobleaching (FRAP) (Gorbsky *et al.*, 1990; Sammak & Borisy, 1986; Saxton *et al.*, 1984). Microtubules in mammalian second meiotic spindles might be highly stable since oocytes are arrested at this stage awaiting fertilization. Surprisingly, as demonstrated in Fig. 4, the microtubules comprising the second meiotic spindle in the mouse oocyte are highly active structures as measured by FRAP analysis (Gorbsky *et al.*, 1990). Recovery rates for turnover of tubulin protein in the mouse second meiotic spindle are similar to the rates measured for somatic cell and echinoderm mitotic spindles (Hamaguchi *et al.*, 1987; Salmon *et al.*, 1984; Gorbsky

Fig. 2. Centrosomes during mouse fertilization. Centrosomes (CENTR, left panels) are found as cytoplasmic foci (A) and at the meiotic spindle poles (A and B) in unfertilized oocytes. Microtubules (MTs, middle panels) extend from the centrosomal material, forming the meiotic spindle and cytoplasmic asters; each focus organizes an aster (arrows) with brighter ones associated with larger asters (triangles). Centrosomes are not detected in mouse sperm or with the entering sperm during incorporation (C and D). They associate with the developing pronuclei (C–G) as microtubules fill the cytoplasm. (Reprinted, with permission, from Schatten *et al.*, 1986*a*.)

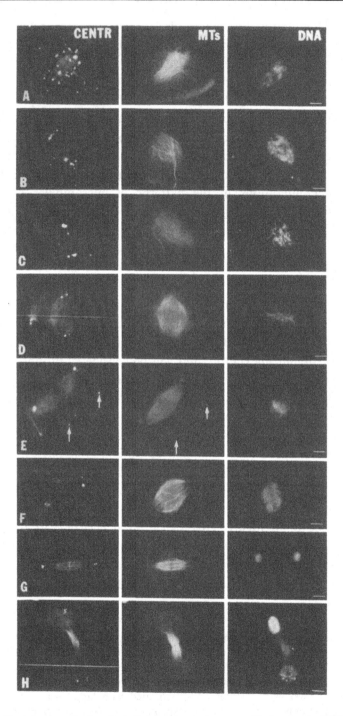

Fig. 3. Centrosomes during first division in mouse eggs. Centrosomes (CENTR, left panels) move as two clusters into the cytoplasm at prophase (A and B), as an irregular mass of microtubules (MTs, middle panels) forms around the aligning

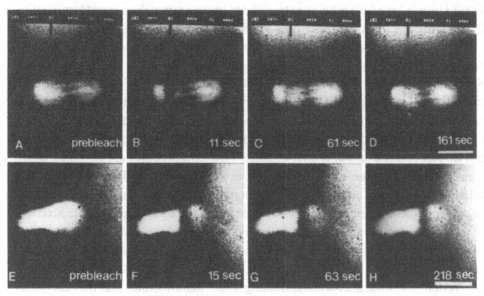

Fig. 4. Fluorescent recovery after photobleaching occurs rapidly in unfertilized mouse oocytes arrested in metaphase of second meiosis but slowly in meiotic midbodies. χ-Rhodamine-tubulin microinjected into metaphase arrested oocytes incorporates into spindle microtubules as detected by live imaging with a cooled charge-coupled device (A, prebleach). Following laser photobleaching of a cylindrical bar across the fluorescent spindle (B), a progression of images after irradiation shows that fluorescent recovery is rapid in the bleached zone (C and D). A prebleach image of a meiotic midbody is shown in E. Following laser photobleaching of a cylindrical bar across the midbody (F), subsequent images (G and H) demonstrate that fluorescent recovery is slow. Times in sec. after photobleaching are indicated in the lower right of frames B–D and F–H. (Bar = 10 μm.) (Reprinted, with permission, from Gorbsky *et al.*, 1990.)

& Borisy, 1989; Wadsworth & Salmon, 1985) and nearly four times the rate measured for telophase midbodies, an incredible rate for a spindle considered arrested! FRAP analysis has advanced our understanding of how changes in microtubule patterns occur during interphase and cell divisions (Mitchison *et al.,*

Caption for fig 3 (*cont.*).
mitotic chromosomes (DNA, right panels). At prometaphase (C) the centrosomes appear as broad clusters on opposing sides of the chromosome mass as a barrel-shaped anastral spindle becomes apparent. At metaphase the centrosomes aggregate into either loose irregular bands (D) or more tightly focused sites (E). Centrosomal foci not associated with spindle poles organize microtubules (arrows, E). During anaphase (F) the centrosomes continue their separation. At cleavage (G and H) the centrosomes are found along the poleward surfaces of the blastomere nuclei and the midbody becomes apparent. All eggs were triple-labelled for centrosomes, microtubules, and DNA. (Bar = 10 μm.) (Reprinted, with permission, from Schatten *et al.*, 1986.)

1986), knowledge which is being extrapolated to the mammalian egg at fertilization by studying the dynamic properties of their microtubules.

The stability of microtubules in the mouse oocyte appears to be influenced by two post-translational modifications of the α-tubulin subunit (for review see Schatten *et al.*, 1988; De Pennart, Houliston & Maro, 1988): the acetylation of the lysine-40 amino acid (LeDizet & Piperno, 1987) and the shuttling of a carboxy-terminal tyrosine residue, a process referred to as detyrosination and tyrosination (Gundersen & Bulinski, 1986; Wehland & Weber, 1987). The mouse oocyte represents a useful model to study how microtubules are modified post-translationally because of the alterations in the appearance, disappearance, and selective stabilization of microtubules during the latter stages of meiotic maturation and during the fertilization process. For instance, the unfertilized oocyte arrested at metaphase can be induced artificially to complete meiosis and the modifications of the microtubules in the spindle, cytasters, and the newly formed midbody structure can be investigated using antibodies specific to acetylated α-tubulin and contrasted with total microtubule staining. Fig. 5 demonstrates that the acetylated form is predominately localized to meiotic poles at metaphase, and to the midbody structure after second polar body formation. The interzonal microtubules are only weakly detected, and the cytoplasmic asters apparently are not acetylated. As shown in Fig. 6, ultrastructural imaging by high voltage electron microscopy (HVEM) of immunogold-labelled meiotic metaphase oocytes supports and extends these observations found by immunofluorescent staining: the majority of acetylated α-tubulin is found at the meiotic poles and only sparse detection of acetylated microtubules can be found within the spindle or near the equator. After fertilization, only the microtubules of the midbody structure remaining from completion of second polar body formation and the incorporated sperm axoneme are found to be acetylated during interphase, although new microtubules fill the cytoplasm nucleated by the cytaster structures. Furthermore, the pattern of acetylated microtubules in the spindles at first mitosis are similar to configurations found at second meiosis (for review see Schatten *et al.*, 1988).

Antibodies specific to detyrosinated and tyrosinated microtubules suggest that the microtubules present during meiosis and mitosis are composed of a combination of these types of post-translationally modified microtubules (De Pennart *et al.*, 1988; for review see Schatten *et al.*, 1988). During interphase, however, unique subsets of microtubules appear to be post-translationally modified: the incorporated sperm axoneme appears to be uniquely detyrosinated while the extensive cytoplasmic microtubule network apparent at late interphase appears to be extensively tyrosinated (unpublished observation). Such observations suggest that highly stable microtubules like those which occur in sperm axonemes are

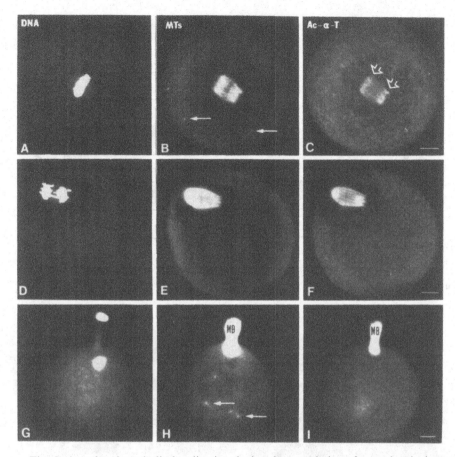

Fig. 5. Acetylated α-tubulin localization during the completion of second meiosis. Mouse oocytes are ovulated-arrested at metaphase (A). Microtubules ((B) Mts) are in the anastral barrel-shaped spindle and cytoplasmic asters ((B) arrows). The acetylated α-tubulin antibody ((C) Ac-a-T) recognizes microtubules at the centrosomes (open arrows) of the spindle. At anaphase (D), the entire meiotic spindle (E) is more heavily acetylated (F). By late telophase (G), the meiotic midbody is acetylated, though the cytasters are not (I). All images triple-labelled for DNA with Hoechst Dye 33258 (left), total tubulin (MTs, either rabbit-affinity-purified antibodies to porcine brain tubulin or rat antitubulin YL1/2) and acetylated α-tubulin antibody (1-6.1, right). (Bars = 10 μm.) (Reprinted, with permission, from Schatten *et al.*, 1988.)

preferentially detyrosinated while those microtubules which actively participate in motility events such as pronuclear apposition remain tyrosinated.

Despite the appearance that detyrosinated microtubules are correlated with the older, more stable microtubule populations, however, the significance of such

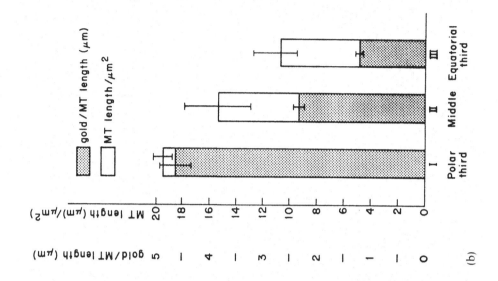

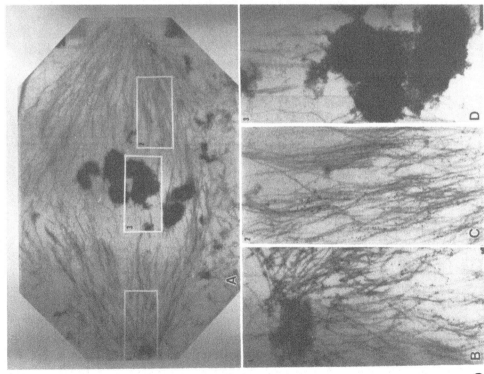

(a)

(b)

post-translational modifications remains unclear. Newer evidence using micro-injected antibodies directed against the tubulin tyrosine ligase responsible for the addition of the c-terminal tyrosine onto the tubulin protomer has clearly demonstrated that detyrosination does not directly result in increased microtubule stability but may occur after the microtubule population has already been stabilized (Webster *et al.*, 1990). Recently, it has been suggested that detyrosination may be crucial in generating unique subsets of microtubules during cell morpho-logical events such as directed motility, neurite outgrowth, and myogenesis (Bulinski & Gundersen, 1991). While the implications of post-translational modifications are not yet fully understood, their presence during meiotic maturation and fertilization in the mouse forces questions regarding their importance to microtubule function in mammals.

Kinetochores, the sites where the spindle microtubules attach to the centromeric region of the chromosome (for review see Rieder, 1982; Brinkley *et al.*, 1989), serve at least three functions during meiosis and mitosis: (a) the capture and stabilization of microtubules *in vitro* (Mitchison & Kirschner, 1985*a*, *b*), (b) congression, the process of alignment of the chromosomes at the spindle equator during prometaphase, and (c) the separation of the chromosomes at anaphase (Mitchison and Kirschner, 1985*b*; Gorbsky *et al.*, 1989; Mitchison, 1989; Nicklas, 1989). The discovery of human autoimmune antibodies from patients with CREST scleroderma (calcinosis, Raynaud's phenomenon, oesophageal dysmotility, sclero-dactyly, and telangiectasia) have pioneered the molecular characterizations of the proteins associated with the kinetochore/centromere complex (for review see Pluta, Cooke & Earnshaw, 1990). The first three specific centromere proteins identified were designated CENP-A (17kD), CENP-B (80 kD), and CENP-C (140 kD), and one of these (CENP-B) has been cloned, sequenced, and proposed as a microtubule binding protein (Earnshaw *et al.*, 1987; Earnshaw, Ratrie & Stetten, 1989; Balczon & Brinkley, 1987). Furthermore, the CREST sera have been localized to the centromere/kinetochore region by immunofluorescent and immunoEM studies (Earnshaw *et al.*, 1987; Cooke, Bernat & Earnshaw, 1990).

Fig. 6(*a*). High voltage electron microscopy of immunogold-labelled thick sections at meiotic metaphase. A Survey image depicting regions shown in (B–D). B Spindle pole region. C Middle of half-spindle. D Spindle equator. E (*b*) Quantitation of gold particles along microtubules as well as total microtubule lengths in the polar third (I), middle third (II), and equatorial third (III) of half-spindles at meiosis. The density of acetylated microtubules is greatest at the poles. (Bars = 100 nm.) (Reprinted, with permission, from Schatten *et al.*, 1988.)

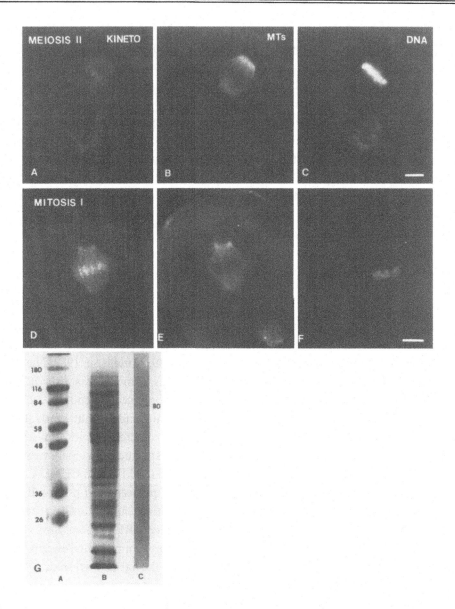

Fig. 7. Serum E.K. detects the centromere/kinetochore complex when microinjected into mouse oocytes and cross-reacts with an 80 kD protein in mouse cells. Microinjected E.K. serum binds to the centromere/kinetochore complex in oocytes naturally arrested at second meiotic metaphase (A) or at first mitotic metaphase (D); the cells are labelled with biotin-streptavidin secondary antibodies following fixation. The centromere/kinetochore complexes (KINETO: A, D) are detected as paired structures at the equator of the spindle detected with antitubulin immunofluorescence microscopy (MTS: B, E). DNA fluorescence (DNA: C, F). (G) E.K. serum (1:1,200) detects a polypeptide of 80 kD in mouse 3T3 cells. Lane c, immunoblot transfer. Lane b, Coomassie blue-stained 12.5% SDS-PAGE gel

In two recent studies, the *in vivo* function of centromere/kinetochore proteins were investigated following microinjection of CREST sera into either mouse oocytes or tissue culture cells (Simerly *et al.*, 1990; Bernat *et al.*, 1990). The mouse oocyte is an especially unique system for exploring the effects of kinetochore antibodies on chromosome motions since the events of chromosome segregation can be investigated independently of chromosome alignment at prometaphase. For instance, mature oocytes arrested at metaphase of second meiosis can be induced to resume anaphase by artificial activation techniques (Kaufman, 1983). Likewise, the use of cytoskeletal drugs at specific points in the cell cycle during meiotic maturation or fertilization will permit congression events to be examined exclusive of chromosome segregation (Wassarman *et al.*, 1976). As demonstrated in Fig. 7, microinjected CREST serum E.K. recognizes the kinetochore/centromere complex in oocytes arrested at metaphase of second meiosis or first mitosis. This sera cross-reacts with an 80 kD protein as analyzed by Western blotting on mouse cells (Fig.7G) and, when injected into prophase-arrested mouse oocytes, interferes with prometaphase congression and anaphase segregation of chromosomes (Fig.8). However, neither microtubule capture nor spindle reformation following recovery from cold or microtubule-disruption drugs were affected by the autoimmune sera. Anaphase segregation in the presence of E.K. serum was also unaffected when injected into metaphase-arrested meiotic or mitotic oocytes (Simerly *et al.*, 1990). Similar findings on chromosome congression were found to occur in tissue culture cells microinjected with autoimmune sera during interphase and examined at first mitosis (Bernat *et al.*, 1990). Although the functioning of the various identified centromere/kinetochore proteins are not well understood, these results are the first demonstration that antibodies produced by CREST patients do interfere with a specific chromosomal motion *in vivo*, namely prometaphase chromosome alignment during congression.

Microtubule organization in bovine oocytes during maturation and fertilization

Although the configurations and dynamics of the cytoskeletal system in the mouse oocyte are surprisingly distinct from most lower animals, investigations of oocytes from domestic species suggest that rodents may be atypical with regard to how

Caption for Fig. 7 (*cont.*).
(125 μg of protein). Lane a, molecular weight standards in kilodaltons. Triple labelled images for kinetochores (A and D), microtubules (B and E), and DNA (C and F). (Bar = 10 μm). (Reprinted, with permission, from Simerly *et al.*, 1990.)

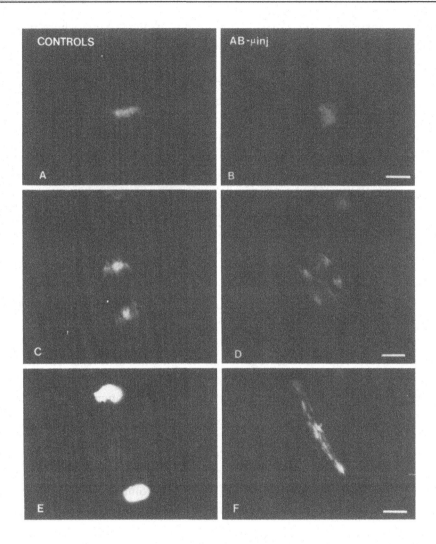

Fig. 8. Antikinetochore/centromere antibodies microinjected into zygotes at first mitosis interfere with prometaphase congression. To explore the possibility that the antibodies were affecting kinetochore maturation at the interphase mitotic transition versus congression, E.K. was microinjected into mitotic oocytes arrested at prometaphase with 5 μM nocodazole. (A, C, and E). Uninjected controls recovering from nocodazole block for an hour. (B, D, and F). Recovery in the presence of anti-kinetochore/centromere antibodies. While control cells can undergo proper chromosome alignment at metaphase (A), microinjected oocytes are unable to complete congression (B). At anaphase controls segregate their chromosomes in an orderly fashion (C), whereas microinjected cells do not (D). After first mitosis, controls display two well-separated nuclei (E) while the injected cells have many chromosomes which remain trapped in the interzonal area of the mitotic spindle (F). Double labelled for DNA (shown) and microtubules (not shown). Bars = 10 μm. (Reprinted, with permission, from Simerly *et al.*, 1990.)

microtubules are assembled during fertilization. For instance, ultrastructural and immunocytochemical analysis of sheep oocytes has suggested that microtubule assembly is initiated by the paternal centrosome shortly after sperm penetration (Le Guen & Crozet, 1989). More recently, work in cows (Long *et al.*, 1993; Navara *et al.*, 1994) indicates that this mammal may undergo fertilization mechanisms more similar to lower vertebrates such as the frog than to the mouse. Consequently, it is unclear if extrapolating the mechanisms involved in fertilization in the mouse would be a reliable indicator of how other mammals such as the human accomplish similar events.

The microtubule patterns which occur during bovine fertilization are shown in Fig. 9 (Navara *et al.*, 1994). As noted in the unfertilized mouse oocyte, the meiotic spindle in the mature bovine oocyte is arrested at metaphase of second meiosis, anastral, and barrel-shaped (A,B). However, unlike the mouse, the cow meiotic spindle is smaller in size, oriented radially to the cell surface, and is the only detectable microtubule staining structure in the unfertilized oocyte (A). Shortly after insemination microtubules assemble around the base of the incorporated sperm head, (C,D). As development continues, this sperm aster structure expands in the cytoplasm, making contact with the female pronucleus and participating in pronuclear apposition during interphase. The first mitotic cow spindle is initially organized without astral microtubules, although the poles are more fusiform than found in the mitotic spindle of the mouse oocyte (E,F). Occasionally, small aster-like wisps of microtubules are organized at the polar MTOCs in the cow metaphase spindle. At anaphase, a dramatic burst of astral microtubule formation occurs and these microtubules increase in density during telophase (G,H) to form the cytoplasmic array in the daughter blastomeres.

The observations on the patterns of microtubules during fertilization in cow and sheep oocytes reinforces the concept that different mammals may accomplish fertilization by varying means. The dominant microtubule organizing centre, or centrosome, may be paternally contributed in the domestic species, and evidence of microtubule organization by the sperm centriolar complex in sheep has been provided (Crozet, 1990). However, in the cow, parthenogenetic activation of the unfertilized bovine oocyte is possible, and these activated oocytes will form a bipolar spindle at first mitosis and undergo equal cleavage without paternal contribution (Navara *et al.*, 1994). Perhaps microtubule assembly during cow fertilization is organized by a heterogenous contribution of centrosomal material from both paternal and maternal sources, as has been recently suggested for the sea urchin (Holy & Schatten, 1991). These findings in the domestic species raise valid concerns about extrapolating the mechanism of fertilization in any lower mammal to the events which occur during fertilization in higher animals such as primates.

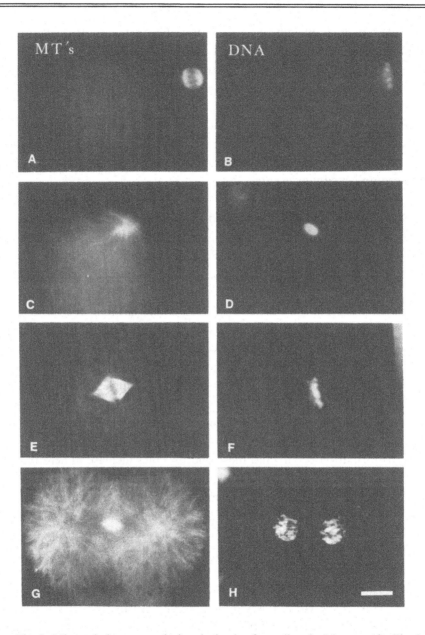

Fig. 9. Microtubule patterns during the bovine first cell cycle. Mature unfertilized bovine oocytes contain small, barrel-shaped, anastral meiotic spindles (A) oriented radially to the cell surface with the maternal chromosomes aligned along the spindle equator (B). No detectable microtubules are found in the cytoplasm of the inactivated oocyte (A). Shortly after sperm penetration, microtubules are organized into a sperm aster structure (C) at the base of the incorporating sperm DNA (D) which participate in male and female pronuclear apposition during first interphase. At the end of first interphase, the microtubule array nucleated by the sperm centrosome disassembles and a tightly focused, anastral mitotic metaphase

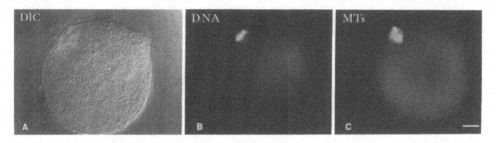

Fig. 10. Detection of microtubules in the unfertilized human oocyte. The mature unfertilized human oocyte arrested at metaphase of second meiosis (B) has a barrel-shaped, anastral meiotic spindle slightly focused at the poles and oriented radially to the cell surface (C). No microtubules are present in the cytoplasm of the inactivated human oocyte (C). Oocyte double labelled for DAPI DNA stain (B) and monoclonal β-tubulin antibody E-7 (C). (A): Differential interference contrast image. Bar = 10 μm.

Microtubule organization in primate oocytes during maturation and fertilization

The configurations of microtubules in primate oocytes and eggs during maturation and following fertilization are beginning to be investigated by modern immunocytochemical techniques. As shown in Fig. 10, the cortical localized spindle in the unfertilized human oocyte arrested at metaphase of second meiosis is anastral, slightly tapered at the poles, and oriented radially to the cell surface, as first demonstrated by antitubulin indirect immunofluorescence by Pickering *et al.* (1988; see also Simerly *et al.*, 1994, 1995). Interestingly, only spindle microtubules are detectable in human oocytes at this stage. Cytoplasmic microtubules can be imaged in spontaneously activated oocytes or in unfertilized oocytes after application of the microtubule-enhancing drug taxol (Pickering *et al.*, 1988) but the patterns of microtubules formed in the cortex are short, linear bundles, surprisingly different from the 'egg aster' structures found in the mouse cytoplasm (Maro *et al.*, 1986*b*; Schatten *et al.*, 1986*a*). Additionally, the microtubules in human meiotic spindles are highly sensitive to temperature variations (Sathananthan *et al.*, 1988), and normal spindle reformation following temperature rescue experiments are minimal (Pickering *et al.*, 1990). These

Caption for fig 9 (*cont.*).

spindle forms (E) with the condensed chromosomes aligned at the equatorial region (F). By telophase, a dramatic assembly of microtubules at the poles of the mitotic apparatus is completed (G) as the segregation of the chromosomes (H) and cytokinesis ensue. Double labelled with monoclonal β-tubulin antibody E-7 (A, C, E, G) and DAPI DNA stain (B, D, F, H). Bar = 20 μm.

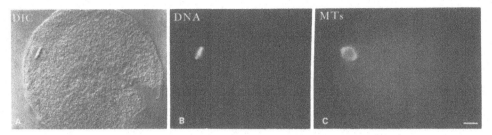

Fig. 11. Detection of microtubules in the unfertilized rhesus monkey oocyte. Microtubules in the mature rhesus monkey oocyte arrested at metaphase of second meiosis (B) are detected only in the second meiotic spindle which is anastral, barrel-shaped, and orientated radially to the cell surface (C). Oocyte double labelled for DAPI DNA stain (B) and monoclonal β-tubulin antibody E-7 (C). (A): differential interference contrast image. Bar = 10 μm.

observations suggest that the architecture and regulation of the cytoskeletal system in the human oocyte drastically differs from that characterized for mice, resembling instead the patterns described for lower animals.

Not surprisingly, the microtubule patterns in fertilized human oocytes are not well documented since the use of human inseminated material for research purposes raises serious ethical questions and runs contrary to the goals of most IVF clinics. Investigations that have been performed suggest that sperm–oocyte fusion and penetration occurs in an analogous fashion to most other mammalian systems examined (Sathananthan *et al.,* 1986). TEM analysis of monospermic or dispermic human oocytes in interphase have demonstrated typical mammalian organization for organelles and pronuclei (Sathananthan, Trounson & Wood *et al.,* 1986; Van Blerkom and Henry, 1991). Interestingly, human mitotic oocytes serial sectioned at metaphase contain spindle poles with sperm-derived centrioles (Sathananthan *et al.,* 1991), a feature comparable to that described for mitotic sheep oocytes (Crozet, 1990). The global organization of the cytoplasmic microtubules responsible for completion of meiosis, pronuclear apposition, and chromosome segregation at first mitosis, however, cannot be inferred from these ultrastructural analyses and must await future research endeavours.

If using human embryos for research purposes is a complicated issue, how can the events of human fertilization be reconciled? One possibility may be in the use of non-human primate animal models such as the old-world monkey, *Macaca mulatta* (Rhesus). As demonstrated in Fig. 11, the rhesus oocyte spindle arrested in metaphase of second meiosis is remarkably similar to the unfertilized human oocyte: barrel-shaped, anastral, with a single pole oriented towards the plasma membrane and no cytoplasmic microtubules. The configurations of microtubules in fertilized monkey eggs leading to the apposition of the male and female pronuclei suggest that the dominant MTOC in this species is obtained from the sperm (Wu *et al.*, 1993). Likewise, preliminary observation on artificially activated monkey oocytes implies that a dense network of linearly arranged microtubules forms in the cytocortex region shortly after stimulation, as have been detected for the bovine and human parthenogenotes (Navara *et al.*, 1994; Johnson *et al.*, 1991). Taken together, these results seem to suggest that primate oocytes and embryos organize their microtubules in a fashion analogous to lower mammals like the cow, sheep, and rabbit. While knowledge of the reproductive physiology and embryology in non-human primates (for review see Bavister *et al.*, 1991) is sufficiently advanced that it is plausible to undertake studies on the cytoskeletal alterations during fertilization, cautious interpretations should be warranted in making direct extrapolation of findings to the other primates such as the human.

Patterns of centrosomal inheritance in mammals: speculations in humans

Centrosomes are the cells' microtubule organizing centres (MTOCs), crucial structures involved in the organization of microtubules which direct meiosis and mitosis, pronuclear development and motility, and many other intracellular events critical to successful fertilization (for review see Schatten & Schatten, 1987). The centrosome remains as one of the great enigmas of the cell since very little is known of its functional or molecular characteristics, despite its long-appreciated importance to cellular functioning. However, unique opportunities to study the origins and behaviour of centrosomes have recently appeared with the discovery of autoimmune antibodies which detect mammalian centrosomal antigens (Calarco-Gilliam *et al.*, 1983) as well as a unique subset of tubulin protein conserved among all known centrosomes, γ-tubulin (Oakley *et al.*, 1990). This section will consider our current knowledge on the configurations and inheritance of centrosomes in mammals, beginning first with the mouse, followed by evidence in domestic species, and ending with speculations in primates.

The centrosome was believed to be typically contributed by the sperm at fertilization (Boveri, 1901) but as first recognized by Lams and Doorme (1907) in the mouse, mammalian fertilization appears to behave differently. Earlier examination of microtubule organization in the unfertilized mouse oocyte demonstrated unusual non-spindle microtubule structures in the cytoplasm (Fig. 2; Schatten, Simerly & Schatten, 1985). As shown in Fig. 2 A and B, human autoimmune antisera which recognize centrosomal epitopes stain both the poles of the second meiotic spindle (Calarco-Gilliam *et al.*, 1983) as well as the cytoplasmic microtubule structures. In addition, no centrosomes have been found in mature sperm (Schatten *et al.*, 1986*a*) nor does the sperm organize a single sperm aster structure following incorporation into the oocyte cytoplasm (Fig.2D–F; Schatten *et al.*, 1986*a*; Maro *et al.*, 1986*b*). Recently, a study has presented evidence suggesting that the non-spindle centrosomes detected at metaphase of second meiosis were derived from centrosomes present during meiotic maturation (Messinger & Albertini, 1991). These observations have led to the hypothesis that the mouse centrosome is of maternal, not paternal, origin (Schatten *et al.*, 1986*a*).

The maternal inheritance theory in the mouse oocyte has been investigated by examining: (i) parthenogenesis, where no paternal contribution is possible; (ii) polyspermy, where multiple paternal contributions are expected; and (iii) recovery from microtubule inhibition, where preferential spindle formation around the male or female chromosomes provides evidence for the source of centrosomal inheritance (Schatten, Simerly & Schatten, 1991). If the hypothesis that the centrosomes are derived from cytoplasmic maternal sources was accurate, then both parthenogenotes and polyspermic oocytes would be expected to divide normally and recovery from microtubule inhibition might be expected to result in spindle formation around both the maternal and paternal sets of chromosomes. If, on the other hand, the mouse sperm were providing the crucial spindle pole organizing material in this species, then parthenogenetically activated oocytes examined at first mitosis would not be able to organize a bipolar mitotic apparatus for chromosome segregation. Likewise, polyspermic insemination would be predicted to form multiple spindle poles at the time of first mitosis. In either case of sperm centrosomal contribution, cell division would not be expected to result in two-cell formation. Furthermore, recovery from microtubule inhibition would show a single bipolar mitotic apparatus surrounding the male chromatin only, as has been demonstrated in invertebrate systems (Sluder & Rieder, 1985). As shown in Fig. 12, unfertilized oocytes parthenogenetically activated in a dilute solution of ethanol and examined at first mitosis form two spindle poles with the haploid chromosomes aligned at the metaphase equator (Fig. 12A,B). The ploidy constitution does not alter the result (Fig. 12c–e), and parthenogenotes divide to form two equal sized blastomeres following chromosome segregation. In polyspermic cases, similar findings have been shown since spindles with two poles and a mass of aligned chromosomes at the metaphase plate are consistently found during mitosis and these cells are able to segregate their chromosomes and cleave normally (Schatten *et al.*, 1991). Recovery from nocodazole, a reversible microtubule inhibitor, has shown that two normal bipolar spindles form in the mitotic cytoplasm, one spindle associated with the condensed set of male chromatin and the other with the condensed set of female chromatin (Schatten *et al.*, 1991). Thus, the unfertilized mouse oocyte contains all the necessary constituents to organize and replicate spindle poles correctly.

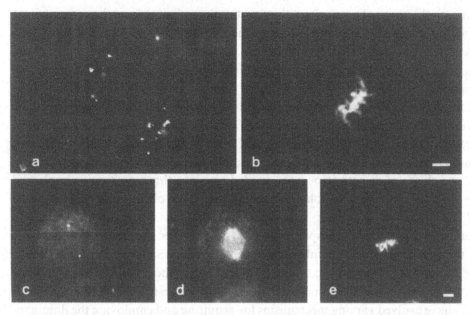

Fig. 12. Centrosomes, microtubules, and chromosome arrangements at first mitosis in haploid and diploid parthenogenotes. (Upper) Haploid parthenogenote. At first mitosis, the centrosomal foci partitioned to form two spindle poles (a), and the chromosomes aligned along a single metaphase plate (b). (Lower) Diploid parthenogenote. The ploidy number did not influence the ability of the oocyte to organize a bipolar spindle containing properly positioned centrosomes (c), and anastral, barrel-shaped spindle (d), and correctly aligned chromosomes on the metaphase equator (e). (a and b) Images were double labelled for centrosomal foci partitioned to form two spindle poles (a), and the chromosomes aligned along a single metaphase plate (b). (Lower) Diploid parthenogenote. The ploidy number did not influence the ability of the oocyte to organize a bipolar spindle containing properly positioned centrosomes (c), and anastral, barrel-shaped spindle (d), and correctly aligned chromosomes on the metaphase equator (e). (a and b) Images were double labelled for centrosomes and DNA. (c–e) Images were triple labelled for centrosomes, microtubules, and DNA. CENTROS, centrosome detection; MTs, microtubule detection; DNA, DNA fluorescence microscopy. Bars = 10 μM. (Reprinted, with permission, from Schatten, Simerly & Schatten, 1991.)

It is premature, however, to extrapolate the findings of centrosomal inheritance in the mouse to other mammalian species. Unfertilized oocytes in domestic species such as the cow and sheep do not have microtubule organizing centres localized in the cytoplasm and sperm incorporation results in the formation of a microtubule aster structure near the neck region which increases in size during pronuclear development and migration (see Fig. 9; Le Guen & Crozet, 1989; Long *et al.*, 1993; Navara *et al.*, 1994). Untrastructural analysis in the sheep has clearly shown a sperm proximal centriole originating from the incorporated neck region lying between the apposed pronuclei with microtubules radiating from the pericentriolar material. Centrioles at a single pole of the first mitotic sheep spindle have been identified as well (Crozet, 1990). In rabbits, TEM analysis, antitubulin immunofluorescence, and antibodies which detect phosphorylated centrosomal epitopes, have identified the assembly of microtubules associated with the base of the sperm head shortly after insemination, although centriolar detection in the cytoplasm of fertilized oocytes is not seen until the blastocyst stage (Longo, 1976; Szöllosi & Ozil, 1991; Yllera-Fernandez, Crozet & Ahmed-Ali, 1992). In primates, an account of the cleavage patterns in triploid human oocytes suggested that up to two-thirds of dispermic oocytes divided one-into-three, a situation explained by the formation of a tripolar spindle as the result of an extra male-donated MTOC (Kola *et al.*, 1989; Van Blerkom, 1991). In a subsequent EM study performed on mono- and dispermic human mitotic eggs, the presence of centrioles at the spindle poles was unambiguously demonstrated (Sathananthan *et al.*, 1991). All of these observations are uniquely different from the centrosomal inheritance patterns seen in the mouse oocyte, and seem to suggest that different mammals may have evolved varying mechanisms for acquiring and employing the dominant microtubule organizing entity for controlling cytoskeletal behaviour within the oocyte.

The mode of centrosomal inheritance in any species cannot be thought of in a strict paternal versus maternal heritage. Instances in which species seem to violate the requirement for the paternal inheritance of the centrosome structure are known throughout the animal kingdom (for review see Schatten *et al.*, 1991, 1994). Even in classical invertebrate species such as the sea urchin, recent investigations are demonstrating a contributing role for the maternal centrosome (Holy & Schatten, 1991). In mammals, including humans (Pickering *et al.*, 1988), oocytes can undergo parthenogenetic activation and development to late pre-implantation stages, although genomic imprinting requires a biparental nuclear contribution to reach full term and birth (Surani *et al.*, 1987). Polyspermic human oocytes can cleave normally, and the birth of triploid infants has been documented (Van Blerkom & Henry, 1991; Uchida & Freeman, 1985). The broad implications of these observations are not yet fully understood. Perhaps the lack of any strict requirements for the mode of centrosomal inheritance would permit variability among mammals, a situation that can now be explored.

Microfilament organization

Microfilaments, 7 nm cytoskeletal elements composed of the protein actin, play an important role in structuring the cell surface and underlying plasma membrane region in mammalian oocytes during meiotic maturation and fertilization. This cytoskeletal element is particularly concentrated in the plasmalemma zone known as the cell cortex region, a 1–5 μm area which contains organelles such as cortical granules, endoplasmic reticulum, ribosomes, and cytoskeletal elements (for review see Longo, 1989). Microfilaments are crucial in oocytes for maintenance of the meiotic spindles near the cortex, the formation of the first and second polar bodies, incorporation cone formation, pronuclear apposition, and cytokinesis following mitotic events. However, in contrast to most other animal systems, the presence of assembled actin does not appear to be required for sperm head penetration (for review see Schatten & Schatten, 1987). This section will briefly review our current understanding of the role of microfilaments and actin-related proteins during mammalian fertilization.

Microfilament organization in rodent species during maturation and fertilization

Microfilament activity in mammals appears to be unique in its organization and functions compared to other non-mammalian fertilization systems (for review see Schatten & Schatten, 1987). Analysis of mammalian oocytes using a variety of modern immunocytochemical and ultrastructural technology has shown that microfilaments predominate in the cortical region of oocytes where this cytoskeletal element can participate in expected cytokinetic functions, such as the extrusion of polar bodies and cell division. Microfilaments have also been shown to assemble in the area of sperm–egg fusion, and to participate in the formation of the incorporation cone after sperm penetration, functions analogous to those described in the invertebrate systems (for review see Schatten, 1982). However, mammals violate expected dogma for microfilament activity. As discussed below, mammalian fertilization may not require direct participation of microfilament assembly for certain aspects of sperm incorporation. Other unique roles for cortical microfilament activity in mammals entail involvement in meiotic spindle events, including peripheral migration of the first meiotic spindle, its anchoring to the cell surface region, and rotation motions during second polar body formation (Webb, Howlett & Maro, 1986; Maro *et al.*, 1984).

In the mouse system, there is a complicated interrelationship between the underlying cortical microfilament system, cell surface modifications and chromosomes which is not well understood (for review see Longo, 1989; Schatten & Schatten, 1987). Microfilaments are crucial to the cortical migration of the first meiotic spindle during maturation, and this event directly restructures the cell surface and cortical region of the maturing oocyte; a prominent microvillus-free zone overlying the meiotic spindle forms which is devoid of underlying cortical granules, enriched in submembraneous actin, and lacks an affinity for the lectin

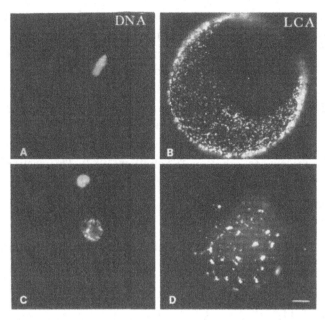

Fig. 13. Detection of cortical granules in unfertilized and artificially activated mouse oocytes. In the mature mouse oocyte arrested at metaphase of second meiosis (A), numerous cortical granules can be detected at the cell cortex except at the site overlying the meiotic spindle region (B). A dramatic reduction in cortical granule numbers (D) occurs in activated oocytes which have entered interphase and formed the female pronucleus (C). All oocytes were double labelled for DAPI DNA stain (A, C) and fluoresceinated-*Lens culinaris* agglutinin (LCA; B, D). Bar = 10 μm.

concanavalin A (Fig. 13, Fig. 14; Johnson *et al.*, 1975; Eager, Johnson & Thurley, 1976; Maro *et al.*, 1984; Longo & Chen, 1985; Schatten *et al.*, 1986*b*; Ducibella *et al.*, 1990). Experiments have demonstrated the reversibility of these spindle-induced changes in the cell cortex, arguing that these alterations are dynamic reorganizations with spatial and temporal characteristics (Van Blerkom & Bell, 1986).

By polarizing the cell surface and cortical regions during meiotic maturation, two crucial events will have occurred by the time of second meiotic arrest in the unfertilized mouse oocyte; the first nuclear reductional division following telophase I through extrusion of the first polar body and the establishment of a region overlying the second meiotic spindle which cannot bind the fertilizing spermatozoa. In the first event, the ploidy status of the oocyte is reduced to 2N prior to insemination while the latter event prevents the potential loss of the paternal genome during second polar body formation (Johnson *et al.*, 1975; Nicosia, Wolf & Inoue, 1977; Longo & Chen, 1985). These key nuclear and plasma membrane modifications mediated by microfilaments are significant prerequisites to the programme of fertilization in the mouse.

Rodent oocytes arrested at metaphase of second meiosis have paratangentially oriented spindles, which must rotate after cell activation to elicit the second polar body (Maro *et al.*, 1984; Okada, Yanagimachi & Yanagimachi, 1986). It has been suggested that spindle orientation may cause actin polarity in rodents since mammals with radially orientated meiotic spindles do not undergo spindle rotation or actin accumulation at the cell surface (Le Guen *et al.*, 1989). Interestingly, preliminary evidence in the mature rat oocyte has shown a uniform distribution of microfilaments in the cortex, and no accumulation of F-actin over the site of the second meiotic spindle (Battaglia & Gaddum-Rosse, 1986). The events of meiotic spindle anchoring to the cell cortex, spindle rotation after second meiotic resumption and second polar body formation, are all dependent on microfilament functioning in the mouse oocyte; evidence of similar microfilament behaviour in other rodent species is not yet known.

Microtubule and microfilament inhibitors along with immunocytochemical technology using antiactin antibodies and phalloidin analogues have provided invaluable information on the action of cortical microfilaments in the unfertilized mouse oocyte (Longo & Chen, 1985; Maro *et al.*, 1984; Schatten *et al.*, 1986*b*). When spindle microtubules are disrupted with a variety of depolymerization drugs, chromosomes of the meiotic spindle scatter along the cortex (Fig. 15A). This elicits a dramatic reorganization in the cell surface and underlying cortex; actin accumulates (Fig.15B) and surface microvilli disappear locally over each chromosome mass as depicted by rhodamine-phalloidin and concanavalin A lectin staining (Longo and Chen, 1985; Schatten *et al.*, 1985; Maro *et al.*, 1986). Microfilament inhibitors alone do not affect chromosome distribution (Fig. 15C). Recovery from microtubule inhibition results in the formation of miniature spindles at each scattered chromosome site, which can rotate and form multiple polar bodies upon oocyte activation (Maro *et al.*, 1986*b*). The process of chromosomal dispersion by microtubule inhibitors is dependent solely on cortical microfilaments since inclusion of cytochalasin (Maro *et al.*, 1986*b*) or latrunculin (Fig. 15D; Schatten *et al.*, 1986*b*) along with the microtubule drug will block this process.

An interesting facet of this microfilament-mediated event is its temporal nature. Once chromosomes have decondensed into nuclei with intact nuclear membranes, the cell surface modifications and regional assembly of cortical actin disappear. Similar observations have been found during the formation of the incorporation cone; sperm chromatin induces a cortical microfilament accumulation and loss of surface microvilli at the site of gametic fusion until the male pronucleus develops a nuclear envelope (Shalgi *et al.*, 1978; Gaddum-Rosse, 1985; Maro *et al.*, 1984).

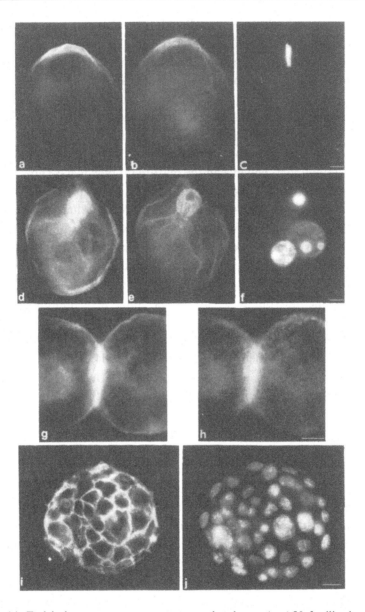

Fig. 14. Fodrin in mouse oocytes, zygotes, and embryos. (a–c) Unfertilized mouse oocyte. In unfertilized oocytes, actin (a) and fodrin (b) are co-localized at the oocyte cortex with a pronounced concentration adjacent to the meiotic spindle. The DNA of the maternal meiotic chromosomes are fluorescently detected at the spindle equator in (c). (d–f) Pronucleate Mouse egg. After insemination, fodrin (e) remains co-localized with cortical actin (d). The intensity of the fluorescence throughout the cortex appears to have increased and there is a concentration of both stains on the cortex of the second polar body. Cytoplasmic actin fluorescence (d) also is apparent. (f) Pronuclei and polar body nucleus detected with Hoechst DNA fluorescence. (g, h) First cleavage. There is a marked accumulation of both

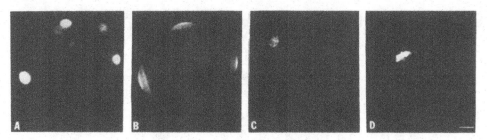

Fig. 15. Latrunculin inhibits colcemid-induced chromosome dispersion and blocks the cortical accumulations of actin adjacent to the dispersed meiotic chromosomes. The meiotic chromosomes of unfertilized mouse oocytes treated with 50 μM colcemid disperse along the egg cortex ((A) Hoechst DNA fluorescence) and the dispersed chromosomes induce regional accumulations of cortical actin ((B) rhodaminyl-phalloidin microfilament fluorescence). This dispersion is prevented by 2.6 μM latrunculin ((C) Hoechst DNA fluorescence). All cells processed at 14 h post-insemination. Bar = 10 μm. × 550. (Reprinted, with permission, from Schatten *et al.*, 1986,)

The underlying mechanism of this transient reorganizational event is not known.

Studies of fertilization in the mouse do not support a required role for microfilaments in sperm head penetration, unlike other non-mammalian animal species (Maro *et al.*, 1984; Schatten *et al.*, 1986*b*; Simerly *et al.*, 1993). Mature mouse spermatozoa do not contain actin at the equatorial site where sperm–egg fusion occurs (Flaherty, Winfrey & Olson, 1986), and SEM investigations of the surface events during sperm incorporation do not suggest active oocyte microvilli participation in the engulfment of the penetrating sperm head (Shalgi, Phillips & Kraicer, 1978). Living studies of sperm penetration in the presence of microfilament inhibitors such as latrunculin reinforce these observations, as shown in Fig. 15. Microfilament inhibition blocks second polar body formation after

Caption for fig 14 (*cont.*).

actin (g) and fodrin (h) at the cleavage furrow during first division. This contrasts to the situation in sea urchin eggs, where little accumulation at the furrow was noted. (i, j) Fodrin in mouse blastocyst. In blastocysts, fodrin is found at each cell border; actin fluorescence (d) also is apparent. (f) Pronuclei and polar body nucleus detected with Hoechst DNA fluorescence. (g, h) First cleavage. There is a marked accumulation of both actin (g) and fodrin (h) at the cleavage furrow during first division. This contrasts to the situation in sea urchin eggs, where little accumulation at the furrow was noted. (i, j) Fodrin in mouse blastocyst. In blastocysts, fodrin is found at each cell border. (i). (j) DNA fluorescence. (a–f): Triple labelling for actin (a, d), fodrin (b, e), and DNA (c, f). (g, h): Double labelling for actin (g) and fodrin (h) at first cleavage. (i, j) Double labelling for fodrin (i) and DNA (j) in a blastocyst. Bars = 10 μm. (Reprinted, with permission, from Schatten *et al.*, 1986.)

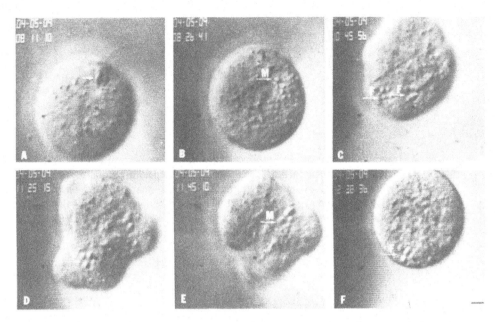

Fig. 16. Time-lapse video microscopy of mouse fertilization *in vitro*. Incorporation
of the sperm head (A) occurs in the presence of 2.6 μM latrunculin, though the
incorporation cone does not enlarge normally at 4 h post insemination (B). The
male pronucleus develops (B: M). Since the formation of the second polar body
is inhibited (B, C), two maternal pronuclei develop, corresponding to a female
pronucleus and the second polar body nucleus. The egg becomes unusually active
at the pronucleate state (D–F) but the pronuclei are not moved from the egg
cortex and further development is arrested. M, Male incorporation cone does not
enlarge normally at 4 h post insemination (B). M, Male pronucleus, F, maternal
pronuclei. Bar = 10 μm. × 500. (Reprinted, with permission, from Schatten *et al.*,
1986.)

sperm incorporation (Fig. 16A), but does not inhibit completion of second meiosis,
as demonstrated by the appearance of two female pronuclei following oocyte
activation (arrows in Fig. 16C). Sperm penetration and pronuclear formation
occur normally (Fig. 16A–C), although pronuclear centration does not proceed
(Fig.16C,D). Surface movements reminiscent of pseudocleavage are also detected
in latrunculin-treated oocytes (Fig. 16D–F), and may be mediated by cortical
microfilaments as observed by rhodamine–phalloidin staining (see Schatten *et
al.*, 1986*b*). These observations are in good agreement with the effects noted for
cytochalasin inhibition during sperm penetration in the mouse (Maro *et al.*, 1984;
Longo & Chen, 1985).

Microfilaments appear to be crucial for the incorporation of the sperm tail, however (Simerly *et al.*, 1993). Time-lapse video microscopy studies of mouse fertilization has shown that tail engulfment into the oocyte is blocked in the presence of microfilament inhibitors. As demonstrated in Fig. 17 by high resolution, low voltage scanning electron microscopy, the plasma membrane of the sperm tail fuses at multiple sites with the oocyte's plasma membrane in normal and microtubule-inhibited eggs (Fig, 17A,B), but only at microvillus-rich sites on the cell surface. Sperm tail incorporation, therefore, does not occur at a single region but rather enters the oocyte laterally along the entire sperm's length. In the presence of cytochalasin (Fig. 17C,D), the number of microvilli is greatly reduced, and the plasma membrane covering the sperm axoneme does not fuse with the oocyte membrane, although multiple depressions in the oocyte surface occur where the axoneme is subjacent to the egg membrane. Sperm head penetration is not affected and the mid-piece portion of the successful spermatozoa remains anchored at the incorporaton site (Fig, 17D).

Microfilament activity is required, post-insemination, for the formation of the incorporation cone (for review see Longo, 1989). At the site of gamete fusion, an extension of cytoplasm forms over the penetrating sperm head which is enriched in actin along its plasmalemma surface (Gaddum-Rosse, 1985; Maro *et al.*, 1984). This transient structure is sensitive to microfilament inhibitors: the presence of cytochalasin will prevent its formation or cause the structure to be reabsorbed, implicating this cytoskeletal element in its formation and maintenance (Maro *et al.*, 1984; Shalgi *et al.*, 1978). Interestingly, the incorporation cone reaches its zenith only after the sperm head has entered the cortex region. Recent experiments by Webster and McGaughey (1990) using isolated cortical preparations from hamster oocytes have used ultrastructure analysis to characterize the organization of the actin network in freshly fertilized oocytes, demonstrating a close association of the penetrating spermatozoa with the loose cortical microfilament meshwork. It is interesting to speculate on the correlation between this sperm-cortex interaction and incorporation cone formation; perhaps this interaction is the crucial step in allowing the developing male pronucleus to migrate away from the cell surface. As noted above, the incorporation cone formation is sensitive to microfilament inhibitors; the male pronucleus develops but remains peripherally localized in the presence of microfilament inhibitors (Maro *et al.*, 1984; Schatten *et al.*, 1986*b*).

Curiously, pronuclear apposition is affected by microfilament activity (for review see Schatten & Schatten, 1987). Microfilaments are detected as a diffuse perinuclear array during the mouse pronuclear centration stage (Maro *et al.*, 1984). This unusual perinuclear microfilament arrangement appears to be required, in addition to the cytoplasmic microtubule matrix, for the movements leading to pronuclear juxtapositioning since cytochalasin (Maro *et al.*, 1984) or

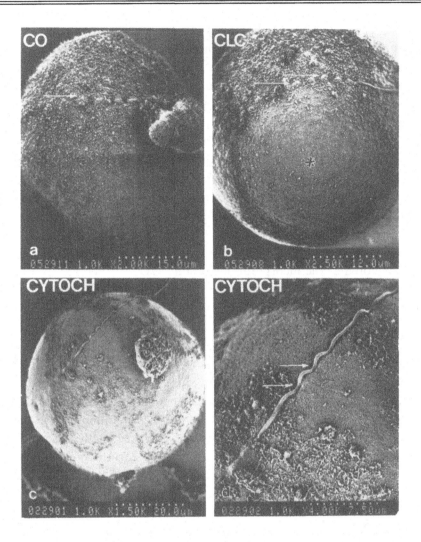

Fig. 17. Low-voltage scanning electron microscopy of sperm penetration in control, colcemid- and cytochalasin-treated oocytes 12 hours post-insemination *in vitro*. A high resolution LVSEM image of sperm penetration in control oocytes demonstrates that the sperm tail of the successful fertilizing spermatoza is completely engulfed into the egg by fusing at multiple sites along the surface of the vitelline membrane (arrow). When oocytes inseminated and cultured continuously in the presence of 50 μM colcemid are processed for LVSEM, multiple fusion sites along the microvillous surface area are observed similar to control oocytes (arrows in b; compare with Fig. 7). Large microvilli-free areas are formed on the oocyte surface membranes as a result of colcemid inhibition (* area in b) but sperm tail penetration never occurs in these denuded zones. Oocytes fertilized in the continuous presence of 10 μM cytochalasin B have a significant reduction of surface microvilli as compared to control eggs (c; compare with a). By 12 hours post-insemination, sperm tail, but not head, engulfment has been blocked in the presence of the microfilament inhibitor (c). The sperm midpiece anchors the tail

latrunculin (Fig. 16; Schatten *et al.*, 1986*b*) will inhibit pronuclear apposition, though not pronuclear development.

Actin-binding proteins such as fodrin have a close association with assembling actin, and are found concentrated in the cortical regions of many types of cells, including the mouse oocyte and fertilized embryo (Sobel & Alliegro, 1985; Damjanov *et al.*, 1986; Reima & Lehtonen, 1985; Schatten *et al.*, 1986*c*). Antibodies to fodrin have detected this protein at the cortical domain adjacent to the second meiotic spindle and co-localized with polymerized actin (Fig, 14A–C). During fertilization, fodrin remains along the entire oocyte and second polar body surface while actin is localized to the both the cortex and perinuclear positions (Fig. 14D–F). Following cleavage, actin and fodrin are found predominately at the cleavage furrow (Fig. 14G,H) and in blastocyst, fodrin circumscribes each cell border (Fig. 14I,J). However, different spectrin-like antibodies are found in different regions at various developmental stages, making the interpretation for their precise role and distribution unclear. Perhaps fodrin participates in the maintenance of the meiotic spindle at the cell cortex, in polar body elicitation, or in creating a gelated cortical region for anchoring the successful sperm to the egg plasma membrane, as has been suggested for lower animals (for review see Schatten & Schatten, 1987). Clearly, the mechanism of actin-binding protein interactions with cytoskeletal-membrane associations during fertilization and early development in mammals warrants further investigation.

Microfilament organization in other mammalian species

In domestic animal species, microfilament patterns are distinct from those reported in the rodents. In unfertilized sheep oocytes, a uniform layer of cortical actin has been observed similar to the distribution found in immature mouse and rat oocytes (Le Guen *et al.*, 1989). Comparable actin staining patterns have been observed in the cow (C. S. Navara, personal communication) but no cortical F-actin has been detected in unfertilized pig oocytes until sperm penetration (Albertini, 1987). A correlation between spindle orientation and F-actin accumulation has been suggested as a possible reason for the lack of microfilament polarity in farm animals: ovine, bovine and porcine oocytes all exhibit radially

Caption for fig 17 (*cont.*).
to the egg surface at the site of incorporation but no fusion between the sperm and oocyte membranes occurs along the length of the axoneme; instead, numerous invaginations of the egg membrane can be seen underlying the bends in the tail structure (d; arrows). 1 Pb = first polar body; 2 Pb = second polar body $V_0 = 1.0$ kV. a: 2000 ×; b: 2500 ×; c: 1500 ×; d: 4500 ×. (Reprinted, with permission, from Simerly *et al.*, 1993.)

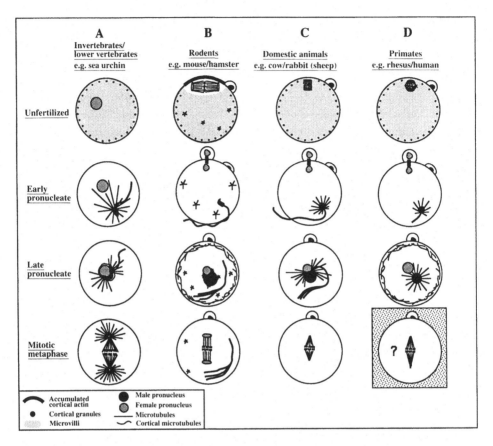

Fig. 18. Comparative summary of microtubule and microfilament patterns during the first cell cycle in sea urchins and various mammals. The model system for understanding the behaviour of the cytoskeletal programme during fertilization has been the sea urchin egg (Column A). The mature unfertilized urchin egg has no assembled cytoplasmic microtubules and displays a uniform distribution of surface microvilli, underlying cortical microfilaments and cortical granules organized at the cell periphery. Sperm penetration, which requires the rearrangement of cortical actin into microfilaments to form the incorporation cone structure responsible for anchoring and drawing the sperm into the egg cytoplasm, brings in the dominate microtubule organizing centre, the centrosome, to direct the organization of the sperm aster. This structure ultimately governs the motions responsible for pronuclear apposition and syngamy during early interphase. The centrosome duplicates and splits during the late pronuclear stage, giving rise to the classical bipolar metaphase spindle at first mitosis with large asters and a pair of centrioles at each pole.

The configurations of the cytoskeletal system in well characterized mammals like the mouse seems to violate most of the dogma characterized for the invertebrates. Unfertilized mouse oocytes are arrested at metaphase of second meiosis and the dominant microtubule structure is the barrel-shaped, anastral meiotic spindle, oriented paratangentially to the cell surface (column B). About a dozen centrosomes are detected in the cytoplasm. Cortical organization in rodents oriented spindles and do not undergo spindle rotation following oocyte activation (Le Guen *et al.*, 1989). Investigations in the sheep, however, do suggest an active role for microfilaments in cortical spindle attachment and second polar body formation since microfilament inhibitors cause a subcortical displacement of the meiotic spindle and inhibit second polar body formation (Le Guen *et al.*, 1989).

Ultrastructural analysis of domestic species also supports evidence demonstrating a lack of polarity in the unfertilized egg. Microvilli distribution is found over the entire surface of the cow oocyte (Navara *et al.*, 1992). TEM analysis of the cortical region in domestic species do not demonstrate a cortical granule-free zone as noted in the mouse oocyte but rather show a uniform distribution of these organelles (Kruip *et al.*, 1983). The first meiotic spindle forms at the cortex of the immature oocyte following germinal vesicle migration to the cell surface (Thibault *et al.*, 1987); microfilaments do not participate in spindle migration and may not, therefore, form a unique relationship with the meiotic chromosomes as has been found in the mouse system. These observations highlight the puzzling variability on the role and action of microfilaments within the mammalian phyla.

Caption for fig 18 (*cont.*).

is highly polarized: surface microvilli and cortical granules are absent at the area occupied by the second meiotic spindle while cortical actin assembly is greatly enhanced at the site where the spindle is anchored to the plasmalemma. Sperm head incorporation does not require the assembly of microtubules or microfilaments and no microtubules amass at the base of the penetrated sperm head. In the absence of any assembled sperm aster structure, the dozen or so cytoplasmic centrosomes nucleate the microtubules responsible for pronuclear apposition during interphase. The first metaphase spindle is anastral, barrel-shaped, and organized without centrioles.

Accumulating knowledge in other mammalian species suggests that rodents may have an atypical oocyte cytoskeletal organization for mammals. Similar to rodents, the infertilized oocyte in domestic species (column C) and primates (column D) are arrested at metaphase of second meiosis. In contrast to rodents, microtubules are detectable only within the small, anastral spindle apparatus oriented radially to the cell surface: no cytoplasmic microtubules are observed in the inactivated cytoplasm of the mature oocyte. Additionally, these species do not demonstrate cortical polarity in the distribution of surface microvilli, cortical microfilaments, and cortical granule organization. Sperm penetration results in a dramatic assembly of microtubules associated with the incorporating sperm DNA and the assembled sperm aster structure plays an analogous role to that in lower animals in participating in pronuclear migration and centration. The mitotic metaphase spindles in domestic animals and primates are anastral and appear more fusiform at the poles than in mice. Sperm-derived centrioles may be an integral part of the morphology of mitotic spindles in these mammals, as shown for human embryos.

As noted for mouse fertilization, sheep insemination in the presence of the microfilament inhibitor cytochalasin did not block sperm head penetration, although sperm tail incorporation appeared delayed. Likewise, the incorporation cone did not form in the presence of cytochalasin as shown for the rodent system (Le Guen *et al.*, 1989). These observations reinforce the notion that mammalian fertilization contrasts sharply with fertilization in lower animal species on the role of microfilaments in sperm-egg interactions. Similar investigations in other domestic species have yet to be explored.

In primates, microfilament organization appears strikingly similar to those reported for the domestic species. Mature rhesus and human oocytes demonstrate a homogeneous polymerized actin layer, uniform cortical granule distribution, and homogeneous surface microvillar organization similar to ovine oocytes (Johnson *et al.*, 1991; Pickering *et al.*, 1988; Sathananthan *et al.*, 1986). In addition, ultrastructural examinations of human fertilization have demonstrated that an incorporation cone forms with a dense aggregate of microfilaments overlying the developing male pronucleus (Zamboni, 1971; Sathananthan *et al.*, 1986). The exact nature of the distribution and role of microfilaments in primate maturation and fertilization awaits future investigation.

Prospective: comparisons of structural alterations during maturation and fertilization among various mammals

Fertilization requires an understanding of the motility and cytoskeletal rearrangements necessary to achieve the union of the sperm and egg nuclei, events which are poorly understood in primates. The vast majority of information in mammals has been derived from studies on rodents, particularly the mouse, but accumulating information is demonstrating that this knowledge cannot simply be extrapolated to higher animals, including the human. Microtubules and microfilaments are at the heart of the motions necessary to achieve correct chromosome segregation, nuclear apposition, and cellular divisions, events which, if inaccurate, can have disastrous consequences on normal development. The limited studies on various mammalian systems seem to suggest that different mammals accomplish fertilization by various means, and these distinctions can be traced by studying the organization and dynamics of their cytoskeletal elements (Fig. 17). Investigations of human oocytes and embryos raise ethical, moral, and practical problems at present, and the short-term solution may be found by studying non-human primate models such as the rhesus monkey. However, given the diversity and complexity of cytoskeletal organization and dynamics in mammals, human fertilization should ultimately be explored.

Note added after submission

Since the submission of this article in 1992, the paternal inheritance of the centrosome has been discovered in all of the studied non-rodent mammals, including marsupials (Breed *et al.,* 1994), non-human primates (Wu *et al.,* 1993) and humans (Simerly *et al.,* 1994, 1995). The implications of these discoveries and the molecular basis of centrosome inheritance has recently been reviewed (Schatten, 1994).

Acknowledgements

We are very grateful to Sara Zoran for help in the preparation of this review, and we also want to thank our many collaborators who have contributed to research reviewed here. The support of the research discussed in this review was sponsored in large measure by the NIH and USDA.

References

Albertini DF. Cytoplasmic reorganization during the resumption of meiosis in cultured preovulatory rate oocytes. *Dev Biol* 1987; **120**: 121–31.

Balczon RD, Brinkley BR. Tubulin interaction with kinetochore proteins: analysis by *in vitro* assemble and chemical cross-linking. *J Cell Biol* 1987; **105**: 855–62.

Battaglia De, Gaddum-Roose P. The distribution of polymerized actin in the rat egg and its sensitivity to cytochalasin B during fertilization. *J Exp Zool* 1986; **1987**: 97–105.

Bavister BD, Boatman DE, Morgan PM, Warikoo PK. Fertilization in the rhesus monkey. In: Dunbar BS, O'Rand MD eds. *Comparative Overview of Mammalian Fertilization.* New York: Planum Press, 1991: 363–83.

Bernat BL, Borisy GG, Rothfield NF, Earnshaw WC. Injection of anticentromere antibodies in interphase disrupts events required for chromosome movement at mitosis. *J Cell Biol* 1990; **111**: 1519–33.

Boveri T. *Zellen-Studien: ueber die Natur der Centrosomen.* Jena: Fischer, 1901: 4.

Breed WG, Simerly C, Navara CS, VandeBerg JL, and Schatten G. Microtubule configurations in oocytes, zygotes and early embryos of a marsupial, *Monodelphis domestica Dev Biol.* 1994; **164**, 230–40.

Brinkley BR, Valdivia MM, Tousson MM, Balczon RD. The kinetochore: structure and molecular characterization. In: Hyams J, Brinkley BR, eds. *Mitosis: Molecules and Mechanisms.* New York: Academic Press, 1989: 77–118.

Bulinski JC, Gundersen GG. Stabilization and post-translational modification of microtubules during cellular morphogenesis. *BioEssays* 1991; **13**: 285–93.

Calarco-Gilliam PH, Siebert MC, Hubble R, Mitchison T, Kirschner M. The effects of aphidicolin, an inhibitor of DNA replication, on sea urchin development. *Cell* 1983; **35**: 621–9.

Cooke CA, Bernat RL, Earnshaw WC. CENP-B: a major human centromere protein located beneath the kinetochore. *J Cell Biol* 1990; **110**: 1475–88.

Crozet N. Fine structure of sheep fertilization *in vitro. Gamete Res* 1988; **19**: 291–303.

Crozet N, Behaviour of the sperm centriole during sheep oocyte fertilization. *Eur J Cell Biol* 1990; **53**: 326–32.

Damjanov I, Damjanov A, Lehto VP, Virtanen I. Spectrin in mouse gametogenesis and embryogenesis. *Dev Biol* 1986; **114**: 132–40.

De Pennart H, Houliston E, Maro B. Post-translational modifications of tubulin and the dynamics of microtubules in mouse oocytes and zygotes. *Biol of Cell* 1988; **64**: 375–8.

Donahue RP. Maturation of the mouse oocyte *in vitro*. I. Sequence and timing of nuclear progression. *J Exp Zool* 1968; **169**: 237–50.

Dulcibella T, Kurasawa S, Rangarajan S, Kopf G, Schultz R. Precocious loss of cortical granules during mouse oocyte meiotic maturation and correlation with an egg-induced modification of the zona pellucida. *Dev Biol* 1990; **137**: 46–55.

Eager DD, Johnson MH, Thurley KW. Ultrastructural studies on the surface membrane of the mouse egg. *J Cell Sci* 1976; **22**: 345–53.

Earnshaw WC, Sullivan KF, Machlin CA *et al.* Molecular cloning of cDNA for CENP-B, the major human centromere autoantigen. *J Cell Biol* 1987; **104**: 817–29.

Earnshaw WC, Ratrie H III, Stetten G. Visualization of centromere proteins CENP-B and CENP-C on a stable dicentric chromosome in cytological spreads. *Chromosoma (Berl)* 1989; **98**: 1–12.

Eichenlaub-Ritter U, Stahl A, Luciani JM. The microtubular cytoskeleton and chromosomes of unfertilized human oocytes aged *in vitro*. *Hum Genet* 1988; **80**: 259–64.

Flaherty SP, Winfrey VP, Olson GE. Localization of actin in mammalian spermatozoa: a comparison of eight species. *Anat Rec* 1986; **216**: 504–15.

Gaddum-Rosse P. Mammalian gamete interactions: what can be gained from observation on living eggs? *Am J Anat* 1985; **174**: 347–56.

Gorbsky GJ, Borisy GG. Microtubules of the kinetochore fiber turn over in metaphase but not in anaphase. *J Cell Biol* 1989; **109**: 653–62.

Gorbsky GJ, Simerly C, Schatten G, Borisy GG. Microtubules in the metaphase-arrested mouse oocyte turn over rapidly. *Proc Natl Acad Sci USA* 1990; **87**: 6049–53.

Gundersen GG, Bulinski JC. Distribution of tyrosinated and nontyrosinated α-tubulin during mitosis. *J Cell Biol* 1986; **102**: 1118–26.

Hamaguchi Y, Toriyama M, Sakai H, Hiramoto Y. Redistribution of fluorescently labeled tubulin in the mitotic apparatus of sand dollar eggs and the effects of taxol. *Cell Struct Funct* 1987; **12**: 43–52.

Holy J, Schatten G. Differential behaviour of centrosomes in unequally dividing blastomeres during fourth cleavage of sea urchin embryos. *J Cell Sci* 1991; **98**: 423–31.

Johnson LD, Mattson BA, Albertini DF *et al.* Quality of oocytes from superovulated rhesus monkeys. *Hum Reprod* 1991; **6**: 623–31.

Johnson MH, Eager D, Muggleton-Harris A, Grave HM. Mosaicism in the organization of concanavalin A receptors on the surface membrane of mouse egg. *Nature, Lond* 1975; **257**: 321–2.

Kaufman MH. *Early Mammalian Development: Parthenogenetic studies* 1st edn. Cambridge University Press, 1983.

Kola I, Trounson A, Dawson G, Rogers P. Tripronuclear human oocytes: altered cleavage patterns and subsequent karyotypic analysis of embryos. *Biol Reprod* 1989; **37**: 395–401.

Kruip TAM, Cran DG, Van Beneden TH, Dieleman SJ. Structural changes in bovine oocytes during final maturation *in vivo*. *Gamete Res* 1983; **8**: 29–47.

Lams MH, Doorme. Nouvelles recherches sur la maturaton et la fécondation. *Arch Biol (Liège and Paris)*. 1907: 18–365.

LeDizet M. Piperno G. Identification of any acetylation site of *Chlamydomonas* α-tubulin. *Proc Natl Acad Sci, USA* 1987; **84**: 5720–4.

Le Guen P, Crozet N. Microtubule and centrosome distribution during sheep fertilization. *Eur J Cell Biol* 1989; **48**: 239–49.

Le Guen P, Crozet N, Huneau D, Gall L. Distribution and role of microfilaments during early events of sheep fertilization. *Gamete Res* 1989; **22**: 411–25.

Long CR, Pinto-Correia C, Duby RT, Ponce De Leon FA, Boland MP, Roche JF, Robl JM. Chromatin and microtubule morphology during the first cell cycle in bovine zygotes. *Mol Reprod Dev* 1993; **36**: 23–32.

Longo FJ. Sperm aster in rabbit zygotes: its structure and function. *J Cell Biol* 1976; **69**: 539–47.

Longo FJ. Egg cortical architecture. In: Schatten H, Schatten G, eds. *The Cell Biology of Fertilization*. San Diego: Academic Press, 1989; 105–38.

Longo FJ, Chen DY. Development of cortical polarity in mouse eggs: involvement of the meiotic apparetus. *Dev Biol* 1985; **107**: 382–94.

Maro B, Johnson MH, Pickering SJ, Flach G. Changes in actin distribution during fertilization of the mouse egg. *J Embryol Exp Morph* 1984; **81**: 211–37.

Maro B, Johnson MH, Webb M. Flach G. Mechanism of polar body formation in the mouse oocyte: an interaction between the chromosomes, the cytoskeleton, and the plasma membrane. *J Embryol Exp Morph* 1986a; **92**: 11–32.

Maro B, Howlett SK, Houliston E. Cytoskeleton dynamics in the mouse egg. *J Cell Sci Suppl* 1986b; **5**:343–59.

Mazia D. The chromosome cycle and the centrosome cycle in the mitotic cycle. *Int Rev Cytol* 1987; **100**: 49–92.

Messing SM, Albertini DF. Centrosome and microtubule dynamics during progression in the mouse oocyte. *J Cell Sci* 1991; **100**: 289–98.

Mitchison TJ. Mitosis: basic concepts. *Curr Op Cell Biol* 1989; **1**: 67–74.

Mitchison T. Evans L, Schulze E, Kirschner M. Sites of microtubule assembly and disassembly in the mitotic spindle. *Cell* 1986; **45**: 515–27.

Mitchison TJ, Kirschner MW. Properties of the kinetochore *in vitro*. I. Microtubule nucleation and tubulin binding. *J Cell Biol* 1985a; **101**: 755–65.

Mitchison TJ, Kirschner MW. Properties of the kinetochore *in vitro*. II. Microtubule capture and ATP-dependent translocation. *J Cell Biol* 1985b; **101**: 766–77.

Navara CS, First NL, Schatten G. Microtubule organization in the cow during fertilization, polyspermy, parthenogenesis and nuclear transfer: the role of the sperm aster. *Develop Biol* 1994; **162**: 29–40.

Nicklas RB. The motor for poleward chromosome movement in anaphase is in or near the kinetochore. *J Cell Biol* 1989; **109**: 2245–55.

Nicosia SV, Wolf DP, Inoue M. Cortical granule distribution and cell surface characteristics in mouse eggs. *Dev Biol* 1977; **57**: 56–74.

Oakley BR, Oakley CE, Yoon Y, Jung MK. Tubulin is a component of the spindle pole body that is essential for microtubule function in *Aspergillus nidulans*. *Cell* 1990; **61**: 1289–301.

Okada A, Yanagimachi R, Yanagimachi H. Development of a cortical granule-free area of cortex and the perivitelline space in the hamster oocyte during maturation and following ovulation. *J Submicrosc Cytol* 1986; **18**: 233–47.

Pickering SJ, Johnson MH, Braude PR, Houliston E. Cytoskeletal organization in fresh, aged and spontaneously activated human oocytes. *Hum Reprod* 1988; **3**: 978–89.

Pickering SJ, Braude PR, Johnson MH, Cant A, Currie J. Transient cooling to room temperature can cause irreversible disruption of the meiotic spindle in the human oocyte. *Fertil Steril* 1990; **54**: 102–8.

Pluta AF, Cooke CA, Earnshaw WC. Structure of the human centromere at metaphase. *Trends Biochem Sci* 1990; **15**: 181–5.

Reima I, Lehtonen E. Localization of nonerythroid spectrin and actin in mouse oocytes and preimplantation embryos. *Differentiation* 1985; **30**: 68–75.

Rieder CL. The formation, structure and composition of the mammalian kinetochore fiber. *Int Rev Cytol* 1982; **79**: 1–48.

Salmon Ed, Leslie RJ, Saxton WM, Karow ML, McIntosh JR. Spindle microtubule dynamics in sea urchin embryos: analysis using a fluorescent-labeled tubulin and measurements of fluorescence redistribution after laser photobleaching. *J Cell Biol* 1984; **99**: 2165–74.

Sammak PJ, Borisy GG. Direct observation of microtubule dynamics in living cells. *Nature Lond* 1986; **332**: 724–6.

Sathananthan AH, Trounson A, Freeman L, Brady T. The effects of cooling human oocytes. *Human Reprod* 1988; **3**: 968–77.

Sathananthan AH, Trounson AO, Wood C. *Atlas of Fine Structure of Human Sperm Penetration, Eggs and Embryos Cultured in vitro*. 1st edn. New York: Praeger Publishers, 1986.

Sathananthan AH, Kola I, Osborne J *et al*. Centrioles in the beginning of human development. *Proc Natl Acad Sci, USA* 1991; **88**: 4806–10.

Saxton WM, Stemple DL, Leslie RJ, Salmon ED, Savortnik M, McIntosh JR. Tubulin dynamics in cultured mammalian cells. *J Cell Biol* 1984; **99**: 2175–86.

Schatten G. Motility during fertilization. *Int Rev Cyt* 1982; **79**: 59–163.

Schatten G. The centrosome and its mode of inheritance: The reduction of the centrosome during gametogenesis and its restoration during fertilization. *Develop Biol* 1994; **145**, 299–335.

Schatten G, Simerly C, Schatten H. Microtubule configurations during fertilization, mitosis, and early development in the mouse and the requirement for egg microtubule-mediated motility during mammalian fertilization. *Proc Natl Acad Sci USA* 1985; **82**: 4152–6.

Schatten H, Schatten G, Mazia D, Balcxon R, Simerly C. Behavior of centrosomes during fertilization and cell division and mouse oocytes and in sea urchin eggs. *Proc Natl Acad Sci USA* 1986*a*; **83**: 105–9.

Schatten G, Schatten H, Spector I *et al*. Latrunculin inhibits the microfilament-mediated processes during fertilization, cleavage, and early development in sea urchins and mice. *Exp Cell Res* 1986*b*; **166**: 191–208.

Schatten H, Cheney R, Balczon R *et al*. Localization of fodrin during fertilization and early development of sea urchins and mice. *Dev Biol* 1986*c*; **118**: 457–66.

Schatten G, Schatten H. Cytoskeletal alterations and nuclear architectural changes during mammalian fertilization. *Current Topics in Developmental Biology* 1987; **23**: 23–54.

Schatten G, Simerly C. Asai DJ, Szöke E, Cooke P, Schatten H. Acetylated α-tubulin in microtubules during mouse fertilization and early development *Dev Biol* 1988; **130**: 74–86.

Schatten G, Simerly C, Schatten H. Maternal inheritance of centrosomes in mammals? Studies on parthenogenesis and polyspermy in mice. *Proc Natl Acad Sci; USA* 1991; **88**: 6785–9.

Schulze E, Asai DJ, Bulinski JC, Kirschner M. Posttranslational modification and microtubule stability. *J Cell Biol* 1987; **105**: 2167–77.

Shalgi R, Phillips DM, Kraicer PF. Observation on the incorporation cone in the rat. *Gamete Res* 1978; **1**: 27–37.

Simerly C, Balczon R, Brinkley BR, Schatten G. Microinjected kinetochore antibodies interfere with chromosome movement in meiotic and mitotic mouse oocytes. *J Cell Biol* 1990; **111**: 1491–504.

Simerly C, Hecht N, Goldberg E, Schatten G. Tracing the incorporation of the spermtail in the mouse zygote and early embryo using an anti-testicular α-tubulin antibody. *Dev Biol* 1993; **158**: 536–48.

Simerly C, Wu G-J, Zoran S, Ord T, Rawlings R, Jones J, Navara CS, Gerrity M, Rinehart J, Binor Z, Asch R, Schatten G. Centrosome inheritance during fertilisation in humans. *Mol Biol Cell* 1994; **5**: 463a.

Simerly C, Wu G.-J, Zoran S, Ord T, Rawlings R, Jones J, Navara CS, Gerrity M, Rinehart J, Binor Z, Asch R, Schatten G. The cell's microtubule organizing center in humans and the implications for infertility. *Nature Medicine* 1995; in press.

Sluder D, Miller FJ, Lewis K, Davison ED, Rieder CL. Centrosome inheritance in starfish zygotes; selective loss of the maternal centrosome after fertilization. *Dev Biol* 1989; **131**: 567–79.

Sluder G, Rieder CL. Centriole number and the reproductive capacity of spindle poles. *J Cell Biol* 1985; **100**: 887–96.

Sobel JS, Alliegro MA. Changes in the distribution of spectrin-link protein during development of the preimplantation mouse embryo. *J Cell Biol* 1985; **100**: 333–6.

Steptoe PC, Edwards RG. Birth after the preimplantation of a human embryo. *Lancet* 1978; **ii**: 366.

Surani MAH, Barton SC, Norris ML. Experimental reconstruction of mouse eggs and embryos: an analysis of mammalian development. *Biol Reprod* 1987; **36**: 1–16.

Szöllosi D, Calarco P, Donahue RP. Absence of centrioles in the first and second meiotic spindles of mouse oocytes. *J Cell Sci* 1972; **11**: 521–41.

Szöllosi D, Ozil JP. *De novo* formation of centrioles in parthenogenetically activated, diploidized rabbit embryos. *Biol Cell* 1992; **72**: 61–6.

Thibault C. Normal and abnormal fertilization in mammals. *Advances in the Biosciences* 1971; **6**: 63–85.

Thibault C, Szöllosi D, Gerard M. Mammalian oocyte maturation. *Reprod Natr Develop* 1987; **27**: 865–96.

Tombes RM, Simerly C, Borisy GG, Schatten G. Germinal vesicle breakdown in mouse oocytes is Ca^2+ independent, while first meiosis, parthenogenetic activation and nuclear envelope breakdown are differentially reliant on Ca^2+. *J Cell Biol* 1992; **117**: 799–811.

Uchida IA, Freeman VC. Triploidy and chromosomes. *Am J Obstet Gynecol* 1985; **151**: 65–9.

Van Blerkom J. Microtubule mediation of cytoplasmic nuclear maturation during the early stages of resumed meiosis in cultured mouse oocytes. *Proc Natl Acad Sci USA* 1991; **88**: 5031–5.

Van Blerkom J, Bell H. Regulation of development in the fully grown mouse oocyte: chromosome-mediated temporal and spatial differentiation of the cytoplasm and plasma membrane. *J Embryl Exp Morph* 1986; **93**: 213–38.

Van Blerkom J, Henry G. Dispermic fertilization of human oocytes. *J Electr Micro Tech* 1991; **17**: 437–9.

Wadsworth P, Salmon ED. Microtubule dynamics in mitotic spindles of living cells. *Ann NY Acad Sci* 1985; **466**: 580–92.

Wassarman PM, Fujiwara K. Immunofluorescent antitubulin staining of spindles during meiotic maturation of mouse oocytes *in vitro*. *J Cell Sci* 1978; **29**: 171–88.

Wassarman PM, Josefowicz WJ, Letourneau GE. Meiotic maturation of mouse oocytes *in vitro*: inhibition of maturation at specific stages of nuclear progression. *J Cell Sci* 1976; **22**: 531–45.

Webb M, Howlett SK, Maro B. Parthenogenesis and cytoskeletal organization in aging mouse eggs. *J Embryo Exp Morph* 1986; **95**: 131–45.

Webster DR, Wehland J, Weber K. Borisy GG. Detyrosination of alpha tubulin does not stabilize microtubules *in vivo*. *J Cell Biol* 1990; **111**: 113–22.

Webster SD, McGaughey RW. The cortical cytoskeleton and its role in sperm penetration of the mammalian egg. *Dev Biol* 1990; **142**: 61–74.

Wehland J, Weber K. Turnover of the carboxy-terminal tyrosine of alpha-tubulin and means of reaching elevated levels of detyrosination in living cells. *J Cell Sci.* 1987; **88**: 185–203.

Wu J-G, Simerly C, Zoran S, Navara C, Gerrity M, Schatten G. Microtubule organization in the rhesus monkey during fertilization, polyspermy, and parthenogenesis and in mature human oocytes *Mol Biol Cell* 1993; **4**: 142a (Suppl.).

Yamada S, Shimazu Y, Kawaji, Nakazawak M, Naito K, Yoyoda Y. Maturation, Fertilization and Development of Dog Oocytes *in vitro*. *Bio of Reprod* 1992; **46**: 853–58.

Yanagimachi R. Mammalian fertilization. In: Knobil E, Neill J *et al.* eds. *The Physiology of Reproduction*. New York: Raven Press, Ltd., 1988; 135–85.

Yllera-Fernandez MDM, Crozet N, Ahmed-Ali M. Microtubule distribution during fertilization in the rabbit. *Mol Reprod Dev* 1992; **32**: 271–6.

Zamboni L. *Fine Morphology of Mammalian Fertilization*. New York: Harper and Row, 1971.

4

Oocyte–genetic aspects

M. PLACHOT

Abnormal embryo development is the major cause of implantation failure, and accounts for the low rate of human fertility *in vivo* and *in vitro*. Chromosome abnormalities are widely involved in this process through meiotic non-disjunctions, fertilization abnormalities and mitotic non-disjunctions.

Oocytes were found to be more sensitive than spermatozoa to non-disjunctions, since when searching for a paternal or a maternal origin for trisomies D and G at birth, the error occurred in 60% of the cases during metaphase I and in 20% of the cases during metaphase II in the oocyte, i.e. in 80% of the cases during female meiosis.

This is why analysing extensively oocyte meiosis and the factors influencing non-disjunctions, enlightens the understanding of the mechanisms leading to embryo or fetal wastage.

Chromosome abnormalities in freshly recovered oocytes

Data on the incidence of chromosome aberrations in freshly recovered human oocytes are scarce for evident ethical reasons.

Martin *et al.* (1986) reported the first series of 50 spare oocytes, i.e. after the three most mature of each cohort had been selected for insemination, according to the guidelines of the University of Calgary. Fourteen were hypohaploid (28%), one was hyperhaploid (2%) and two had a structural abnormality (4%) leading to a total incidence of chromosome anomalies of 34%.

However, the formation of disomy during meiotic division, should, at the same time, result in the formation of nullosomy. The independent segregation of the chromosomes between the oocyte and the polar body should therefore yield an equal incidence of hypohaploid and hyperhaploid oocytes. This excess of hypohaploidy could be attributed to artificial loss owing to the cytogenetic procedures, or to anaphase lag, which seems to occur more frequently in the female than in the male. Indeed, in a large study comparing human sperm and hamster oocyte chromosome complements in a zona-free hamster egg–human sperm IVF test, Martin (1984) showed that male pronuclei are as often hyperhaploid as hypohaploid, whereas female pronuclei show a significant excess of hypohaploid complements. Nevertheless, the incidence of aneuploidy is usually calculated by doubling the rate of hyperhaploidy, leading to so-called 'conservative estimates' of only 8% chromosome anomalies (Martin *et al.*, 1986).

Similar conclusions were reached by Van Blerkom and Henry (1988) who reported 8% aneuploidy, without any difference between spare oocytes from women having either fertilized eggs or repeated fertilization failure.

A higher incidence of chromosomal disorders was noted by Warmsby, Fredga and Liedholm (1987) who concluded that on a small series of 23 oocytes, nearly 50% had an abnormal karyotype, mainly hypohaploidy.

Facing these discrepancies, several groups started to use large series of oocytes from fertilization failures.

Chromosome abnormalities in inseminated-unfertilized human oocytes

Since the first report on meiosis in human oocytes (Edwards, 1968), a large number of publications deals with the cytogenetical analysis of inseminated oocytes that failed to fertilize in the framework of an IVF programme.

So far, nearly 3000 oocytes have been analysed. Data on 2434 oocytes, reported by 12 groups having studied at least about 100 oocytes, and giving detailed data, are shown in Table 1.

The total incidence of chromosome anomalies ranges from 8.1 to 54.2% with an average of 26.5%: 13.3% hypohaploidy, 8.1% hyperhaploidy, 1.6% structural anomalies, 3.5% diploidy. By doubling the rate of hyperhaploidy, the conservative estimates of chromosome imbalance reaches 21.3%.

The most represented anomaly is therefore non-disjunction. The process of non-disjunction should produce an equal number of hypohaploid (<23 chromosomes) and hyperhaploid (>23) oocytes. Although a hypohaploid metaphase II plate is generally attributed to a loss of chromosomes during fixation, other mechanisms could also be involved such as anaphase lag (Martin, 1984), anomalies in the structure or distribution of microtubules (Van Blerkom and Henry, 1988) or alterations in the cytoskeleton.

All chromosome groups are represented among aneuploidies, but non-disjunction is not a random event in female meiosis. In particular, there is a significant excess of non-disjunction in the acrocentric D and G groups (Pellestor, 1991), as already reported in spontaneous abortuses and liveborns (Boué, Boué & Lazar, 1975).

A different finding was reported by Angell *et al.* (1991) who observed that 13%

of the analysable haploid metaphases were hyperhaploid but none contained extra whole chromosomes. The extra components were a single chromatid (one case), or two single chromatids replacing a whole chromosome (4 cases). The authors suggested that the chromatids arose as a result of premature centromere division at meiosis I, this anomaly being a major mechanism for trisomy formation, rather than non-disjunction of whole bivalents at meiosis I, as generally believed.

The reasons for chromosomal non-disjunctions are still unclear. They could include reduced chiasma formation, persistence of nucleolar membranes, the absence of true centrioles in meiotic oocytes, inadequate tubulin polymerization in meiotic spindles, and defective hormonal mechanisms regulating follicular growth and oocyte maturation (Dyban & Baranov, 1987).

The second most represented anomaly is diploidy resulting from an anomaly in the maturational process: the failure of the first meiotic division. The observation of diploid oocytes was also tentatively explained by either sperm entry into the oocyte with no pronuclear formation nor subsequent cleavage, or by retention of the first polar body (Bongso *et al.*, 1988; Selva *et al.*, 1991).

Structural aberrations are reported in only 5 out of the 12 reports, probably because of the difficulty to detect minor deletions or translocations, due to the particular aspect of meiotic chromosomes that appear curly and contracted. The most obvious chromosomal breaks are observed, the incidence ranging from 0.7% to 8.3%. It may depend on different factors such as culture conditions, handling of the oocytes, light exposure or early degeneration of ageing oocytes.

An interesting study was reported by Van Blerkhom and Henry (1988) in which oocyte chromosome complements and location were examined by fluorescence microscopy after staining living oocytes with DNA-specific probes. Specifically, this approach identified living oocytes that contained no apparent chromosomes in the ooplasm, or contained chromosomes not associated with the metaphase II spindle, or had weak or not detectable chromosomal fluorescence in the first polar body. These findings demonstrated that about 8% of the oocytes were aneuploid, another 6.5% displaying anomalies in chromosome structure or distribution that could lead to aneuploidy. Taken together, these results strongly suggest that, in spite of the great discrepancy between different teams, there is no increase in the incidence of aneuploidy in oocytes that fail to fertilize when compared with preovulatory oocytes.

When comparing with other mammalian species in which the incidence of aneuploidy in oocytes ranges from 2.4% in mice (Zackowski & Martin Deleon, 1988) to 5.5% in horse (King *et al.*, 1990), 8.9% in squirrel monkey (Asakawa & Dukelow, 1982) and 10.1% in rabbit (Asakawa *et al.*, 1988), the rate observed in humans is very high.

Several clinical parameters can explain these findings. They will be studied in detail.

M. Plachot

Table 1. *Review of the literature concerning the incidence of chromosome anomalies in human oocytes*

Authors	No. of oocytes	Hypohaploidy	Hyperhaploidy	Struct. anomalies
Veiga *et al.*, 1987	117	3	9	5
Plachot *et al.*, 1988*b*	316	38		n.m.
Van Blerkom & Henry, 1988	135	9	2	n.m.
Bongso *et al.*, 1988	251	33	20	1
Djalali *et al.*, 1988	96	18	2	n.m.
Delhanty & Penketh, 1990	155	67	4	n.m.
De Sutter *et al.*, 1991	171	48	23	n.m.
Pieters *et al.*, 1991	86	13		n.m.
Tejada *et al.*, 1991	334	31	33	n.m.
		27.3%		
Pellestor, 1991	413			0.7%
Tarin *et al.*, 1991	228	38	5	18
Selva *et al.*, 1991	132	21	19	11

n.m.: not mentioned.

Effect of type of sterility

It has been suggested that the occurrence of meiotic disorders leading to chromosome anomalies in oocytes could be related to the type of sterility. More precisely, tubal or male infertility (not involving ovarian pathology) were thought to be less prone to oocyte chromosomal non-disjunctions than idiopathic infertility. Among the six groups having checked this parameter, three reported a correlation between type of sterility and oocyte abnormality and confirmed the former hypothesis. De Sutter *et al.* (1991) observed a difference in oocyte normality between male (58/100 normal oocytes) and non-male infertility groups (25/67 normal oocytes), as determined by sperm morphology, suggesting that lack of

Diploidy	% of anomalies		PCC %	Treatment
	Total	2 × hyper		
8	21.4	26.5		Cl/hMG
6		26.0		Cl/hMG: 24% ⎫
				hMG : 24% ⎬ NS
				FSH : 20% ⎪
				Gn RHa/hMG: 36% ⎭
n.m.	8.1	3		Cl: 7% ⎫
				Cl/hMG: 10% ⎭
5	23.5	18.3		FSH/hMG
11	32.3	15.6		hMG ou Cl/hMG
13	54.2	13.6	4.5	Bus/hMG
12	48.5	33.9	6.3	Cl/hMG ⎫
				Gn RHa/hMG ⎭
n.m.		30.2	12	Cl/hMG: 31.2%
				Gn RH-a/hMG: 29.6%
13	23	23.7	11.1	Gn RH-a/hMG: 22.4% ⎫
				LA/FSH/hMG: 23.6% ⎭
n.m.	28			
				Gn RH-a/hMG ⎫
18	26.8	12.3		hMG ou Cl/hMG ⎭
				Cl/hMG ⎫
n.m.	30.3	28.8	5.6	Gn RH-a ⎬
				hMG ⎭

fertilization with good sperm may be due to oocyte factors. It is, however, still not clear to what extent the genetic constitution is involved.

The same conclusions were reached by Pellestor and Sèle (1988) who reported a higher rate of aneuploidy in idiopathic infertility (22.5%) than in male infertility (10.2%), and by Selva *et al.* (1991) who observed more abnormalities in tubal (60%) and idiopathic infertility (52%) than in male infertility (34%).

Effect of stimulation treatment

The effect of stimulation treatment alone on the incidence of chromosome disorders in human oocytes is unknown because of the lack of control (unstimulated patients) series.

It is, however, possible to compare different stimulation protocols. Although individual small series sometimes show differences between stimulation protocols, when pooling data of the literature (mentioned in Table 1), no difference appears in the rate of chromosome anomalies in 348 oocytes recovered after C1/hMG (29%), 537 oocytes recovered after hMG and/or FSH (27.7%) and 857 oocytes analysed after the Gn RH-a/hMG stimulation protocol (27.9%).

In the same way, a high ovarian response to gonadotropins did not increase the incidence of chromosome imbalance in oocytes, which ranged from 26.1% when 1 to 5 oocytes were recovered, to 17.3% for 6 to 10 oocytes and 18.3% for > 11 oocytes. However, an increased incidence of diploid metaphase II was observed when more than 11 oocytes were recovered (Tarin & Pellicer, 1990).

The doses of hMG required to promote an optimal follicle growth do not correlate with the incidence of non-disjunctions, which is 24% when 6 to 20 ampules of hMG were given, and 35% for 21 to 46 ampules ($p > 0.05$) (Plachot *et al.,* 1988*b*).

These data allow the conclusion that aneuploidy rates are not influenced by the type of hormonal stimulation in humans.

In other species, there are conflicting reports concerning the effect of superovulation treatments when assessed on preimplantation embryos.

No adverse effect on the chromosomal integrity of pre-implantation embryos was reported in PMSG-treated hamsters (2.2% vs 1.2% in natural cycles) (Sengoku & Dukelow, 1988) nor in FSH-LH treated rabbits. Conversely, PMSG was found to be correlated with an increased rate of chromosome anomalies, mainly triploidy, in rabbit blastocysts (9.7% vs 0% in natural cycles), as well as in early mouse embryos (Takagi & Sasaki, 1976).

The mechanisms of polyploidy induction in such treated oocytes could be the consequence of cortical granules reaction impairment (leading to dispermy) or the normal fertilization of a diploid oocyte (leading to digyny), the incidence of which increasing after exogenous gonadotropin treatment in mice.

When comparing a stimulation protocol using PMSG alone or PMSG/GRF (growth releasing factor) in mice, no difference was noted in the rate of aneuploidy (4.4% and 5.8% respectively) showing that GRF has no deleterious effect at the chromosomal level (Aran *et al.,* 1991).

Regarding the doses of gonadotropins, a drastic effect was reported in mice where the incidence of triploidy was proportional to the dose of PMSG given, the dose response being linear, with the level of polyploidy rising from 8% with a PMSG dose of 1.5 i.u./female to 20.8% with 10 i.u./female. In all cases, polyploidy was the result of polyspermy, or fertilization by diploid spermatozoa (Maudlin & Fraser, 1977).

Thus, exogenous gonadotropins seem to have a detrimental action on oocytes at the cytoskeleton level (microfilaments of actin) rather than at the meiotic level (microtubules).

Effect of oocyte maturity

Oocyte maturity is correlated with follicle hormonal environment. In humans, steroid analysis in the follicular fluid of preovulatory follicles did not show significant differences for chromosomally normal or abnormal oocytes except for 17-β estradiol levels which were higher in follicles containing imbalanced oocytes. Moreover, it was found that cytogenetic normality was not related to oocyte maturity (De Sutter *et al.*, 1991).

The effect of oocyte immaturity on the incidence of chromosome anomalies in the resulting embryos has been studied in mice using immature oocytes recovered 2 to 4 h before ovulation. After insemination, a decrease in the fertilization rate (65.5% and 16.6% for 2–3 h- and 3–4 h-immature oocytes, respectively) when compared with control (78.2%) was reported. When no difference in the incidence of aneuploidy and parthenogenetic activation was noted, an increased rate of polyploidy was observed in the experimental group (31.2%) when compared with control (14.6%) suggesting either the fertilization of nonreduced oocytes or the failure of the cortical reaction (Badenas *et al.*, 1989).

Effect of maternal age

Although the influence of advanced maternal age on meiotic non-disjunction is well documented – the estimated rate of all clinically significant cytogenetic abnormalities in live births rising from about 1 per 500 at the youngest maternal ages (< 30) to 1 per 20 at age 45 (Hook, 1981) – data are conflicting regarding oocytes.

Indeed, among the nine groups having checked this parameter, only three reported an increased incidence of chromosome imbalance in older women (> 35 years of age), either because the age of patients showing aneuploidy was above the mean for the entire group of patients in the study (36.7 versus 33.5 years, respectively) (Bongso *et al.*, 1988), or because the incidence of aneuploidy was higher in patients > 35 years (34.8 to 38%) when compared with younger patients (18.4 to 24%) (Plachot *et al.*, 1988*b*; Macas *et al.*, 1990).

In mice, Maudlin and Fraser (1978) reported a significantly higher incidence of aneuploidy in the aged group, solely due to a higher proportion, in females, of trisomies at first cleavage, while there is no difference in the incidence of monosomies.

It has been shown that chiasma frequency declines with increasing maternal age, and that the frequency of bivalents showing terminal chiasmata was much higher in older oocytes. The reduction in chiasma frequency is accompanied by the production of univalents, probably at the origin of non-disjunctions (Henderson & Edwards, 1968).

The sperm premature chromosome condensation

Although not a chromosome abnormality, sperm premature chromosome condensation (PCC) was discovered on fixed preparations of oocytes for cytogenetic purpose. The phenomenon of PCC was first reported in human oocytes by Schmiady *et al.* (1986) and Plachot *et al.* (1987).

It is characterized by the presence of sperm chromatids in inseminated mature or immature oocytes that failed to form pronuclei and therefore were considered as unfertilized. By inducing PCC by experimental fusion of mitotic and interphase nuclei, it has been shown that chromosomes vary according to the stage of the interphase nucleus at the time of fusion. PCC of G1-phase cells are single chromatids, those of S-phase have a pulverized appearance, and those of G2-phase, after DNA synthesis have two chromatids.

In human oocytes, chromatids and not chromosomes are most often observed, since chromosome condensation occurs before the S-phase which usually takes place in fully grown pronuclei (Fig. 1).

In IVF programmes, 4.5 to 28% oocytes showing prematurely condensed sperm chromosomes, near a set of maternal metaphase I or II chromosomes have been described (Table 1) (Zenzes *et al.*, 1990; Angell *et al.*, 1991; De Sutter *et al.*, 1991; Calafell *et al.*, 1991), with a higher incidence in immature oocytes (34%) than in mature oocytes (14%) (Plachot & Crozet, 1992).

Normally, after sperm penetration, the development of male and female pronuclei is under the control of oocyte cytoplasmic factors, mainly the maturation promoting factor (MPF) the concentration of which decreases after fertilization. In immature oocytes (metaphase I) or non-activated (cytoplasmically immature) metaphase II, PCC of the male nucleus may occur, owing to the presence of MPF in the ooplasm.

Using a murine model, a high incidence of PCC at the G1-phase (45.4%) was observed when immature oocytes were immediately fertilized *in vitro*. A small incidence of PCC at the S-phase (3.3%) was noticed when inseminating *in vitro* matured oocytes. Neither G-1 or S-PCC were found in the control group of *in vivo* matured oocytes (Calafell *et al.*, 1991).

The rate of sperm PCC in oocytes seems to depend on the stimulation treatment: it was found to be lower after GnRH-a/hMG (7 to 22%) than after Cl/hMG, FSH/hMG or leuprolide acetate (21 to 39%) showing that in the former, more oocytes are inactivated by sperm and therefore arrested in their development (Janny *et al.*, 1990; Tejada *et al.*, 1991; Selva *et al.*, 1991; Plachot & Crozet, 1992).

According to Angell *et al.* (1991) the frequency of PCC varies according to the stimulation protocol, those oocytes maturing longer *in vivo* showing less propensity to abnormal fertilization.

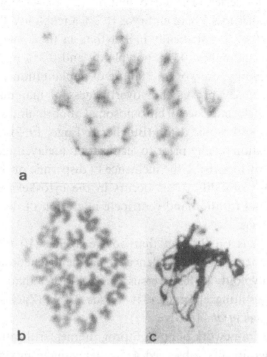

Fig. 1a, b, c. Different sets of chromosomes observed in 9% of supposed unfertilized oocytes recovered after Bus/hMG; (a) polar body, (b) metaphase II chromosomes, (c) sperm chromatids). (Plachot & Crozet, 1992) (With the permission of G. Hartshorne.)

The effect of the type of sterility on the occurrence of PCC is controversial. The incidence of PCC has been found to be decreased in idiopathic infertility (Janny *et al.,* 1990), or increased (Selva *et al.,* 1991) or unchanged (Plachot & Crozet, 1992).

This phenomenon has to be taken into account when considering oocytes with no pronuclei or no cleavage as unfertilized, mainly in case of deficient semen where sperm is generally suspected to be responsible for fertilization failure, hiding the role of oocyte quality and maturity.

Effect of oocyte ageing

Since it is well known that oocyte maturation and fertilization have a clockwork precision, any oocyte ageing induces chromosome anomalies and abnormal embryonic development.

Oocyte ageing, before fertilization, can occur as a result of delayed ovulation or postovulation ageing.

In rats, on a large series, delayed ovulation (24 or 48 hours) resulted in chromosomal anomalies in 4.3% of embryos (1.2% aneuploidy, 0.7% polyploidy and 2.4% mosaics), that is statistically higher than in the control group, where they observed 1.4% anomalies (0.7% polyploidy and 0.7% mosaics). A higher incidence of degenerating embryos and failure of implantation was found in the treated group. This study proves that overripeness of mammalian ova is an important factor in the occurrence of chromosomal abnormalities as well as being responsible for early embryonic death (Butcher & Fugo, 1967).

In mice, postovulation ageing prior to fertilization (delayed mating) decreases the size of the litter by increasing the incidence of dispermic or digynic triploidy.

Indeed, degenerative modifications occurs in the cytoskeleton organization, including an abnormal rotation and centripete migration of the meiotic spindle in the centre of the egg.

There is a consensus on the fact that oocyte ageing (10 to 14 hours after ovulation) in mice increases the incidence of parthenogenetic activation (44% versus 0%), and polyploidy (31.6% versus 14.6%), rather than the incidence of aneuploidy in the resulting embryos (3% versus 2.4%) (Zackowski & Martin Deleon, 1988; Badenas *et al.*, 1989).

In humans, in the framework of an IVF programme, fertilization is sometimes delayed as pronuclei are first observed 42 h after gamete mixing and cleavage 24 h later. This delayed fertilization of mature oocytes induces oocyte ageing *in vitro* resulting in a drastically high rate of chromosome abnormalities (87%) as compared with timely fertilization (29.2%). This is mainly due to an increase in the rate of mosaicism (30% versus 10.6%). In view of these results, we do not replace untimely fertilized oocytes in order to decrease the incidence of chromosomally abnormal fetuses (Plachot *et al.*, 1988*a*).

Chromosome abnormalities and reproduction

When the incidence of aneuploidy is relatively high in human inseminated unfertilized oocytes from infertile women, it seem to be very low in the fertile population. Indeed, only a 3.6% incidence of chromosome anomalies was found in a small series of 56 oocytes recovered from fertile women undergoing laparoscopy for surgical sterilization.

Differences, in these two populations, in the incidence of two chromosome anomalies (diploidy and oocytes with fragmented chromosomes) may be explained by a natural selection at fertilization against these oocytes. However, any gametic selection against aneuploid oocytes is likely to be very weak or non-existent, leading to the conclusion that the high incidence of aneuploidy in infertile patients reported in previous papers may be an artefact introduced by sample collection (Tarin, Gomez & Pellicer, 1991).

When classifying 35 patients according to their oocyte chromosome status, it was demonstrated that 15 patients have all their oocytes chromosomally normal, 5 have all their oocytes abnormal and 15 have a mixture of normal and abnormal oocytes, showing that the production of normal or aneuploid oocytes is patient specific. Patients with multiple aneuploid oocytes may be therefore predisposed to recurrent failure (Zenzes, Wang & Casper, 1991).

Finally, no difference was found in the incidence of chromosome anomalies in oocytes from patients having either a total failure of fertilization or one or more fertilized oocytes (De Sutter *et al.*, 1991).

Conclusion

To conclude, several lines of evidence indicate that oocyte meiosis is very sensitive to endogenous or exogenous factors. Synchrony of gamete meeting is a prerequisite condition to avoid any gamete ageing liable to increase the incidence of cytogenetic defects, all of which impair embryonic development. The fact that a high incidence of chromosome anomalies was found in pre-implantation embryos (about 29%) indicates that there is probably no selection at fertilization against aneuploid oocytes. However, the fact that 'only' 0.6% of liveborns carry chromosomal disorders shows that a drastic selection is supposed to occur probably in two steps: during the pre-implantation period, and during the first trimester of pregnancy (Plachot *et al.*, 1988*a*).

References

Angell RR, Ledger W, Yong EL, Harkness L, Baird DT. Cytogenetic analysis of unfertilized human oocytes *Hum Reprod* 1991; **6**: 568–73.

Aran B, Moragas M, Torello MJ *et al.* Chromosomal studies in mouse zygotes after GRF (growth releasing factor) treatment. Abstracts from the seventh meeting of the European Society of Human Reproduction and Embryology. *Hum Reprod* 1991.

Asakawa T, Dukelow R. Chromosomal analyses after *in vitro* fertilization of squirrel monkey (saimiri sciureus) oocytes. *Biol Reprod* 1982; **26**: 579–83.

Asakawa T, Ishikawa M, Shimizu T, Dukelow WR. The chromosomal normality of *in vitro* fertilized rabbit oocytes. *Biol Reprod* 1988; **38**: 292–5.

Badenas J, Santalo J, Calafell JM, Estop AM, Egozcue J. Effect of the degree of maturation of mouse oocytes at fertilization: a source of chromosome imbalance. *Gam Res* 1989; **24**: 205–18.

Bongso A, Ng SC, Ratnam S. Sathananthan H, Wong PC. Chromosome anomalies in human oocytes failing to fertilize after insemination *in vitro*. *Hum Reprod* 1988; **3**: 645–9.

Boué JG. Boué A. Lazar P. Retrospective and prospective epidemiological studies of 1500 karyotyped spontaneous human abortions. *Teratology*. 1975; **12**: 11–26.

Butcher RL, Fugo NW. Overripeness and the mammalian ova. *Fertil Steril* 1967; **18**: 297–302.

Calafell JM, Badenas J. Egozcue J, Santalo J. Premature chromosome condensation as a sign of oocyte immaturity. *Hum Reprod* 1991; **6**: 1017–21.

Delhanty JA, Penketh RJA. Cytogenetic analysis of unfertilized oocytes retrieved after treatment with the LH-RH analogue, Buserelin. *Hum Reprod* 1990; **5**: 699–702.

De Sutter P, Dhont M, Vanluchene E, Vandekerckhove D. Correlations between follicular fluid steroid analysis and maturity and cytogenetic analysis of human oocytes that remained unfertilized after *in vitro* fertilization. *Fertil Steril* 1991; **55**: 958–63.

Djalali M, Rosenbusch B, Wolf M, Sterzik K. Cytogenetics of unfertilized human oocytes. *J Reprod Fert* 1988; **84**: 647–52.

Dyban AP, Baranov VS. *Cytogenetics of Mammalian Embryonic Development. Oxford Science Publications.* 1987.

Edwards RG. Meiosis in oocytes and the origin of mongolism and infertility in older mothers. Proceedings of the Sixth World Congress on Fertility and Sterility, Tel Aviv 1968; 64–71.

Henderson SA, Edwards RG. Chiasma frequency and maternal age in mammals. *Nature, Lond* 1968; **218**: 22–8.

Janny L, Ben Khalifa M, Pouly JL *et al.* La condensation prématurée des chromosomes, facteur fréquent d'échec de fécondation *in vitro*? *Contraception Fertilité Sexualité* 1990; **18**: 536–7.

King WA, Desjardin M, Xu KP, Bousquet D. Chromosome analysis of horse oocytes cultured *in vitro*. *Genet Sel Evol* 1990; **22**: 151–60.

Macas E, Floersheim Y, Hotz E *et al.* Abnormal chromosomal arrangements in human oocytes. *Hum Reprod* 1990; **5**: 703–7.

Martin RH. Comparison of chromosomal abnormalities in hamster egg and humam sperm pronuclei. *Biol Reprod* 1984; **31**: 819–25.

Martin RH, Mahadevan MM, Taylor PJ *et al.* Chromosomal analysis of unfertilized human oocytes. *J Reprod Fert* 1986; **78**: 673–8.

Maudlin I, Fraser LR. The effect of PMSG dose on the incidence of chromosomal anomalies in mouse embryos fertilized *in vitro*. *J Reprod Fert* 1977; **50**: 275–80.

Maudlin I, Fraser LR. Maternal age and the incidence of aneuploidy in first-cleavage mouse embryos. *J Reprod Fert* 1978; **54**: 423–6.

Pellestor F. Sèle B. Assessment of aneuploidy in the human female by using cytogenetics of IVF failures. *Am J Hum Genet* 1988; **42**: 274–83.

Pellestor F. Differential distribution of aneuploidy in human gametes according to their sex. *Hum Reprod* 1991; **6**: 1252–8.

Pieters MHEC, Dumoulin JCM, Engelhart CM *et al.* Immaturity and aneuploidy in human oocytes after different stimulation protocols. *Fertil Steril* 1991; **56**: 306–10.

Plachot M, Grouchy de J, Junca AM *et al.* From oocyte to embryo: a model, deduced from *in vitro* fertilization, for natural selection against chromosome abnormalities. *Ann Genet* 1987; **30**: 22–32.

Plachot M. Grouchy de J, Junca AM *et al.* Chromosome analysis of human oocytes and embryos: does delayed fertilization increase chromosome imbalance? *Hum Reprod* 1988a; **3**: 125–7.

Plachot M, Veiga A, Montagut J *et al.* Are clinical and biological IVF parameters correlated with chromosomal disorders in early life: a multicentric study. *Hum Reprod* 1988b; **5**: 627–35.

Plachot M. Crozet N. Fertilization abnormalities in human IVF. *Hum Reprod* 1992 suppl. 1, 89–94.

Schmiady H, Sperling K, Kentenich H, Stauber M. Prematurely condensed human sperm chromosomes after *in vitro* fertilization (IVF). *Hum Genet* 1986; **74**: 441–3.

Selva J, Martin-Pont B, Hugues JN *et al*. Cytogenetic study of human oocytes uncleaved after *in vitro* fertilization. *Hum Reprod* 1991; **6**: 709–13.

Sengoku K, Dukelow WR. Gonadotropin effects on chromosomal normality of hamster pre-implantation embryos. *Biol Reprod* 1988; **38**: 150–5.

Takagi N, Sasaki M. Digynic triploidy after superovulation in mice. *Nature (Lond)* 1976; **264**: 278–81.

Tarin JJ, Pellicer A. Consequence of high ovarian response to gonadotropins: a cytogenetic analysis of unfertilized human oocytes. *Fertil Steril* 1990; **54**: 665.

Tarin JJ, Gomez E, Pellicer A. Chromosome anomalies in human oocytes *in vitro. Fertil Steril* 1991; **55**: 964–9.

Tejada MI, Mendoza R, Corcostegui B, Benito JA. Chromosome studies in human unfertilized oocytes and uncleaved zygotes after treatment with gonadotropin-releasing hormone analogs. *Fertil Steril* 1991; **56**: 874–80.

Van Blerkom J, Henry G. Cytogenetic analysis of living human oocytes: cellular basis and developmental consequences of perturbations in chromosomal organization and complement. *Hum Reprod* 1988; **3**: 777–90.

Veiga A, Calderon G, Santalo J, Barri PN, Egozcue J. Chromosome studies in oocytes and zygotes from an IVF programme. *Hum Reprod* 1987; **5**: 425–30.

Wramsby H, Fredga K, Liedholm P. Chromosome analysis of human oocytes recovered from preovulatory follicles in stimulated cycles. *N Engl J Med* 1987; **316**: 121–4.

Zackowski JL, Martin Deleon PA. Second meiotic non-disjunction is not increased in postovulatory aged murine oocytes fertilized *in vitro*. In vitro *cell dev biol* 1988; **24**: 133–7.

Zenzes MT, Geyter C, Bordt J, Schneider HPG, Nieschlag E. Abnormalities of sperm chromosome condensation in the cytoplasm of immature human oocytes. *Hum Reprod* 1990; **5**: 842–6.

Zenzes MT, Wang P, Casper RF. Chromosome status of unfertilized oocytes may help predict reproductive outcome in the IVF procedure. Communication at the 8th International Congress of Human Genetics, Washington, October, 1991.

5

Genetic control of ovarian development

J . L . SIMPSON

Although presumed to be under genetic control, the elucidation of ovarian development has proved more difficult than the analogous search for control of testicular development. It is clear, however, that separate processes govern initial ovarian development and later ovarian (germ cell) maintenance. Development further is governed by loci on both the X and on autosomes. Perhaps it is this complexity that has slowed molecular elucidation of ovarian determination.

In this communication we shall summarize current knowledge concerning genes directing the indifferent embryonic gonad into a functional ovary, specifically considering location and numbers of these ovarian-maintenance determinants. Finally, we shall offer a few caveats concerning the strategy of applying molecular technology to identify and clone X-linked and autosomal genes controlling ovarian determination.

Ovarian development is constitutive

In the absence of a Y chromosome, the indifferent embryonic gonad develops into an ovary. Germ cells exist in 45,X human fetuses (Jirasek, 1976); thus, the pathogenesis of germ cell failure in humans can be presumed to involve increased germ cell attrition. If two intact X chromosomes are not present, 45,X ovarian follicles usually degenerate by birth. The second X chromosome is therefore responsible for ovarian maintenance, rather than ovarian differentiation. Further supporting constitutive ovarian differentiation are observations of oocyte development in infants with XY gonadal dysgenesis (Cussen & McMahon, 1979) or genito-palato-cardiac syndrome (Greenberg et al., 1987). Oocyte development in the presence of a Y chromosome is well documented in mice (Evans et al., 1977).

108

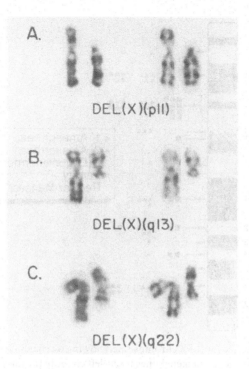

Fig. 1. Schematic diagram of X chromosome abnormalities used to deduce locations of genes responsible for normal ovarian development. (From Simpson & Le Beau, 1981.)

Location of ovarian maintenance determinants

Although for decades efforts have gone into localizing those regions of the X chromosome important for ovarian maintenance, these have of necessity been restricted to deducing ovarian maintenance determinants on the basis of phenotypic-karyotypic correlations (Simpson, 1986, 1987*a, b*). Figure 1 shows examples of X structural abnormalities that are potentially informative for localizing regions integral for ovarian function. Analysis of terminal deletions are the most straightforward structural aberration. Each arm has more than one region (? loci) of importance for ovarian development.

Genes on the X short arm (Xp)

Of 24 reported terminal [del(X)(p11.2-11.4)] cases, 11 (45.8%). show primary amenorrhea (Simpson, 1986, 1987*a, b*) (Fig. 2). The 13 other individuals showed

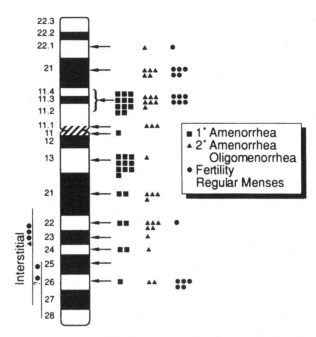

Fig. 2. Schematic diagram of X chromosome, showing ovarian function as function of terminal deletion. The bracketed lines to the left connote the interstitial deletions as reported by Krauss *et al.* (1987) and also observed by our team Tharapel *et al.* (1993) (Modified from Simpson, 1988.)

secondary amenorrhea. Pregnancy has occurred, albeit rarely. One locus in region Xp11.2–11.4 is thus important for ovarian maintenance. Separate telomeric determinants exist, but their function is less integral because all reported [del(X)(p21)] women have menstruated. However, five of the ten reported [del(X)(p21)] women were infertile, manifesting secondary amenorrhea.

Genes on the X long arm (Xq)

Similar topography appears to exist on the X long arm (Fig. 2). Terminal deletions arising at Xq11.3 or proximal Xq21 are usually (10 of 11 reported cases) associated with complete ovarian failure (Simpson 1986, 1987*a, b*). However, a second locus in region Xq25 or Xq26 also exists. Terminal or interstitial deletions in this region lead to secondary amenorrhea. In several cases a mother and her daughters have shown either an interstitial or terminal deletion (Krauss *et al.*, 1987; Tharapel *et al.*, 1993). Although two or more regions on Xq must play roles in ovarian maintenance, these regions differ in importance, the proximal region being more important.

Conclusion and possible homologies to other species

Multiple genes (regions) on the X are obviously necessary for ovarian maintenance. In fact, this cascade is reminiscent of *Caenorhabditis elegans* (Hodgkin, 1987) and *Drosophila melanogaster* (Nöthiger & Steinmann-Zwicky, 1987). The temptation to postulate evolutionary conservatism with respect to general framework is almost irresistible, although DNA sequences presumably have diverged greatly.

Autosomal control of ovarian differentiation

In addition to ovarian maintenance determinants located on the X, existence of autosomal determinants can be deduced on the basis of various disorders of gonadal development.

XX Gonadal dysgenesis

Gonadal dysgenesis histologically similar to that detected in individuals with an abnormal sex chromosomal complement occurs in 46,XX individuals. Mosaicism can be reasonably excluded in adults, but embryonic mosaicism can never be excluded. None the less, the term XX gonadal dysgenesis can be applied to these individuals (Simpson *et al.*, 1971; Simpson, 1979). Most individuals with XX gonadal dysgenesis are normal in stature (mean height 165 cm) (Simpson, 1979). Turner stigmata are usually absent.

XX gonadal dysgenesis is inherited in autosomal recessive fashion. Of further interest are several families in which one affected sibling had streak gonads, whereas another had primary amenorrhea and extreme ovarian hypoplasia (presence of a few oocytes) (Simpson, 1979; Boczkowski, 1970; Portuonodo *et al.*, 1987). These families suggest that the mutant gene responsible for XX gonadal dysgenesis is capable of exerting a more variable effect. Possibly the XX gonadal dysgenesis mutation is also responsible for some sporadic cases of premature ovarian failure.

The mechanism underlying failure of germ cell persistence is unknown; however, one reasonable possibility is perturbation in meiosis. In plants and lower mammals meiosis is known to be under genetic control. If similar mutants exist in human females, one would expect infertility in otherwise normal women. It is reasonable to hypothesize that perturbation of meiosis could well be the mechanism responsible for XX gonadal dysgenesis or germ cell failure in both sexes. Other possibilities include interference with germ cell migration or abnormal connective tissue milieu.

XX gonadal dysgenesis with somatic anomalies

XX gonadal dysgenesis may or may not coexist with distinctive patterns of somatic anomalies. The combination of XX gonadal dysgenesis and neurosensory deafness (Perrault syndrome) has been observed in several sibships (Christakos *et al.,* 1969; Pallister & Opitz, 1979; McCarthy & Opitz, 1985). Other syndromes include XX gonadal dysgenesis and myopathy (Lundberg, 1973); XX gonadal dysgenesis and cerebellar ataxia (Skre *et al.,* 1976); and XX gonadal dysgenesis, microcephaly and arachnodactyly (Maximilian, Ionescu & Bucur, 1970).

Germ cell failure in both sexes

In five sibships, male and female sibs have each shown germ cell failure. Affected females had streak gonads, whereas affected males had testicular germ cell aplasia (Sertoli-cell only syndrome or del Castillo phenotype). In two of these families, parents were consanguinous, and in neither did somatic anomalies coexist (Smith, Fraser & Noel, 1979; Granat *et al.,* 1983). In three other families, characteristic patterns of somatic anomalies coexisted. Hamet *et al.,* (1973) reported germ cell failure, hypertension and deafness. Al-Awadi *et al.,* (1985) reported germ cell failure and alopecia. Mikati *et al.,* (1985) reported germ cell failure, microcephaly, short stature and minor anomalies.

These five families demonstrate that several different autosomal genes are capable of affecting germ cell development in both sexes, presumably acting at a site common to early germ cell development. Elucidation of these genes could have profound implications for understanding normal developmental processes.

Conclusion

The inheritance of the disorders discussed above makes it clear that autosomal loci must be intact for normal ovarian maintenance. This raises the possibility that determinants on the X and Y act in regulatory fashion. Structural loci for directing the indifferent gonad into testis or ovary would then of necessity be autosomal.

Premature ovarian failure

Up to 1% of women are estimated to undergo (premature) ovarian failure (POF) before age 40 (Coulam, Adamson & Annegers, 1986). Premature ovarian failure can result from several genetic mechanisms, two of which have already been discussed. 1) X-chromosomal abnormalities like mosaicism or deletions; and 2) 46,XX gonadal dysgenesis. A third mechanism involves mutant autosomal genes.

X-chromosomal abnormalities

Of 45,X/46,XX individuals, at least 10–15% menstruate; less than 5% of 45,X individuals menstruate (Simpson, 1975). Some mosaic individuals may be so mildly affected that they are never even detected clinically, or show secondary amenorrhea only beginning in their third or fourth decade.

Similar to monosomy X, deletions of the X short arm or X long arm have traditionally been associated with complete ovarian failure (primary amenorrhea). However, deletions may also be associated with premature ovarian failure. Spontaneous menstruation, albeit often leading thereafter to amenorrhea, occurs in almost 40% of 46,X,del(X)(p11) individuals (Simpson, 1987a,b). Almost all 46,X,del(X)(p21 or 22) individuals are fertile (Simpson, 1987a,b). Deletions or X-autosomal translocations involving the region Xq13 or Xq26 also are as likely to be associated with premature ovarian failure as with sterility (Simpson, 1987a, b; Mattei *et al.*, 1981; Maden, 1983).

In conclusion, X-chromosomal abnormalities do not always produce complete ovarian failure. Premature ovarian failure or only anovulation may be manifested.

Mutant recessive genes

Of relevance with respect to premature ovarian failure are data previously cited indicating that varied expressivity may occur in XX gonadal dysgenesis. Dissimilar gonadal development may be observed in affected siblings. One affected sibling had streak gonads, whereas another had extreme ovarian hypoplasia (Boczkowski, 1970; Guisti *et al.*, 1966; Malkova *et al.*, 1974).

Overall, we can conclude that individuals carrying the autosomal recessive mutation for XX gonadal dysgenesis need not have complete absence of oocytes, but rather sometimes manifest less severe pathology. The mutant gene may thus sometimes be responsible for familial premature ovarian failure.

Mutant dominant genes

Because individuals in more than one generation have been reported (Starup & Sele, 1972; Austin, Coulam & Ryan, 1979) to have premature ovarian failure, autosomal dominant genes influencing POF have been postulated. Mattison *et al.*, (1984) found no ovarian antibodies in five families studied, for which reason the authors postulated a mutant autosomal or X-linked dominant gene. However, these families could have been drawn from a very large population base, in which case familial aggregates could have been observed merely by chance or on the basis of polygenic factors.

Molecular strategy: pitfalls and potential approaches

Molecular technology has now localized, isolated and characterized genes responsible for testicular differentiation. One might thus wonder why less molecular progress has been accomplished toward elucidating ovarian differentiation. Actually, several pitfalls caution against assuming the approach to this problem will be straightforward.

Ascertainment biases

One unavoidable problem is that absence of population-based studies inevitably dictates selection biases, which secondarily carry consequences for molecular delineation of ovarian development. No individuals with X deletions were recovered among series totalling over 50 000 consecutively born neonates (Hook & Hamerton, 1977). All reported individuals with del(Xp) and del(Xq) were identified because they manifested clinical abnormalities. Moreover, there is surely a greater tendency for less severely affected individuals to escape detection. Conversely, biases in reporting favour unusual cases. Although selection and reporting biases are inescapable, investigators should still be cognizant of their existence. Mode of ascertainment should also be considered. For example, data derived from deletions transmitted from a parent with an X-autosome translocation should be analysed separately from data derived from individuals with *de novo* terminal or interstitial deletions.

Cytogenetic pitfalls

Molecular studies should be restricted to cytogenetically well-studied individuals in whom mosaicism is reasonably excluded and chromosomal composition unequivocally determined utilizing high-quality banding techniques. Analysis of individuals with unstable aberrations (rings, dicentrics) should be eschewed because monosomy X and other cell lines may arise secondarily, perhaps in tissues (e.g. gonads) inaccessible to study. Analysis of translocations is also hazardous because of vicissitudes of X-inactivation.

Molecular isolation of X-linked genes

The obvious first step in the molecular elucidation of ovarian development is to determine precise composition of deleted or rearranged X chromosomes associate with a given phenotype. This approach has been used to show that at least two apparent terminal deletions were in fact interstitial deletions. The approach is

Table 1. *Table illustrating the approach that shows an apparently terminal deletion shown in Fig. 3 actually to be interstitial, Data from Tharapel et al., 1993*

	Probe locus	Chromosome location	Result and interpretation
DNA markers	DXS3	Xq21.3	Present on two X chromosomes (two alleles)
	DXS17	Xq22	Present (two alleles)
	DXS11	Xq24-25	Present (two alleles)
	DXS42	Xq25	Present (two alleles)
	DXS86	Xq26.1	Deleted on one X chromosone (hemizygous)
	DXS105	Xq27.1→q27.2	Deleted (hemizygous)
	DXS304	Xq28	Deleted (hemizygous)
	DXS52	Xq28	Deleted (hemizygous)
Fluorescent *in situ* hybridization *(FISH)*			
Total human telomere	Xq telomere		Present deletion interstitial not terminal

DNA markers on Xq26.1 through proximal Xq28 show hemizygosity, i.e. one rather than the expected two alleles. However, FISH with a telomeric probe resulted in hybridization. Thus, the deletion is interstitial.

illustrated in Table 1 and Fig. 3. First, fluorescent *in situ* hybridization (FISH) for telomeric DNA showed that a telomere was indeed present. Next, the combination of RFLP analysis and densitometric studies showed that regions distal Xq26→proximal Xq28 were missing. Deletion of this interval thus has some deleterious effect on ovarian development, characterized by premature ovarian failure.

Especially useful would be detection of interstitial deletions involving Xq13 or Xp11, the key regions for ovarian maintenance. If a relatively small region is shown to be integral, one could hope to localize and sequence the DNA, followed by use of transgenic models to determine function of the gene product.

Molecular isolation of autosomal genes

If molecular dissection of X-ovarian determinants poses problems, identifying autosomal sex-determining genes is even more daunting. This would hold true for dissecting autosomal recessive genes known to cause XX gonadal dysgenesis

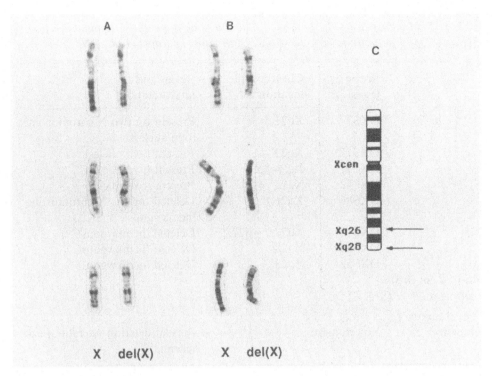

Fig. 3. GTG-banded partial karyotype of X chromosomes from the proband panel A and her mother panel B. A diagram of X chromosome, ISCN (1985) showing the deleted region (Xq26→Xq28) appears in panel C.

or the syndrome of germ cell aplasia in both sexes. A realistic attempt to identify and later clone such genes is likely to await clues concerning chromosomal location. One could then attempt to identify a DNA sequence close to the locus, using family studies involving segregation of restriction fragment length polymorphrisms (RFLPs). Realistically, investigation is likely to await the fortuitous family in which a translocation (autosomal, X/autosomal or Y/autosomal) is detected in a family also showing XX gonadal dysgenesis. Although sporadic cases of gonadal dysgenesis have shown reciprocal translocations, no consistent autosome has been involved.

A final possibility would become available if a relevant non-human mammalian gene integral for ovarian development was isolated. If so, this cDNA probe could be used to identify a homologous human sequence.

References

Al-Awadi SA, Farag WTI, Geebie AS *et al.* (1985). Primary hypergonadism and partial alopecia in three sibs with Mullerian hypoplasia in the affected females. *Am J Med Genet* 1985; **22**: 619–22.

Austin GE, Coulam CB, Ryan JR. A search for antibodies to luteinizing hormone receptors in premature ovarian failure. *Mayo Clin Proc* 1979; **54**: 3945–4000.

Boczkowski K. Pure gonadal dysgenesis and ovarian dysplasia in sisters. *Am J Obstet Gynecol.* 1970; **106**: 626–62.

Christakos AC, Simpson JL, Younger JB, Christian CD. Gonadal dysgenesis as an autosomal recessive condition. *Am J Obstet Gynecol.* 1969; **104**: 1027–30.

Coulam CB, Adamson SC, Annegers JT. Incidence of premature ovarian failure. *Obstet Gynecol.* 1986; **67**: 604–6.

Cussen LK, McMahon R. Germ cells and ova in dysgenetic gonads of a 46,XY female dizygote twin. *Arch Dis Child.* 1979; **133**: 373–5.

Evans EP, Ford CE, Lyon MF. Direct evidence of the capacity of the XY germ cell in the mouse to become an oocyte. *Nature, London.* 1977; **267**: 430–1.

Granat M. Amar A, Mor-Yosef S, Brautbar C, Schenker JG. Familian gonadal germinative failure: Endocrine and human leukocyte antigen studies. *Fertil Steril.* 1983; **40**: 215–19.

Greenberg F, Gresik MW, Carpenter RJ, Law SW, Hoffman LP, Ledbetter DH. The Gardner–Silengo–Wachtel or Genito-Palato-Cardiac syndrome: male pseudohermaphroditism with micrognathia, cleft palate, and conotruncal cardiac defects. *Am J Med Genes.* 1987; **26**: 59–64.

Guisti G, Borghi A, Salti M, Bigozzi U. 'Disgenesia gonadica pura, con cariotipo 44A + XX in sorelle figlie di cugni'. *Acta Genet Med Gemellol.* 1966; **15**: 51–71.

Hamet P, Kuchel O, Nowacynski JM, Rojo Ortega JM, Sasaki C, Genest J. Hypertension with adrenal, genital, renal defects, and deafness. *Arch Intern Med.* 1973; **131**: 563–9.

Hodgkin J. Primary sex determination in the nematode C. elegans. *Development.* 1987; **101** (Suppl.): 5–16.

Hook EB, Hamerton JL. The frequency of chromosome abnormalities detected by consecutive newborn studies – differences between studies – results by sex and by severity of phenotypic involvement. In Hook EB, Porter IH, eds. *Population Cytogenetic Studies in Humans.* New York: Academic Press, 1977: 63–72.

Jirasek J. Principles of reproductive embryology. In Simpson JL, ed. *Disorders of Sexual Differentiation,* New York: Academic, 1976: 51–111.

Krauss CM, Turkray RN, Atkins L, McLaughlin C, Brown LG, Page DC. Familial premature ovarian failure due to interstitial deletion of the long arm of the X chromosome. *N Engl J Med.* 1987; **317**: 125–31.

Lundberg PO. Hereditary myopathy, oliophrenia, cataract, skeletal abnormalities and hypergonadotropic hypogonadism: a new syndrome. *Eur Neurol.* 1973; **10**: 261–80.

McCarthy DJ, Opitz JM. Perrault syndrome in sisters. *Am J Med Genet.* 1985; **22**: 629–31.

Maden K. Balanced structural changes involving the human X: effect on sexual phenotype. *Hum Genet.* 1983; **63**: 216–21.

Malkova J, Chrz R, Motik K, Starka L, Kobilkova J, Silinkova-Malkova E. 46,XX gonadal dysgenesis and ovarian hypoplasia. *Humangentik.* 1974; **23**: 205–11.

Mattison DR, Evans MI, Schwimmer WB, White BJ, Jensen B, Shulman JD. Familial premature ovarian failure. *Am J Hum Genet.* 1984; **36**: 1341–8.

Mattei M, Mattei JF, Vidal I, Giraud F. Structural anomalies of the X chromosome and inactivation center. *Hum Genet.* 1981; **56**: 401–8.

Maximilian C, Ionescu B, Bucur A. Deux soeurs avec dysgenesie gonadique majeure, hypotrophic staturale, microcehalie, arachnodactylie et caryotype 46,XX *J de Genetique Humain.* 1970; **18**: 365–8.

Mikati MA, Samir SN, Sahil IF. Microcephaly, hypergonadotropic hypogonadism, short stature and minor anomalies. A new syndrome. *Am J Med Genet.* 1985; **22**: 599–608.

Nöthiger R, Steinmann-Zwicky M. Genetics of sex determination: What can we learn from Drosophila? *Development.* 1987; **101** (Suppl.): 17-24.

Pallister PD, Opitz JM. The Perrault syndrome: autosomal recessive ovarian dysgenesis with facultative, non sex-limited sensorineural deafness. *Am J Med Genet.* 1979; **4**: 239–46.

Portuonodo JA, Neyro JL, Benito JA, de la Rioa A, Barral A. Familial 46,XX gonadal dysgenesis. *Int J Fertil.* 1987; **32**: 56–8.

Simpson JL. Gonadal dysgenesis and abnormalities of the human sex chromosomes: current status of phenotypic karyotypic correlations. *Birth Defects Orig Artic Ser.* 1975; **11(4)**: 23–59.

Simpson JL. Gonadal dysgenesis and sex chromosome abnormalities. Phenotypic/karyotypic correlations. In Vallet HL, Porter IH, eds. *Genetic Mechanisms of Sexual Development.* New York: Academic Press, 1979; 365–405.

Simpson JL. Phenotypic–karyotypic correlations of gonadal determinants: current status and relationship to molecular studies. In Sperling K, Vogel F, eds. *Proceedings 7th International Congress Human Genetics* (Berlin, 1968), Heidelberg: Springer-Verlag, 1987*a*; 224–32.

Simpson JL. Genetic control of sexual development. In Ratnam SS, Teoh ES, eds. In *Advances in Fertility and Sterility: Releasing Hormones and Genetics and Immunology in Human Reproduction,* Vol III, *Proceedings 12th World Congress on Fertility and Sterility,* 1986, Singapore, Lancaster UK: Parthenon Press, 1987*b*; 165–73.

Simpson JL. Genetics of sex determination: In Iizuka R, Semm K, eds. *Human Reproduction: Current Status Future Prospect. Proceedings of VIth World Congress on Human Reproduction, 1987, Tokyo.* Amsterdam: Elsevier Scientific Publishing, 1988, 19–33.

Simpson JL, Christakos AC, Horwith M, Silverman F. Gonadal dysgenesis associated with apparently chromosomal complements. *Birth Defects.* 1971; **7(6)**: 215–18.

Simpson JL, LeBeau MM. Gonadal and statural determinants on the X chromosome and their relationship to *in vitro* studies showing prolonged cell cycles in 45, X; 46, X, del(X) (p11); 46, X, del(X) (q13); and 46, X, del(X) (q22) fibroblasts. *Am J Obstet Gynecol* 1981; **141**: 930.

Skre H, Bassoe HH, Berg K, Frovig AG. Cerebellar ataxia and hypergonadism in the two kindreds. Chance occurrence, pleiobokism or linkage? *Clin Genet.* 1976; **9**: 234–44.

Smith A, Fraser IS, Noel M. Three siblings with premature gonadal failure. *Fertil Steril.* 1979; **32**: 528–30.

Starup J, Sele V. Premature ovarian failure. *Acta Obstet Gynecol Scand.* 1972; **52**: 259–68.

Tharapel AT, Anderson KP, Simpson JL, Martens PR, Wilroy RS, Llerena JC, Schwartz CE. Deletion (X) (q26.1→q28) in a proband and her mother: molecular characterisation and phenotypic–karyotopic deductions. *Am J Hum Gen* 1993; **52**: 463–71.

6

Ovulation 1: Oocyte development throughout life

R. G. GOSDEN

Prologue

The life history of the oocyte is as intriguing as that of any cell, and a good deal more complex than the majority. Although germ cells are not essential for the survival of the body, they hold the key to the life cycle and the generation of new individuals. The oocytes assume even greater importance than spermatozoa for, although they both transmit genetic information, they contribute virtually all the cytoplasm to the early embryo. These are good reasons, then, for the close attention that has been paid to the origin, growth and maturation of oocytes.

In the past, germ cells have sometimes assumed almost as much mystical significance as they generated pure scientific interest. This was partly because they do not pass on a burden of age changes to the next generation as somatic cells do to their progeny: babies are not born 'old'. This privilege clearly has adaptive value for the species, although it is evidently not absolute because older oocytes are less fertile and more likely to undergo chromosomal non-disjunction. Our understanding of age changes in these cells is still rudimentary, but we presume that cell selection and highly efficient repair mechanisms play important roles in minimizing the transmission of genetic and cytoplasmic damage to the next generation (Medvedev, 1981).

Towards the end of the nineteenth century there was a debate raging between Waldeyer, who argued that germ line cells are formed continuously, and Nussbaum's school, which taught that they are derived from a special patch of cytoplasm in the egg which does not contribute to the somatic parts of the body. The influential German biologist, August Weismann, developed the second hypothesis into his expansive and influential 'germplasm theory' to explain early development and ageing. These ideas are mainly of historical interest nowadays, but they illustrate early recognition of the importance of the early history of cells for understanding the biology of adult characteristics.

This chapter is an account of the origins and early stages of germ cell development, folliculogenesis and the manner in which the follicle population is utilized throughout life. For a discussion of molecular and cellular aspects of oocyte development the reader should consult the chapter by Gosden & Bownes (page 23).

The early history of germ cells

The germplasm theory, which held sway for more than 50 years, was eventually swept away by comparative embryology which showed that the germ cell lineage does not originate from a special region of the egg's cytoplasm in higher animals. Mammalian oocytes are not compartmentalized in this sense and the fact of totipotency of the blastomeres in early embryos clearly supports this conclusion.

The stage of embryonic life when germ cell and somatic cell lineages diverge is not yet known, although there is experimental evidence showing that it is not later than the peri-implantation stage in mouse embryos. Epiblast cells isolated from mouse blastocysts can give rise to germ cells after microinjection into host blastocysts to make chimaeras. Unfortunately, there are no specific cytochemical markers for identifying and tracing germ cells at such early stages, although alkaline phosphatase is a useful, if not absolutely specific, tracer from the primitive streak stage onwards in human embryos and some other species. For practical reasons, most of our knowledge about the cell biology of these so-called primordial germ cells (PGCs) has been derived from experimental work in the mouse as the few studies of humans have been primarily microanatomical in nature.

Germ cells become detectable by histochemical staining on the 8th day of mouse development when they are immediately posterior to the primitive streak in the extraembryonic mesoderm of the yolk sac (Ginsburg, Snow & McLaren, 1990). The extraembryonic phase is one of the most striking and general features of the early history of germ cells in vertebrate animals. Towards the end of gastrulation, the PGCs move into the embryo via the allantois and temporarily settle in both the mesoderm and endoderm of the primitive streak.

Although the initial transport of PGCs may depend on mass movement of surrounding tissues, their subsequent migration depends mainly on an inherent capacity for independent movement. They pass into the developing hind gut and dorsal mesentery and move progressively closer to the nephrogonadoblastic ridge which will form the future gonad (Fig. 1). PGCs reach this destination on or around day 10 in mouse embryos and after day 26 in humans (Witschi, 1948). It is generally agreed that few, if any, PGCs are carried by the fetal circulation in mammals, although this is the principal route taken in avian embryos. PGCs are well adapted for self-propulsion and tissue invasion and when observed by

Development of human ovary

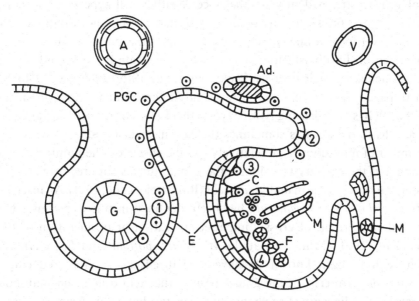

Fig. 1. Diagrammatic illustration of the route taken by primordial germ cells (PGC) along the gut (G) mesentery (1) to the gonadal ridge (2). The germ cells multiply during migration and continue to increase in number after entering the ridge where they become associated with cortical cords (C) (3). In contrast to germ cells in the testis which become relatively quiescent within seminiferous cords, oogonia begin meiosis and become enveloped within follicles (F) (4). The figure also shows the adrenal gland (Ad), aorta (A), cardinal vein (V), coelomic epithelium (E) and mesonephric tubules and duct (M).

time-lapse videomicrography on lawns of cultured fibroblasts they become elongated and migrate at speeds of approximately $50\,\mu m\,h^{-1}$. At their leading edges they carry lamellipodia, filopodia and frequently a distinct uroid with retraction fibres which are typical features of amoeboid-like cells (Kuwana & Fujimoto, 1983; Stott & Wylie, 1986). Male and female PGCs appear identical but they are distinguishable from neighbouring somatic cells by their fine structure as well as alkaline phosphatase staining. They are large cells possessing a round nucleus with one or more conspicuous nucleoli and many glycogen granules, ribosomes and mitochondria and a few lipid droplets in the cytoplasm. PGCs proliferate during migration and have undergone six or more divisions by the time they colonize the future gonad.

There are interesting parallels between the phenotypes of PGCs and metastatic tumour cells. Both are mitotically active, migratory and undifferentiated cell types, though these characteristics are shared with many other embryonic cells.

More significantly, however, some of the mechanisms involved in the control of normal growth are evidently in abeyance. Neither cell type exhibits contact inhibition of growth *in vitro*, interactions with underlying substratum tend to be weak and fewer focal contacts are produced than in less motile or immotile cells. When plated on fibroblast monolayers, PGCs penetrate between and underlap the cells, mimicking their invasive behaviour *in vivo* (Stott & Wylie, 1986). Such ability to penetrate extracellular matrices and disrupt cellular adhesion indicates either that PGCs are releasing lytic enzymes themselves or inducing neighbouring somatic cells to do so, as is sometimes the case in metastases.

A number of mutations have relatively specific effects on the number of PGCs surviving and their ability to colonize the gonad, just as suppressor genes affect the metastatic phenotype in malignant cells (Birchmeier *et al.*, 1991). An insertional mutation, *gcd* (*germ-cell deficient*), has been identified in transgenic mice which are infertile as a result of grossly impaired migration or proliferation of PGCs (Pellas *et al.*, 1991). Mutations at the *W* (*White-spotting*) and *Sl* (*steel*) loci in mice have long been known to have similar effects, severely reducing the population of germ cells in the gonad besides the stem cells of haematopoietic and melanoblast lineages. Their molecular genetics have now been clarified and shown to involve complementary effects. The *W* locus encodes the cellular proto-oncogene, c-*kit*, a transmembrane receptor protein with tyrosine kinase activity for which the natural ligand is the product of the *Sl* locus, a polypeptide growth factor that is known by several names but will be called stem cell factor here (Fig. 2). PGCs and a number of other cell types express c-*kit* in a developmentally regulated manner, but they do not produce its ligand. Stem cell factor is, however, expressed by embryonic cells along their migration route. It was anticipated that stem cell factor would turn out to be either a mitogen or a chemotropic substance, but neither activity could be demonstrated. Maintenance of the cell cycle of PGCs, as of other cell types, probably depends on a complex mixture of growth factors and inhibitors which remain to be discovered. A principal role of stem cell factor in both sexes appears to be promoting the survival of germ cells and thereby ensuring that sufficient stem cells reach the gonad to provide for future fertility (Godin *et al.*, 1991; Dolci *et al.*, 1991).

Once the extragonadal source of PGCs was recognized it was assumed that the subsequent migration is orientated by chemotactic substances diffusing from the gonadal ridge. Recent evidence suggests that a known growth factor, transforming factor $beta_1$, produced by the anlage is chemotactic for PGCs as well as having inhibitory effects on their growth (Godin & Wylie, 1991). At present it is unclear how the chemotactic factor acts: whether by setting up a concentration gradient it polarizes the cells or by affecting the production of extracellular matrix, such as fibronectin or its receptors, it helps to guide cells to their destination.

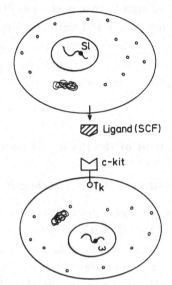

Fig. 2. Primordial germ cell survival in mouse fetuses is enhanced by stem cell factor (SCF), a product of the *steel* (*Sl*) gene in somatic cells. This growth factor binds to c-*kit*, a membrane receptor with tyrosine kinase activity (Tk) expressed by the *W* gene in migrating germ cells and at later stages of development.

Mechanisms guiding PGC migration to the gonadal ridge are not infallible however. Some PGCs form associations with somatic cells *en route* whereas others wander off-course, though the extent of such errant behaviour and its pathophysiological significance are conjectural. Ectopic germ cells have been observed occasionally in human embryos and in one prosimian, the bushbaby, as much as half the PGC population fails to reach the gonad. In the mouse, small numbers of cells end up in the wrong organ, such as the adrenal gland, where they rapidly differentiate into meiotic oocytes irrespective of whether their karyotype is XX or XY (Upadhyay & Zamboni, 1982).

The possibility of PGC survival in extragonadal sites has occasionally been invoked to explain occasional claims of ovarian 'regeneration' after oophorectomy, though it is safer to assume incomplete ablation of the organs is normally responsible. There is a possibility that PGC 'rests' give rise to extragonadal teratomas later in life because of certain resemblances, namely, pluripotentiality, expression of alkaline phosphatase activity and derivation from mitotic precursor cells (Friedman, 1987). By contrast, ovarian teratomas typically develop from oocytes which have undergone meiosis and parthenogenesis (Linder *et al.*, 1975). The similarities have not been reinforced, however, with firm experimental foundations, and teratogenesis could otherwise emerge by dedifferentiation and transformation of other cell types.

While the numbers, fate and significance of ectopic PGCs require clarification, the majority are evidently short-lived and represent the first of several waves of germ cells that die. The survival and function of these cells that successfully colonize the gonad depends on their interactions with somatic cells, specifically those deriving from the common lineage giving rise to either pre-granulosa or pre-Sertoli cells.

Establishment of the germ cell population

Growth and death of germ cells

The phenotype of PGCs changes once they become established in the gonad, becoming more spherical with fewer cytoplasmic organelles and staining less intensely with alkaline phosphatase. The cells lose their ability to elongate and spread on a culture vessel surface or to move in an amoeboid-like manner, perhaps as a result of changes in cell surface macromolecules involved in substrate adhesion (Donovan *et al.*, 1986).

Germ cells in the mouse ovary, commonly called oogonia at this stage, undergo approximately four mitotic cycles before entering meiosis between days 14 and 16 of a 20-day gestation period. Human oogonia undergo many more rounds of division over a period of several months until shortly before birth (Fig. 3). At mid- and late gestation, the human ovary is packed with germ cells at different stages of development spread throughout the organ which still lacks a distinctive cortex and tunica albuginea (Fig. 4). Cytoplasmic cleavage may be incomplete and results in daughter cells sometimes remaining linked by cytoplasmic bridges allowing the transfer of macromolecules and even cytoplasmic organelles (Fig. 5). 'Nests' of syncytial germ cells tend to develop synchronously until associations begin to break down at meiosis. Binucleate oogonia form when cleavage fails completely, and they can potentially give rise to polyploid embryos.

The scheduling of the mitotic phase has a crucial bearing on the long-term functional capacity of the ovary because oogonia are the stem cells from which all oocytes in the postnatal ovary are derived. The absence of oogonial activity after birth is one of the cornerstones of ovarian biology and is now established beyond any reasonable doubt. There is an inexorable decline in the numbers of ovarian oocytes with age (see below) because, once the oogonia have disappeared, no mechanism exists for replacing them. Some of the most convincing experimental evidence has been obtained by injecting tritiated thymidine into pregnant laboratory rodents for several days at the beginning of the third and final week of gestation. We anticipate that cells

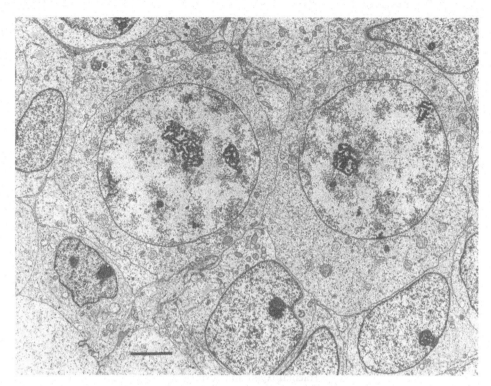

Fig. 3. Fine structure of two oogonia in a human fetus (crown-rump length 41 mm). These cells are larger and more spheroidal than neighbouring somatic cells, have a high nucleo-cytoplasmic ratio and are relatively deficient in cytoplasmic organelles. Bar = 3 μm. (Courtesy of Dr Daniel Szollosi, INRA, France.)

entering the synthetic (S-) phase of the mitotic cycle will incorporate the label into their nuclei, and those continuing in mitosis after withdrawing treatment dilute the label at each successive division. The results showed that germ cells in postnatal ovaries at any age remained labelled, indicating that they had been formed before birth when they had already completed their quota of divisions (Peters, Levy & Crone, 1962). Oogonia do persist to adulthood in a few mammals (e.g. lemurs) but it is doubtful whether any new oocytes are formed at these ages. The restricted period of oogenesis in mammals contrasts with amphibians, reptiles and teleost fish in which oogenesis continues throughout life and egg numbers may actually increase with age.

Germ cell numbers

These reach a peak of nearly 7 million at mid-gestation in normal human fetuses and fall dramatically during the third trimester when the rate of

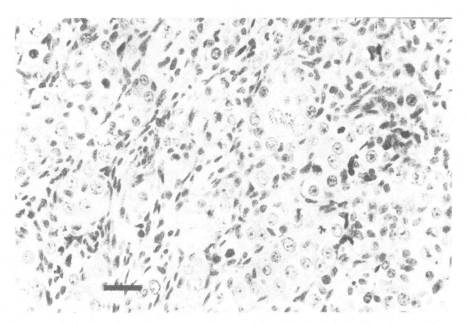

Fig. 4. The ovary of a human fetus at approximately 16 weeks gestation is packed with oogonia and oocytes at early stages of prophase I of meiosis. Follicles are formed later in gestation once oocytes have reached diplotene. Bar = 38 μm. Haematoxylin and eosin.

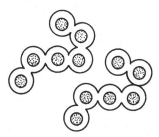

Fig. 5. Diagrammatic illustration of cytoplasmic bridges persisting between oogonia when cytoplasmic cleavages after mitosis are incomplete.

death exceeds that of replacement (Fig. 6). Cell death is therefore a major factor determining the composition of the postnatal ovary, as it is for many other developing organs.

Few moribund germ cells are observed in the early stages of oogenesis but they become increasingly frequent in the third month of gestation when three types are present: 1) large numbers of oogonial cells dying in mitosis ('atretic divisions') rather than during interphase; 2) an even larger

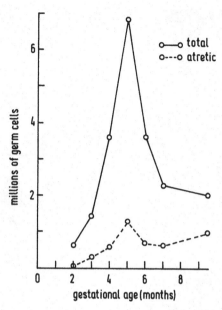

Fig. 6. Variation in the total numbers of germ cells and the numbers of degenerating ('atretic') germ cells in human fetal ovaries. (Reproduced with permission from Baker, 1963.)

proportion of cells (20–30%) dying at pachytene after chromosomal synapsis ('Z' cells); 3) a somewhat smaller number of deaths occurring at diplotene (Baker, 1963; Speed, 1985, 1988). It is interesting that the majority of deaths are associated with the timing of genetic recombination and that many synaptic errors occur between homologous chromosomes (e.g. see Fig. 9). The overall incidence of meiotic anomalies in human fetal ovaries is remarkably high and ten times greater than in mice, a difference roughly corresponding to the different frequencies of aneuploid conceptuses in the two species. The incidence of meiotic anomalies is also much higher in oocytes than in male germ cells. Why these differences exist is not understood.

The hypothetical possibility of a mechanism for selectively eliminating defective oocytes is attractive on evolutionary grounds of the advantages that it could confer on individuals by maximizing reproductive success and reducing pregnancy wastage (Burgoyne & Baker, 1984). Although this theory is speculative, it is supported by evidence from humans and animals with abnormal karyotypes which are deficient in germ cells, e.g. X0 and autosomal trisomy (Carr, Haggar & Hart, 1968; Russell & Altschuler, 1975; Hojager *et al.*, 1978; Burgoyne & Baker, 1984). Whether the variable and generally more complete loss of cells in Turner's syndrome than in

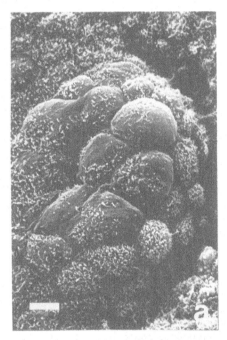
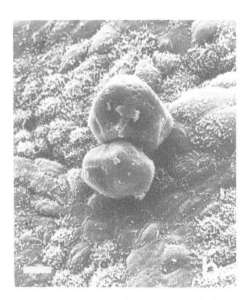
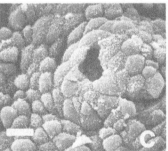

Fig. 7. Scanning electron micrographs of the human fetal ovary at 36 weeks gestation. (*a*) Germ cells, recognisable by their larger size and paucity of microvilli bulge through the surface epithelium (Bar = 1.7 μm); (*b*) two oocytes have emerged through the surface epithelium, from which they are readily detached (Bar = 2 μm); (*c*) after emergence of a germ cell, a space has been left between epithelial cells (Bar = 5 μm) (Reproduced with permission from Makabe, Nottola & Motta, 1989.)

X0 mouse ovaries is due to more meiotic pairing errors or to fewer oogonial mitoses requires investigation.

Moribund germ cells are normally removed by phagocytes but apparently healthy cells disappear too. Significant numbers of oogonia and oocytes pass between epithelial cells at the ovarian surface leaving a temporary 'crater' and entering the peritoneal cavity where they presumably degenerate (Fig. 7). The early cytologists knew that germ cells are sometimes located within the epithelium and drew the erroneous conclusion that they originated there. Unfortunately, the misnomer they introduced, 'germinal epithelium', is still widely used. Cellular extrusion is all the more remarkable because the emerging cells may be actively involved by altering shape and even extending pseudopod-like structures. Such observations raise interesting questions. Is the migratory capacity of at least some germ cells retained? Are cells eliminated simple by virtue of chance location in superficial layers? Do the cells being eliminated appear defective in some way? Only a few cells can be observed emerging at the ovarian surface at the same time, but continual wastage at a low level for several weeks accounts for many of the cells disappearing in immature mouse ovaries. In human ovaries, the situation is less clear and it is unlikely that many cells are lost in this way once they have been captured within follicles and the fibrous tunica albuginea has formed.

Prophase of meiosis

After a number of rounds of oogonial divisions, germ cells begin to leave the mitotic cycles to enter meiosis (Fig. 8). This early milestone in the sexual differentiation of the ovary, occurring at about 6 weeks post-fertilization, contrasts with the situation in the testis in which germ cells become arrested at preleptotene stage and do not proceed to reduction divisions until puberty. Whereas in some species significant quantities of steroid hormones are produced in advance of meiosis and follicle formation, in humans and laboratory rodents this is not the case (Byskov, 1986).

Chromosomal threads become visible as oogonia pass from interphase to leptotene of prophase I, after having duplicated their DNA for the last time (Baker & Franchi, 1967). They shorten during zygotene and the 23 sets of maternally- and paternally-derived chromosomes zipper together to form tripartite ribbons called synaptonemal complexes at the next stage, pachytene (Fig. 9). The fuzzy outlines of these structures superficially resemble lampbrush chromosomes of amphibian and fish oocytes which superactively transcribe RNA from thousands of lateral chromatin loops, but it is doubtful if parallels should be drawn between oocytes of these species and the much less active ones of mammals (see p. 29).

It is not until several weeks after the initiation of meiosis that the first diplotene cells are found (Figs. 8, 10). These oocytes are larger, have more cytoplasmic organelles and, most significantly, have undergone genetic recombination of maternally and paternally derived segments of DNA at the sites of chiasmata. No further nuclear development normally occurs until oocytes have grown to full size in a follicle that has been stimulated by gonadotrophic hormones,

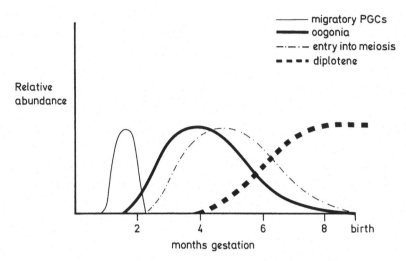

Fig. 8. Diagrammatic illustration of the scheduling of germ cell migration, oogonial multiplication and prophase I of meiosis in human fetal ovaries.

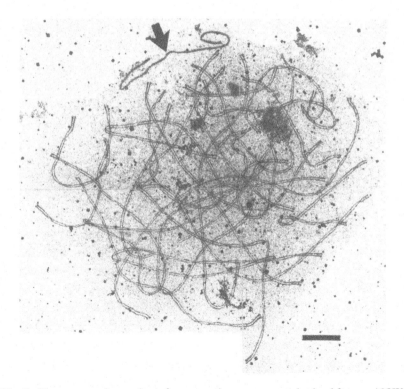

Fig. 9. Synaptonemal complexes from a pachytene oocyte obtained from a 46,XX human fetus. In addition to the twenty-three normal complexes there is a univalent with a thickened axial element (arrow). Bar = 7 μm. Silver stained (Reproduced with permission from Speed, 1988.)

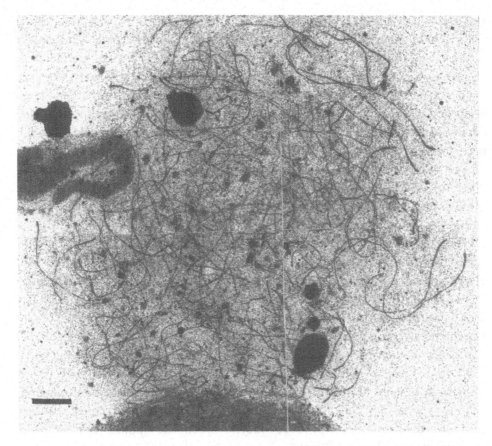

Fig. 10. At diplotene of meiosis, the chromosomes of human fetal oocytes, although considerably lengthened, are still visible. Bar = 10 μm. Silver stained. (Reproduced with permission from Speed, 1988.)

follicle-stimulating hormone (FSH) and luteinizing hormone (LH). Some cells will wait fifty or more years suspended at diplotene still carrying the same DNA that was synthesized before birth during the last S-phase before meiosis. The low fertility of oocytes in older women is not surprising in view of this long history (Navot *et al.*, 1991), yet the molecular nature of the age changes is completely unknown.

Gonadotrophins in the fetal bloodstream. FSH, LH and hCG, do not appear to trigger the initiation of meiosis. This role has been ruled out on the grounds that oogenesis continues in the absence of significant amounts of hormones when fetal ovaries are maintained in culture as well as in anencephalic fetuses (Baker & Scrimgeour, 1980). It is suspected that meiosis depends on the balance of stimulatory and inhibitory factors present within the gonad and differences in the balance and time of expression of these factors could explain the distinctive scheduling of meiosis in females and males. A meiosis-inducing substance(s) (MIS) has been detected in the culture medium of gonads of either sex containing germ cells undergoing meiosis. On the other hand, a meiosis-preventing substance(s) (MPS) is produced by testes at fetal ages when meiosis is inhibited (Byskov & Saxen, 1976). It seems therefore that the developmental schedule of germ cells is determined more by the intragonadal production of diffusible substances from somatic cell types than by an intrinsic 'clock' within germ cells. This theory is consistent with the aforementioned observation that female *and* male germ cells wandering into the adrenal gland both enter meiosis precociously. The molecular characters of MIS and MPS has yet to be elucidated.

There is no clear-cut cortical-medullary boundary in fetal ovaries, but some topographic organization evidently exists because the first cells to enter meiosis in the third month of gestation are generally found nearer the centre of the organs. More peripheral cells do not reach the same stage until several months later, further indicating an influence of the local environment on development. The centrifugal pattern of maturation in the ovary is consistent with the theory that the medullary mesonephric cells drive meiosis and are the source of MIS. The mesonephros is an embryonic system of renal structures, though lacking a filtration function in most species. Its role is inferred from the failure of fetal mouse ovaries either to differentiate or produce oocytes when the tubules are removed at an early stage (Byskov, 1974).

The differentiation of primitive germs cells to form oocytes rather than spermatozoa is not determined by the presence of two X chromosomes or the absence of a Y chromosome. This conclusion is counter-intuitive but it rests on a substantial weight of evidence, including the observations that oocytes can form from precursors with XO or even XY karyotypes. It is not the genetic sex that determines whether a cell will become either an oocyte or a sperm so much as the time of onset of meiosis and the somatic cell environment. In the testis, the primary event in sexual differentiation is the expression of the sex-determining gene encoded on the short arm of the Y chromosome, which has been designated *SRY* (called *Sry* in mice). Consistent with theory, *Sry* is expressed only briefly and in the somatic cells of the gonadal ridge just at the time when sexual differentiation is beginning (Koopman *et al.,* 1990). The site of expression is the supporting cell lineage and genes on other chromosomes downstream of *Sry* action are responsible for differentiation of Sertoli cells and, hence, morphogenesis of the testicular cords. In the absence of this gene in female gonads, cords fail to form and the same lineage is evidently the source of the granulosa cells. Thus, the ovary is formed as the "default" phenotype in the absence of *Sry* (McLaren, 1991).

Reprogramming the genome

Shortly after implantation, one of each pair of X chromosomes in embryonic cells is inactivated to adjust the dose of active genes to that of the normal male karyotype. Each daughter cell inherits the same pattern of sex chromosome expression as its progenitor. In PGCs, however, the second X chromosome is reactivated shortly before the cells enter meiosis and so both Xs are active during oogenesis. This has been demonstrated in women who were heterozygous for isozymal variants of the X-linked enzyme, glucose-6-phosphate dehydrogenase (G6PD), the presence of a hybrid electrophoretic band indicating that both chromosomes were transcriptionally active in the same cell (Gartler, Liskay & Gant, 1973). While normal oocytes contain double the quantity of X-encoded products at XO cells, the deficiency does not, however, render the latter infertile.

PGCs are derived from the epiblast which is a developmentally restricted population and unable to form either primary endoderm or trophectoderm cells. They require reprogramming of their genome in order to restore totipotency to the egg. The marked undermethylation of DNA is one of the notable features of PGCs of both sexes because methylation of the pyrimidine base, cytosine, is associated with inhibition of specific genes, chromosome domains and even whole chromosomes, such as the X chromosome (Monk, Boubelik & Lehnert, 1987). Another interesting finding is that the gene *Oct-3*, which encodes a transcription factor, is expressed only in the germ line and in pluripotent embryonic stem cells (Rosner *et al.*, 1990). Uncovering the molecular foundations of totipotency and dedifferentiation are as important goals for developmental biology as they are crucial for cancer research.

Formation and development of ovarian follicles

Folliculogenesis

Rapid proliferation of somatic cells contributes to the enlargement of fetal ovaries and among this population is a group that associates with diplotene oocytes to form the rudiments of future primordial follicles. Follicles are the lifeboats of the ovary because they nourish and control the development of oocytes: any oocytes remaining naked are doomed to die. Follicles are the ovarian equivalents of the testicular cords and their granulosa cells are homologous to Sertoli cells and probably share a common origin (Fig.

Germ cell - somatic cell interactions

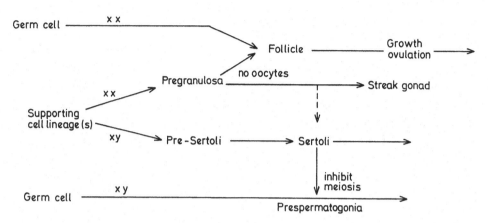

Fig. 11. The fates of germ cells and their supporting cells are interdependent. Survival of oocytes depends on interactions with pregranulosa cells, but when they are absent the resulting streak gonad is afollicular and has little capacity for steroidogenesis.

11). Follicles and cords isolate their germ cells from systemic influences by sequestering them behind layers of epithelial-like granulosa or Sertoli cells where a special environment is created. The structure of follicles contrasts with that of cords in many respects, however, and not least because the former possess a single, non-renewing germ cell (except for occasional binovular and polyovular follicles) and have the capacity to produce most of the gonadal sex steroids. Moreover, the follicle wall is a much coarser sieve and allows molecules (including potential toxins) of up to 500 kilodaltons to gain ready access to the oocyte.

The origins of the supporting cell lineage are still not firmly settled because, in the absence of reliable cell markers, they can only be traced by morphology and fine structure (Makebe, Nottola & Motta, 1989). The cortex of the human ovary at seven weeks of gestation, shortly after becoming sexually differentiated, is packed with so-called ovigerous or sex cords consisting of both somatic and germ cells. Since these cords appear to be confluent with ingrowths from the surface epithelium and the basement membranes are often continuous, it has been assumed that the former may derive from the latter. Alternatively, the cords may be derived wholly or in part from the rete ovarii, which emerges from mesonephric elements in the medulla of the gonadal ridge (Byskov, 1975). Other potential origins exist. It is difficult to

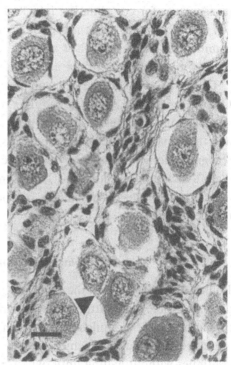

Fig. 12. Human ovary at birth. (*a*) A low-power field shows that small follicles are very abundant and widely scattered; the tunica albuginea is poorly developed. Growing follicles are commonly found in infant ovaries, though absent in this specimen (Bar = 340 μm). (*b*) At higher magnification the density of primordial follicles is more evident, some of them being joined in 'nests' (arrow). The contraction of oocytes from their flattened pregranulosa cells is an artefact of either fixation or *post-mortem* change or both. Bar = 20 μm. Haematoxylin and eosin.

distinguish the boundaries of the proliferating cords at mid-gestation because they intermingle, but fairly convincing morphological evidence shows that, at least in some mammals, mesonephric cells are the precursors of the granulosa cells.

The process of folliculogenesis, like entry of oocytes into meiosis before it, begins in the medullary region and continues while oogonia are still active in the more peripheral parts of the ovary. Follicles first become recognizable in human fetuses at approximately 22 weeks of gestation. Oocytes have lost any intercellular bridges by this stage and are enveloped by a single layer of flattened or polyhedral cells resting on a delicate basement membrane. These are so-called primordial follicles and they number approximately one million at birth (Fig. 12). Junctional apparatus form between the oocyte and the follicular cells but it is not known whether they are simply pathways for nutrient transport or for coordinating follicle development or both. The third follicular cell type, the theca, is not morphologically recognisable until follicle growth has commenced and, although it appears to be derived from mesenchymal cells in the stroma, its precise origin also requires clarification.

The germ and somatic cell compartments of the follicle are interdependent. On the one hand, oocytes require granulosa cells for growth and survival whereas, on the other, granulosa cells do not differentiate in sterile individuals and the gonad becomes a functionless 'streak' organ (Fig. 11). This principle was recognised long ago, as the pioneering cytologists stated, 'Ohne Ei, kein Follikel' (Seitz's dictum). We should not, therefore, expect to find anovular follicles except under the unusual circumstances of oocytes dying within an otherwise healthy follicle.

Follicle recruitment and growth

Follicle recruitment is the process by which a primordial follicle makes an irreversible commitment to growth. The first signs are a slow increase in numbers of pregranulosa cells, which become more cuboidal, and secretion of zona proteins and enlargement of the oocyte. Once this process has started it continues without halting until ovulatory maturity is attained or, in the majority of cases, until the follicle dies (atresia). This is one of the most important yet most poorly understood phenomena in ovarian biology. The first follicles begin growing in the human ovary shortly after they are formed and by the time of birth a few multilaminar follicles are usually present. Primordial stages are the vast majority of follicles present though at this and all ages. Follicles are recruited continuously until the original store is exhausted shortly after menopause in mid-life.

Far more follicles than the single one required for ovulation are recruited each month. The fate of the surplus is atresia, a process that apparently begins with the programmed cell death (apoptosis) of the granulosa and theca cells (Tilly *et al.*, 1992). The actual numbers of follicles that begin growing each day is an exponential function of numbers of stored follicles remaining and, hence, declines with age. The dynamics of the follicle population as a whole can be illustrated by a mathematical model which predicts the flow of follicles between successive stages from primordial (stage I) to Graafian (stage V+) in mouse ovaries (Table 1). Although a comparable model for human ovaries does not yet exist, it is likely that the situation is probably similar, albeit with much slower rates of growth and accelerated disappearance of follicles in mid-life (see below).

The fate of the first cohorts of primordial follicle recruits is atresia (Table 1). Thus, the majority of follicles disappear even before animals are physiologically

Table 1. *Mean numbers of follicles in CBA mouse ovaries leaving and entering five stages[a] at specified ages througout life[b]*

Age scan (calendar months)	Movement of follicles from and to successive groups								
	I→	→II	II→	→III	III→	→IV	IV→	→V+	V+→
0–1	5657	593	366	366	182	182	155	155	84
1–2	1342	348	185	185	204	204	209	209	255
2–3	859	223	224	224	212	212	210	210	207
3–4	549	143	203	203	214	214	215	215	215
4–5	352	91	164	164	190	190	194	194	200
5–6	225	58	125	125	155	155	159	159	169
6–7	144	37	96	91	119	119	123	123	132
7–8	92	24	64	64	87	87	91	91	99
8–9	59	15	45	45	62	62	65	65	71
9–10	38	10	31	31	44	44	46	46	50
10–11	24	6	21	21	30	30	31	31	35
11–12	15	4	14	14	21	21	21	21	24
12–13	10	3	9	9	14	14	14	14	16

[a] Follicle stages were from primordial (I) to Graafian (V+) (Gosden, 1985).
[b] Follicle dynamics were estimated from fitted mathematical model.

ready for ovulation at pubertal age (c. 35 days in mice). This is not because the follicles are incapable of developing fully but a result of inadequate gonadotrophic stimulation. The frequencies of atresia vary markedly between follicle stages and ages, and the numbers dying are indicated in the Table by the differences between those flowing out of one stage and into the next (horizontal rows). The highest rates of depletion are found among primordial follicles before puberty which either die *in situ* or are extruded through the surface of the ovary into the peritoneal cavity. Few primordial follicles die at adult ages in most strains of mice, the CBA strain depicted in the Table being peculiar. On the basis of cytology, the same appears to be true for human ovaries but such small structures may be cleared quickly and a low death rate could contribute significantly to the overall attrition over the long lifespan. Atresia is rarely observed in preantral follicles before the antrum forms but is common afterwards, suggesting that it is at the latter stages when follicle selection for ovulation is occurring. In the human ovary, at the beginning of the menstrual cycle, there are about 20 small antral follicles available for selection but only one normally survives to mid-cycle.

At later ages (vertical columns), fewer follicles start to grow each day because of the dwindling size of the store and the rate at which follicles progress from stage-to-stage slows after puberty. This slow-down may seem paradoxical just at the time when ovulatory cycles are being established, but there is an excess number at most ages and there are indications that mature follicles exert inhibitory influences over the progression of growing ones.

The rate at which primordial follicles disappear and the time taken for those surviving to reach ovulation are scaled according to the lifespan of the species (Gosden, 1990). The time for the population to halve is three months in the mouse and seven years in humans. This is not unexpected in view of our 30-fold longer lifespan. Furthermore, it takes follicles in a mouse ovary less than a month to reach full maturity but the corresponding time in humans is more than six months. Follicular 'clocks' in humans run at much slower paces than in smaller, shorter-lived animals.

Follicle growth can be classified in two stages according to the stage of oocyte development. The first stage involves the growth of the oocyte to almost full size (120 μm) and is reached when several layers of granulosa cells are present and the fluid-filled antrum is appearing (Fig. 13). The second stage is the formation and expansion of the antrum in the Graafian follicle which grows to more than 2 cm in diameter with a fertile oocyte and achieving maximal steroidogenic activity.

The appearance of the follicular population is one of impressive order. Primordial follicles in the ovarian cortex give rise to successive growing stages which are found at progressively deeper levels in the ovary (Fig. 14). Finally, the swelling antrum forces them to bulge at the ovarian surface in preparation for ovulation. Does the apparent orderliness of oogenesis and follicle utilization imply that some sort of production line exists in the ovary? And what factors determine whether a given primordial follicle will begin to grow at one year of age or 20 or 50?

According to the production line hypothesis, the environment in which the first oocytes are formed affects the scheduling of later development. The first formed are the first to be recruited for growth, and the last formed are last to be ovulated. This hypothesis was originally based on indirect evidence from cytogenetic studies of mouse oocytes and provided an important, though still unproven, theory for the aetiology of chromosomal non-disjunction in the oocytes of older mothers (Henderson & Edwards, 1968). More recently, experimental support has been obtained from other sources. When pregnant rats were given tritiated thymidine during the later stages of pregnancy a small number of germ cells in the female fetuses were labelled 'late-formed', but these cells were not within the group of follicles which were first to begin growing near the medulla

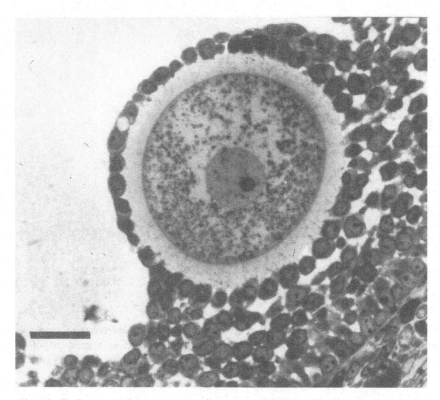

Fig. 13. Fully grown human oocyte in an antral follicle. The oocyte contains a prominent nucleolus in the germinal vesicle nucleus and is surrounded by a zona pellucida and layers of granulosa cells. Bar = 33 μm. (Reproduced with permission from Zamboni, 1972.)

after birth (Hirshfield, 1992). Additional support for the hypothesis has been obtained by radio-labelling of oocytes in culture followed by grafting (Polani & Crolla, 1991). It is unlikely, however, that follicle recruitment is quite as rigidly predetermined as a production line. Although it is not possible on morphological or topographical criteria to predict which follicle will begin growing next, this need not imply that the chances of growing are strictly growing next, this need not imply that the chances of growing are strictly random either. The numbers of primordial follicles are distributed according to an exponential function of age and the great majority have disappeared at the age when chiasma frequency has fallen and aneuploidy has risen. If, for the sake of argument, we assume that mouse oocytes are formed at a constant rate on each of the four days of oogenesis, the potentially defective ones would be among those formed after 9.30 pm on the last day. It is doubtful whether substantial differences in oocyte quality would occur within such a narrow time-frame in

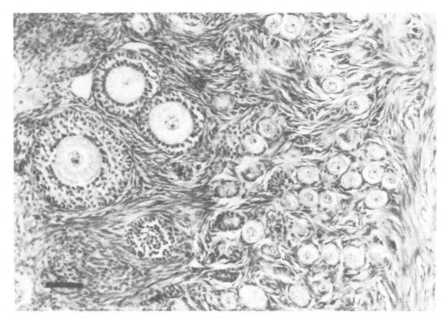

Fig. 14. The ovarian cortex of the young adult rhesus monkey contains many primordial follicles underlying the tunica albuginea. There is a gradient of progressively more advanced follicle stages towards the medulla. Bar = 63 μm. Haematoxylin and eosin. (Reprinted from Gosden, 1985.)

this species, but this hypothesis is more plausible during the protracted process of human oogenesis.

In conclusion, therefore, we have found that the dynamics of the primordial follicle population have characteristics of both orderly and stochastic processes. The unsatisfactory state of knowledge about this important stage is due to our ignorance of the cell biology. On present evidence, there is little indication that substances secreted by Graafian follicles have any feedback effects on follicle recruitment (Hirshfield, 1991). Neither should we be surprised because follicles are overabundant and regulation can and does occur at later stages. Recruitment evidently continues regardless of the state of reproductive endocrinology for, if it were otherwise, variations in pituitary gonadotrophins or ovarian hormones with reproductive history or steroidal contraception would affect menopausal age. To date, no consistent effect has been detected and, apart from a possible priming action of gonadotrophins at fetal ages (Baker & Scrimgeour, 1980), the early stages of follicle growth seem to be independent of hormones. The evidence of slower follicle depletion in hypophysectomized mice may not be a specific effect of hypogonadotrophism but to general metabolic effects (Jones & Krohn, 1961). The possible effects of hypergonadotrophism on follicle growth and recruitment during the perimenopausal years cannot be ruled out however.

The basic answers to the question of follicle recruitment probably lie within the ovary itself. Local growth-promoting factors presumably play a role and the expression of *c-kit* on the surfaces of small and growing oocytes after birth suggests that it may have a second function in the ovary for promoting growth and survival (Manova *et al.*, 1993; Packer *et al.*, 1994). A search for a 'trigger' substance may be misguided, however, because, we might expect on *a priori* grounds that inhibitory factors are equally if not more important that growth factors. The clinical risks of over-recruiting follicles are well known and the theoretical possibility that natural inhibitory mechanisms exist as safeguards is attractive.

Dynamics of the follicular population from birth to menopause

The peak number of germ cells in human ovaries at mid-gestation falls to approximately 1 million at birth when virtually all are diplotene oocytes invested in primordial follicles. The follicle population is divided more-or-less evenly between each pair of ovaries, in contrast to the dramatic regression of the right organ in birds.

During childhood, the ovary contains growing follicles at virtually all stages of development apart from dominant ones which secrete large amounts of oestradiol. It is not therefore a quiescent organ, as had long been supposed, and the extent of follicle growth is reminiscent of the activity we have noted in immature animals. Most of the early histological studies were based on small numbers of specimens obtained *post-mortem* from children who had been chronically ill, many having been suffering with wasting diseases and treated with cytotoxic drugs and/or ionizing radiations. Subsequent studies of specimens obtained from accidental deaths or after a short acute illness indicated that ovaries during infancy and childhood are not normally quiescent, with the possible exception of abnormal conditions such as Down's syndrome (Peters, Himelstein-Braw & Faber, 1976). In addition to preantral stages, there are almost always a few antral follicles measuring > 2 mm in diameter as well as atretic forms. The follicles are larger and more abundant in older children as puberty approaches and are responsible for the increasing urinary excretion of oestrogen. The state of the prepubertal ovary is therefore reminiscent of that of domesticated animals during the non-breeding season. The sheep ovary, for example, possesses follicles of several mm in diameter during anoestrus and these are capable of secreting oestrogen and ovulating when stimulated by a single injection of gonadotrophin. The child's ovary is also in a state of latent readiness to respond as soon as the gonadotrophic environment becomes favourable.

As a result of continuing recruitment and an unknown contribution of atresia, the numbers of primordial follicles dwindle to about 25% of the numbers at birth during the years before puberty. The onset of cyclical follicle maturation and ovulation does not affect the steady rate of decline in follicle numbers, neither does the rate change during the following two decades of adult life. This is not surprising since fewer than 0.1% of the total numbers are ovulated.

There have been few quantitative studies of the total follicle population in human ovaries because whole organs are rarely available from healthy young people and can yield two thousand or more histological sections, representing a colossal effort for microscopical analysis. A recent study of data that had been collected from individuals at different ages up to about 50 years showed that the rate of decline of follicle numbers is not constant throughout life but increases more than two-fold after age 37 when about 25 000 remain (Fig. 14). Since primordial stages represent the great majority of follicles at all ages, this result implies that they disappear faster during the final 10–15 years of menstrual life. Because the dynamics of small follicles are very difficult to study in humans, it is not yet clear whether this change reflects a higher rate of death within the surviving population of primordial follicles or at later stages as a result of a higher rate of recruitment. A rising fraction of growing follicles of the total (Block, 1952) suggests that recruitment is increased, perhaps to compensate for a dwindling store, but alternative interpretations of the data are possible. Whatever the explanation, it is interesting to speculate whether rising serum concentrations of FSH in the decade before menopause affect the rate of recruitment and/or growth of small follicles despite the lack of any concrete evidence that lowering gonadotrophin levels affects the rate of follicle attrition.

Estimating the numbers of follicles present at menopause is difficult because the last menstrual cycle is identified retrospectively and normally only after a full year of amenorrhoea. Few remain and the perimenopausal ovary is in transition between full activity and senescence (Fig. 15). Extrapolating the decline in follicle numbers in Fig. 14 suggests that a threshold number of about 1000 remain at age 51, the median age of menopause in the population from which the subjects were obtained. Had the rate of follicle disappearance not accelerated after age 37 this threshold would not have been reached until age 70. The threshold should only be regarded as an approximation, however, as we have no information about the normal range of values at menopause. Some middle-aged women evidently continue cycling when only a few hundred follicles remain (Richardson, Senikas & Nelson, 1987).

Since the single dominant follicle contributes about 90% of the oestradiol produced during the menstrual cycle, it is puzzling that cycles do not continue until the last follicle disappears. This is partly explained by the continuing wastage of follicles, but it is possible that each small follicle promotes the development

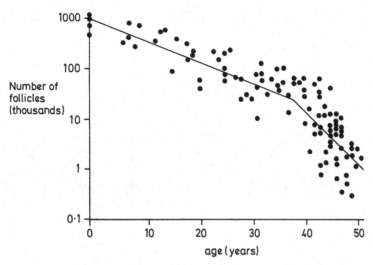

Fig. 15. Variation in total numbers of follicles in human ovaries from neonatal age to 51 years old showing a fitted bi-exponential model with accelerated depletion after age 37. (Reprinted from Faddy *et al.*, 1992.)

of others by secreting growth-promoting factors, rather like preimplantation embryos influence the growth of others in culture. A reduction in paracrine influences as a result of the rarefication of follicles throughout the cortex could then be responsible for the failure of residual follicles to undergo normal growth and differentiation after the menopause (Fig. 16, Fig. 17). In addition, follicular cells may have accumulated damage during the course of life and, since neither oocytes nor pregranulosa cells are multiplying, selection to weed out defective cells and maintain the vigour of the unit may not occur. Cytological changes have been observed in the primordial follicles of older ovaries, but it is not known whether they reflect actual cellular injury or if this is related purely to the passage of biological time or to a history of exposure to toxic influences, such as tobacco products, ethanol, medications or even occupational hazards (Mattison, Shiromizu & Nightingale, 1983). Relatively little attention has been paid to the exposure of oocytes during their long lives to potentially hazardous agents or to the ability of these cells to detoxify them. Attention should now be paid to these questions because it is important to determine the extent to which they can account for reduced fertility and premature menopause.

Perspective

The life history of oocytes is a complex series of stages requiring molecular signals and cellular interactions at the right times in order for the progeny of primordial

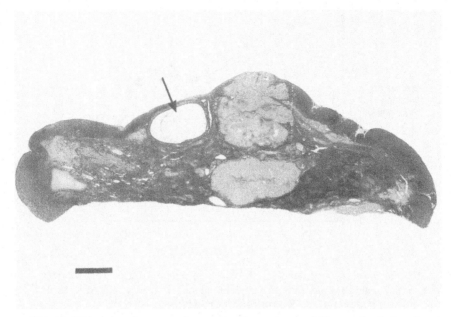

Fig. 16. This ovary from a perimenopausal woman aged 51 contained abundant stromal tissue, two corpora albicantia and one cystic follicle (arrow). The cortex is almost completely depleted of small follicles. Bar = 1740 μm. Haematoxylin and eosin. (Reprinted from Gosden, 1985.)

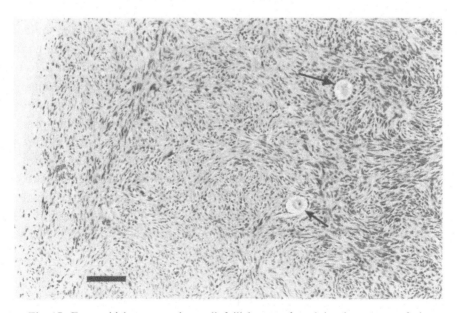

Fig. 17. Few, widely scattered, small follicles are found in the cortex of the postmenopausal ovary which consists mainly of stromal tissue and remnants of former follicles and corpora lutea. Bar = 80 μm. Haemotoxylin and eosin.

Life history of the mammalian oocyte

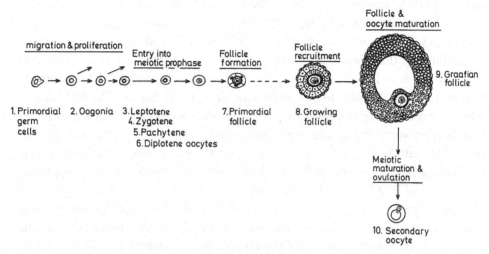

Fig. 18. Diagrammatic illustration of the life history of the mammalian oocyte from its genesis as a primordial germ cell (1) to ovulation at metaphase II of meiosis (10). All the stages up to diplotene in primordial follicles (7) occur exclusively at fetal ages. These oocytes do not undergo further development until growth (8) is initiated after 'resting' for a variable period lasting weeks to decades. Only a small fraction of follicles will eventually attain preovulatory maturity when nuclear development is resumed (9).

germ cells to produce mature oocytes in Graafian follicles (Fig. 18). The crucial question of whether oocytes are formed continuously from stem cell precursors in the 'germinal epithelium' or once and for all in fetal life was still being hotly argued only 40 years ago. The answer made a permanent impact on the research agenda. Questions of high priority became: What is the origin of germ cells and their supporting cell lineages? What controls their growth and migration to the future gonad? Does the genetic sex of the germ cells or the somatic cells enveloping them determine whether the indifferent stage gonad will differentiate as an ovary or testis? What are the molecular hallmarks of totipotency in germ cells? To what extent is the wastage of germ cells a result of meiotic errors? Do primordial follicles have an intrinsic timing mechanism for triggering recruitment into the population of growing follicles? How vulnerable are oocytes to environmental dangers and what is their capacity for repairing cellular injury during the extended diplotene phase?

While many of these questions still figure prominently on the agenda, much progress has been made. The first germ cells detected in embryos are located in the yolk sac. An explanation for this extraembryonic stage is still elusive and tracing their earlier history will have to wait until suitable markers of primordial germ cells become available. The character of gene expression and undermethylation of DNA indicate that germ cells are undifferentiated, yet they evidently still need to undergo genetic reprogramming in oogenesis in order to guarantee totipotency of the oocyte. We can expect to see further progress towards understanding the molecular genetics of these cells in the near future now that their scarcity is no longer a serious hindrance to progress because of the increasing sensitivity and sophistication of molecular biology techniques. The incidence of meiotic errors during oogenesis is of high importance because of the possibility that oocytes surviving to adulthood may contribute to pregnancy wastage and even birth defects. It is a moot point whether the wave of cell deaths selectively eliminate abnormal genotypes by switching on mechanisms that induce apoptosis.

The role of PGCs in establishing fecundity depends on sequential changes in the phenotype. They have to make their way to the target organ, become stationary, continue multiplying and enter meiosis. The nature of the cues guiding the cells to their destination and the fate of those wandering from the proper path needs to be clarified. And when the molecules and their respective genes responsible for triggering the onset of meiosis are identified we shall be able to verify whether mesonephric cells are in fact their source. A related question concerns the origin of the supporting cell lineage which, it is assumed, gives rise to either granulosa or Sertoli cells according to the expression of sex-determining genes. There is good morphological evidence that the rete ovarii is the origin of these cells, at least in some species, but until reliable cell markers are available conflicting claims cannot be settled.

The primordial follicle is the simplest type of follicle consisting of a small, non-growing oocyte and a single ring of granulosa cells, but this is a stage we know least about. It is more than a matter of theoretical interest to discover whether its recruitment is random or orderly and to identify stimulatory or inhibitory factors involved. These questions have a bearing on the origins of chromosomally abnormal oocytes and the feasibility of postponing menopause. In this respect, the observed acceleration of follicle loss in the decade before menopause may be significant. At present, however, it is far from clear whether it will ever be possible to slow down the rate of follicle disappearance.

Acknowledgements

The author gratefully acknowledges support from The Wellcome Trust, The Medical Research Council and The Galton Institute (London).

References

Baker TG. A quantitative and cytological study of germ cells in human ovaries. *Proc Roy Soc B* 1963; **158**: 417–33.

Baker TG, Franchi LL. The fine structure of oogonia and oocytes in human ovaries. *J Cell Sci* 1967; **2**: 213–24.

Baker TG, Scrimgeour JB. Development of the gonad in normal and anencephalic human fetuses. *J Reprod Fert* 1980; **60**: 193–9.

Birchmeier W, Behrens J, Weidner KM, Frixen UH, Schipper J. Dominant and recessive genes involved in tumor cell invasion. *Curr Opin in Cell Biol* 1991; **3**: 832–40.

Block E. Quantitative morphological investigations of the follicular system in women: variations at different ages. *Acta Anat* 1952; **14**: 108–23.

Burgoyne PS, Baker TG. Meiotic pairing and gametogenic failure. In: Evans CW, Dickinson HG. *Controlling Events in Meiosis. Symp Soc Exp Biol* 1984; **38**: 349–62.

Byskov AG. Does the rete ovarii act as a trigger for the onset of meiosis? *Nature, London* 1974; **252**: 396–7.

Byskov AG. The role of the rete ovarii in meiosis and follicle formation in the cat, mink and ferret. *J Reprod Fert* 1975; **45**: 201–9.

Byskov AG. Differentiation of mammalian embryonic gonad. *Physiol Rev* 1986; **66**: 71–117.

Byskov AG, Saxen L. Induction of meiosis in fetal mouse testes *in vitro*. *Dev Biol* 1976; **52**: 193–200.

Carr DH, Haggar RA, Hart AG. Germ cells in the ovaries of XO female infants. *Am J Clin Path* 1968; **49**: 521–6.

Dolci S, Williams DE, Ernst MK, Resnick JL, Brannan CI, Lock LF, Lymans SD, Boswell HS, Donovan PJ. Requirement for mast cell growth factor for primordial germ cell survival in culture. *Nature, London* 1991; **352**: 809–11.

Donovan PJ, Stott, D, Cairns LA, Heasman J, Wylie CC. Migratory and postmigratory mouse primordial germ cells behave differently in culture. *Cell* 1986; **44**: 831–8.

Faddy MJ, Gosden RG, Gougeon A, Richardson SJ, Nelson JF. Accelerated disappearance of ovarian follicles in mid-life: implications for forecasting menopause. *Hum Reprod* 1992; **7**: 1342–6.

Friedman NB. The function of the primordial germ cell in extragonadal tissues. *Int J Androl* 1987; **10**: 43–9.

Gartler SM, Liskay RM, Gant N. Two functional X-chromosomes in human fetal oocytes. *Exp Cell Res* 1973; **82**: 464–6.

Ginsburg M, Snow MHL, McLaren A. Primordial germ cells in the mouse embryo during gastrulation. *Development* 1990; **110**: 521–8.

Godin I, Wylie CC. TGF*beta*₁ inhibits proliferation and has a chemotropic effect on mouse primordial germ cells in culture. *Development* 1991; **113**: 1451–7.

Godin I, Deed R, Cooke J, Zsebo, K, Dexter M, Wylie CC. Effects of the *steel* gene product on mouse primordial germ cells in culture. *Nature, London* 1991; **352**: 807–9.

Gosden RG. *Biology of Ageing: The Causes and Consequences of Ovarian Ageing*. London: Academic Press, 1985.

Gosden RG. Control of recruitment of preantral follicles in mammalian ovaries. In: Dale B, ed. *Mechanisms of Fertilization*. NATO ASI, H45. Berlin, Heidelberg: Springer-Verlag, 1990: 101–13.

Henderson SA, Edwards RG. Chiasma frequency and maternal age in mammals. *Nature, London* 1968; **218**: 22–8.

Hirshfield AN. Development of follicles in the mammalian ovary. *Int Rev Cytol* 1991; **124**: 43–100.

Hirshfield AN. Heterogeneity of cell populations that contribute to the formation of primordial follicles in rats. *Biol Reprod* 1992; **47**: 466–72.

Hojager B, Peters H, Byskov AG, Faber M. Follicular development in ovaries of children with Down's Syndrome. *Acta Paediat Scand* 1978; **67**: 637–43.

Jones EC, Krohn PL. The effect of hypophysectomy on age changes in the ovaries of mice. *J Endocr* 1961; **21**: 497–509.

Koopman P, Munsterberg A, Capel B, Vivian N, Lovell-Badge R. Expression of a candidate sex-determining region gene during mouse testis differentiation. *Nature, London* 1990; **248**: 450–2.

Kuwana T, Fujimoto T. Active locomotion of human primordial germ cell *in vitro*. *Anat Rec* 1983; **205**: 21–6.

Linder D, Hecht F, McCaw BK, Campbell JR. Origin of extragonadal teratomas and endodermal sinus tumours. *Nature, London* 1975; **254**: 597–8.

McLaren A. Development of the mammalian gonad: the fate of the supporting cell lineage. *Bioessays* 1991; **13**: 151–6.

Makabe S, Nottola SA, Motta PM. Life history of the human germ cell: ultrastructural aspects. In: Van Blerkom J, Motta PM, eds. *Ultrastructure of Human Gametogenesis and Early Embryogenesis*. Kluwer Academic, 1989: 33–60.

Manova K, Huang EJ, Angeles M, De Leon V, Sanchez S, Pronovost SM, Besmer P, Bachvarova RF. The expression pattern of the c-*kit* ligand in gonads of mice supports a role for the c-*kit* receptor in oocyte growth and in proliferation of spermatogonia. *Dev Biol* 1993; **157**: 85–99.

Mattison DR, Shiromizu K, Nightingale MS. Oocyte destruction by polycyclic aromatic hydrocarbons. In: Mattison DR, ed. *Reproductive Toxicology*. New York: Alan R. Liss 1983: 191–202.

Medvedev ZA. On the immortality of the germ line: genetic and biochemical mechanisms – a review. *Mech Ageing Dev* 1981; **17**: 331–59.

Monk M, Boubelik M, Lehnert S. Temporal and regional changes in DNA methylation in the embryonic, extraembryonic and germ cell lineages during mouse embryo development. *Development* 1987; **99**: 371–82.

Navot D, Bergh PA, Williams MA, Garrisi GJ, Guzman I, Sandler B, Grunfield L. Poor oocyte quality rather than implantation failure as a cause of age-related decline in female fertility. *Lancet* 1991; **337**: 1375–7.

packer A, Hsu YC, Besmer P, Bachvarova RF. The ligand of the c-*kit* receptor promotes oocyte growth. *Dev Biol* 1994; **161**: 194–205.

Pellas TC, Ramachandran B, Duncan M, Pan SS, Marone M, Chada K. Germ-cell deficient (*gcd*), an insertional mutation manifested as infertility in transgenic mice. *Proc Natl Acad Sci, USA* 1991; **88**: 8787–91.

Peters H, Himelstein-Braw R, Faber M. The normal development of the ovary in childhood *Acta Endocr* 1976; **82**: 617–30.

Peters H, Levy E, Crone M. DNA synthesis in oocytes of mouse embryos. *Nature, London* 1962; **195**: 915–6.

Polani PE, Crolla JA. A test of the production line hypothesis of mammalian oogenesis. *Hum Genet* 1991; **88**: 64–70.

Richardson SJ, Senikas V, Nelson JF. Follicular depletion during the menopausal transition: evidence for accelerated loss and ultimate exhaustion. *J Clin Endocr Metab* 1987; **65**: 1231–7.

Rosner MH, Vigano MA, Ozato K, Timmons PM, Poirer F, Rigby PWJ, Standt LM. A POU-domain transcription factor in early stem cells and germ cells of the mammalian embryo. *Nature, London* 1990; **345**: 686–92.

Russell P, Altschuler G. The ovarian dysgenesis of trisomy 18. *Pathology* 1975; **7**: 149–55.

Speed RM. The prophase stages in human foetal oocytes studied by light and electron microscopy. *Hum Genet* 1985; **69**: 69–75.

Speed RM. The possible role of meiotic pairing anomalies in the atresia of human fetal oocytes. *Hum Genet* 1988; **78**: 260–6.

Stott D, Wylie CC. Invasive behaviour of mouse primordial germ cells *in vitro*. *J Cell Sci* 1986; **86**: 133–44.

Tilly JL, Kowalski KI, Schomberg DW, Hsueh AJW. Apoptosis in atretic ovarian follicles is associated with selective decreases in messenger ribonucleic acid transcripts for gonadotropin receptors and cytochrome P450 aromatase. *Endocrinology* 1992; **131**: 1670–6.

Upadhyay S, Zamboni L. Ectopic germ cells: natural model for the study of germ cell sexual differentation. *Proc Natl Acad Sci USA* 1982; **79**: 6584–8.

Witschi E. Migration of the germ cells of human embryos from the yolk sac to the primitive gonadal folds. *Contributions to Embryology of the Carnegie Institution of Washington* 1948; **32**: 67–80.

Zamboni L. Comparative studies on the ultrastructure of mammalian oocytes. In: Biggers JD, Schuetz AW, eds. *Oogenesis*. Baltimore: University Park Press, 1972: 5–45.

7

Ovulation 2: Control of the resumption of meiotic maturation in mammalian oocytes

S. M. DOWNS

Introduction

In mammals, mitotically active oocyte precursor cells, called oogonia, populate the primitive ovary during prenatal development. At about the time of birth, meiosis is initiated, and these cells, now called (primary) oocytes, progress through most of prophase I and become arrested at the diplotene stage. Coincident with initiation of meiosis, a single flattened layer of somatic follicle cells encompasses each oocyte, forming a primordial follicle. It is from this pool of resting primordial follicles that oocytes are periodically recruited during the reproductive life of the female.

The recruitment signal for initiation of follicle development is unknown, but in response to it, dramatic changes occur leading to growth and differentiation within the follicle. The prophase I-arrested oocyte is characterized by a prominent nucleus, termed the germinal vesicle, containing decondensed chromatin that is transcriptionally active. During the growth phase, the germinal vesicle-stage oocyte prepares itself for later development by stockpiling mRNA, proteins and other macromolecules needed for the completion of meiosis, fertilization and early embryonic development. The oocyte is aided by nutritional and regulatory contributions from the somatic component of the follicle, with which it is coupled via gap junctions. The oocyte undergoes a tremendous increase in size (from a diameter of 20 μM to 70–80 μM in the mouse) and develops the competence to resume meiotic maturation. While some studies suggest that gonadotropins from the pituitary gland may contribute to the acquisition of meiotic competence, others have indicated little role for gonadotropins in this physiological process (Eppig & Downs, 1984). Recent work has implicated cAMP in facilitating the development of meiotic competence in mouse oocytes grown *in vitro* (Carroll, Whittingham & Wood, 1991; Chesnel, Wigglesworth & Eppig, 1994). Although acquisition of meiotic competence is usually associated with attainment of a certain oocyte size, it has been shown that mouse oocytes, when removed from the ovary and cultured *in vitro*, become meiotically competent as a result of an intrinsic clock that is not dependent upon cell volume (Canipari *et al.*, 1984). Despite the ability to resume meiosis, the competent oocyte remains in the germinal vesicle stage due to constraints imposed on it by the surrounding follicular tissue.

In the somatic compartment of the recruited follicle, the epithelial follicle cells assume a more cuboidal shape in response to the recruitment signal and begin to proliferate mitotically and, in most species, follicular fluid accumulates in the intercellular spaces. Eventually a Graafian follicle forms, comprising a pseudo-stratified layer of membrana granulosa cells surrounding a fluid-filled antrum. Within the antrum is situated a fully grown, germinal vesicle-stage oocyte encompassed by a specialized mass of follicle cells, called the cumulus oophorus, which is anchored to the membrana granulosa by a stalk of connecting cells.

Oocytes within Graafian follicles resume meiotic maturation, manifested by germinal vesicle breakdown (GVB), in response to a preovulatory gonadotropin surge or as a result of follicle degeneration, or atresia. Since only a limited number within the available pool of primordial follicles successfully progresses to ovulation, the fate of the majority of oocytes is that of degeneration. After the resumption of meiosis, the oocyte completes meiosis I and extrudes the first polar body to become a secondary oocyte and progresses to metaphase II, where it encounters a second meiotic block. After ovulation and successful fertilization of the secondary oocyte within the oviduct, meiosis is completed with release of the second polar body (Fig. 1). Strictly speaking, a true haploid 'ovum' never exists in mammals because the reduction division is not completed until after sperm entry.

This review will address possible mechanisms by which 1) meiotic arrest is maintained and 2) the resumption of meiotic maturation is stimulated in mammalian oocytes. Oocyte maturation is often defined as that period of development between the two meiotic blocks, from GVB to the metaphase II arrest. For the purpose of this review, an oocyte will be considered to be mature when it has undergone GVB.

Spontaneous versus ligand-induced maturation

If fully grown oocytes are removed from mature Graafian follicles and cultured in a simple buffered medium, they will spontaneously undergo GVB and progress meiotically to metaphase II in the absence of hormonal inducement. Such behaviour led to the idea that components of the follicle imposed a constraint upon the oocyte that maintained it in meiotic arrest. Accordingly, release from

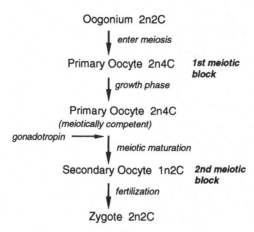

Fig. 1. Developmental scheme for oocyte maturation *in vivo*. For each type of germ cell the chromosomal (n) and DNA (C) content are given.

the follicular environment would eliminate this inhibitory influence and allow meiosis to proceed unimpeded. Supporting this idea is the finding that the prophase I state is maintained when individual intact Graafian follicles are cultured in hormone-free medium.

Two principal types of *in vitro* model systems have been employed for the examination of meiotic control mechanisms. The first involves isolation of denuded or cumulus cell-enclosed oocytes and an analysis of the effects of various inhibitory agents on spontaneous GVB. Oocytes are removed from the natural inhibitory constraints of the follicle and released into permissive conditions that lead to resumption of meiotic maturation. This is an obvious departure from the intrafollicular environment and, therefore, spontaneous maturation of the oocyte may be considered to be artifactual, because under normal conditions GVB requires hormonal stimulation. Furthermore, the response of the oocyte to inhibitory agents may be altered owing to severed communication with the cumulus cells or membrana granulosa, and the possibility exists that this response does not mimic that occurring *in vivo*. On the other hand, the use of isolated oocytes greatly simplifies conditions in that conflicting or competing interactions are not manifested during the experiment. As a result, direct actions of agents on the oocyte or cumulus cell-enclosed oocyte can be examined.

The second model system involves stimulation of maturation by various ligands either in follicle-enclosed oocytes or in cumulus cell-enclosed oocytes maintained in the germinal vesicle stage by meiotic inhibitors. This system more closely approximates conditions *in vivo* because oocytes maintained in meiotic arrest *in vitro* are induced to undergo GVB by a stimulatory ligand. This approach enables the examination of interactions between the ligands and the somatic compartment of the follicle or oocyte–cumulus cell complex as it relates to the subsequent meiotic response of the oocyte. Studies of this nature have established that the somatic follicular cells mediate the action of the stimulatory ligands on oocyte maturation and thus are important participants in meiotic control mechanisms.

Cyclic adenosine monophosphate and meiotic arrest

Many studies have provided evidence in support of a role for cyclic nucleotides in mediating meiotic arrest in mammalian oocytes. Spontaneous maturation of oocytes from several mammalian species can be prevented by supplementing culture medium with compounds that maintain elevated cyclic adenosine mono-phosphate (cAMP) levels, including cAMP analogues such as dibutyryl cAMP (dbcAMP) and inhibitors of the cAMP-degrading enzyme, phosphodiesterase (PDE), such as 3-isobutyl-1-methylxanthine (IBMX) (Eppig & Downs, 1984; Schultz, 1986). The gonadotropin FSH and pharmacological agents like forskolin, which generate increased cAMP through activation of adenylate cyclase, have also been shown to block GVB *in vitro* (Eppig & Downs, 1984; Schultz, 1986). In one particularly novel study, invasive adenylate cyclase from *Bordatella pertussis* increased cAMP in rat oocytes and prevented GVB (Aberdam, Hanski & Dekel, 1987). Bornslaeger, Wilde & Schultz (1984) demonstrated that the relative efficacy of different cAMP PDE inhibitors in suppressing cAMP catabolism was directly proportional to their meiosis arresting potency. Further-more, microinjection of PDE into prophase I-arrested oocytes induced GVB (Bornslaeger, Mattei & Schultz, 1986). Finally, microinjection of oocytes with an inhibitor of the catalytic subunit of cAMP-dependent protein kinase (PKA) overcame meiotic arrest maintained by dbcAMP or IBMX (Bornslaeger *et al.*, 1986). Thus, activation of PKA and subsequent phosphorylation of specific proteins are important processes involved in the control of meiotic maturation (Schultz, 1986).

Measurement of cAMP levels has shown that a drop in oocyte cAMP is associated with GVB and that preventing this drop blocks oocyte maturation (Schultz, Montgomery & Belanoff, 1983*a*; Schultz *et al.*, 1983*b*; Vivarelli *et al.*, 1983; Aberdam *et al.*, 1987). In fact, if mouse oocytes are cultured in inhibitor-free medium, thereby allowing a decrease in cAMP, the oocytes become committed to mature such that transfer of these germinal vesicle-stage oocytes to medium containing normally inhibitory concentrations of cAMP analogues or PDE inhibitors does not prevent spontaneous GVB (Schultz *et al.*, 1983*a*). Specific protein dephosphorylations that occur during this period are evidently responsible for mediating the oocyte's irreversible commitment to resume meiotic maturation (Schultz, 1986).

Demonstration of active adenylate cyclase within the oocyte has been a controversial area of research. The enzyme has been identified in the oolemma of bovine oocytes by cytochemical localization (Kuyt, Kruip & DeJong-Brink, 1988). In addition, forskolin has been shown to stimulate cAMP production in follicle cell-free (denuded) oocytes from several species and coincidentally, to prevent meiotic maturation (Olsiewski & Beers, 1983; Schultz *et al.*, 1983*a*; Urner *et al.*, 1983; Racowsky, 1985*a*, *b*). However, Racowsky (1984) reported a lack of effect of forskolin on GVB or cAMP in denuded rat oocytes, and concluded that the rat oocyte does not possess ample adenylate cyclase to influence meiotic maturation. Cholera toxin, which ADP-ribosylates the stimulatory G-protein for adenylate cyclase and thereby constitutively activates the enzyme, failed to affect the maturation of denuded rodent oocytes in inhibitor-free medium (Schultz *et al.*, 1983*a*; Olsiewski & Beers, 1983), but if a partial arrest of meiosis was maintained by other cAMP-elevating agents, the toxin produced an inhibitory effect (Vivarelli *et al.*, 1983; Downs *et al.*, 1985; Downs, Buccione & Eppig, 1992). Also, elevation of oocyte cAMP by cholera toxin was observed but only if FSH or IBMX was included in the medium (Vivarelli *et al.*, 1983; Olsiewski & Beers, 1983). We have shown that microinjection of GTPγS into denuded mouse oocytes transiently maintains meiotic arrest (Downs *et al.*, 1992). This is consistent with activation of the stimulatory G-protein and elevation of oocyte cAMP, although other mechanisms are certainly possible.

The inconsistent data regarding the presence of functional oocyte adenylate cyclase may be due to a combination of low enzyme activity and rapid hydrolysis of cAMP by PDE (Bornslaeger *et al.*, 1984). Preventing PDE activity with inhibitors or augmenting cAMP levels with cyclic nucleotide analogues, when combined with cholera toxin or forskolin, may elevate cAMP above the threshold required for meiotic arrest. The possibility that adenylate cyclase activity in denuded oocytes was an artefact resulting from residual cumulus cell processes embedded within the zona pellucida was dispelled by Bornslaeger & Schultz (1985*a*), who showed that forskolin still stimulated cAMP synthesis in mouse oocytes after zona pellucida removal.

Cells within the ovarian follicle are closely associated with one another through gap junctions. These membrane specializations produce a syncytium through which the oocyte and follicle cells are metabolically coupled to one another (Larsen & Wert, 1988). The follicle cells can communicate directly with the oocyte because cellular processes from the cumulus oophorus traverse the zona pellucida to form small gap junctions at the oolemma. Therefore, informational signals from the somatic compartment could conceivably travel through gap junctional channels to impose regulatory control on meiotic maturation. It has been hypothesized that cAMP originating in the somatic compartment of the follicle is transferred to the oocyte through gap junctions and is responsible for maintaining meiotic arrest (Dekel & Beers, 1978, 1980). Studies aimed at demonstrating this phenomenon have involved stimulation of cAMP production within the oocyte–cumulus cell complex by FSH, forskolin, or cholera toxin followed by comparison of cAMP levels in denuded and cumulus cell-enclosed oocytes. Thus, if the theory is valid, cAMP should increase within the oocyte. When examined in the rat, pig, hamster and mouse systems, an increase in cyclic nucleotide was observed in the cumulus cell-enclosed oocyte (Racowsky, 1984, 1985a,b; Bornslaeger & Schultz, 1985b; Salustri *et al.*, 1985; Sherizly, Galiani & Dekel, 1988). In the mouse, supraphysiological levels of cAMP were often required in the oocyte–cumulus cell complex before the increase in oocyte cAMP occurred, and, even under these conditions, equilibration of cAMP between the two cell types was not always achieved (Bornslaeger & Schultz, 1985b; Salustri *et al.*, 1985). Also, many of the studies were formed with forskolin, a non-physiological activator which may have a direct effect on denuded oocytes. Nevertheless, evidence is consistent with the idea that cyclic nucleotide can be transferred from the follicle cells to the oocyte. But an increase in cAMP levels in the cumulus cell-enclosed oocyte in response to activators of adenylate cyclase should be interpreted with caution. Although cAMP increases in the cumulus cell-enclosed oocyte, one cannot assume that it originated in the somatic compartment. Products of cumulus cell metabolism could influence the oocyte to maintain higher levels of cAMP by modulating cAMP synthesis and/or catabolism within the germ cell itself. Such a mechanism could explain why a higher frequency of cumulus cell-enclosed than denuded mouse oocytes is maintained in meiotic arrest by a given concentration of dbcAMP (Schultz *et al.*, 1983b). In this latter study it was proposed that the cumulus cells produced a factor other than cAMP in response to dbcAMP exposure that somehow acts on the oocyte in an inhibitory capacity. A similar finding was reported for pig and hamster oocytes treated with forskolin (Racowsky, 1985a,b).

All cAMP analogues do not produce the same effect on oocyte maturation. While dbcAMP is a potent inhibitor of spontaneous maturation in rat and mouse oocytes, 8-bromo-cAMP (8BrcAMP) has little inhibitory activity (Tornell *et al.*, 1984; Eppig, 1989). Interestingly, 8BrcAMP is more potent than dbcAMP in blocking GVB in bovine oocytes (Homa, 1988). Also, whereas dbcAMP prevents gonadotropin-induced GVB in follicle-enclosed rat oocytes, persistent exposure to 8BrcAMP stimulates GVB in the absence of gonadotropin (Hillensjo *et al.*, 1978). Furthermore, although 8BrcAMP has little inhibitory action on the meiotic maturation of cumulus cell-enclosed rodent oocytes, it nevertheless is more effective than dbcAMP in stimulating cumulus cell progesterone production (Tornell *et al.*, 1984) or expansion of the cumulus oophorus (Eppig, 1989). Because dbcAMP and 8BrcAMP have differential affinities for binding to the regulatory subunit of cAMP-dependent protein kinase (PKA), the above data likely reflect the presence of different PKA isozymes in the germ and somatic compartments of the follicle. This idea has been borne out in preliminary experiments with mouse oocytes using site-selective analogues of cAMP that preferentially stimulate either the type I or type II isozyme of PKA. Treatments that stimulate type I PKA are inhibitory to oocyte maturation, whereas those that stimulate type II PKA promote cumulus expansion and trigger GVB, the latter response following transient exposure of cumulus cell-enclosed oocytes to high concentrations of analogues (Downs, unpublished observations).

It is important to emphasize that many of the studies implicating cAMP in the regulation of mammalian oocyte maturation have been carried out with rodent oocytes, which are particularly sensitive to this cyclic nucleotide. The spontaneous maturation of oocytes from some species may be difficult to suppress persistently with agents that elevate cAMP (cf. Jagiello, Ducayen & Goonan, 1981). For example, several studies have shown that high levels of cAMP-elevating agents exert only a transient suppression of GVB in bovine oocytes (Homa, 1988; Sirard & First, 1988; Sirard, 1990). Findings such as these may question the universality of cAMP as the primary meiotic regulator. While cAMP is likely involved in at least some capacity in most species, there may be species differences in the relative contribution of other inhibitory factors to meiotic regulation. One such possibility for the bovine is a thecal cell contribution that modulates granulosa cell-mediated meiotic arrest (Kotsuji, Kubo & Tominaga, 1994; see below).

Follicular components and meiotic arrest

The accumulation of follicular fluid during follicle growth results from secretions of follicular origin as well as contributions from the thecal vasculature. Since the developing oocyte is exposed to this antral fluid, it is logical to address the possibility that factors present within the fluid participate in maintaining meiotic arrest. Indeed, Chang (1955) reported that follicular fluid from rabbits prevented spontaneous meiotic maturation of rabbit oocytes *in vitro*. Follicular fluid was subsequently shown to suppress maturation in hamster, rat, pig, and mouse oocytes in a species-independent manner (see Tsafriri, Dekel & Bar-Ami, 1982; Eppig & Downs, 1984). The efficacy of follicular fluid as a suppressor of meiosis is related to the stage of follicular development. Studies indicate that, as a follicle matures, the inhibitory activity within the antral fluid declines (Channing *et al.,* 1983).

The meiosis-arresting activity of follicular fluid alone in oocyte cultures can be somewhat limited. Supplementing culture medium with 50% porcine follicular fluid or low molecular weight fractions thereof arrested the spontaneous maturation of about 25% of pig oocytes after 43–48 hours of culture (Tsafriri & Channing, 1975) and delayed the spontaneous maturation of mouse oocytes by less than 30 minutes (Downs & Eppig, 1984). This limited effect may explain why several laboratories have failed to demonstrate an inhibitory action of follicular fluid on oocyte maturation. For example, when the effects of porcine follicular fluid were tested on rat oocyte maturation, no suppression of GVB was observed after 10 hours of culture (Fleming, Khalil & Armstrong, 1983). Since only several hours are required for GVB in rat oocytes, a transient inhibitory effect if present would likely be missed. That a delay in meiosis resumption did occur was suggested by decreased polar body formation in oocytes treated with follicular fluid (Fleming *et al.,* 1983). Thus, the importance of kinetics experiments when testing potential inhibitory agents cannot be over-emphasized. Other possible reasons for discrepancies in the reported inhibitory potency of follicular fluid include differences in oocyte isolation procedures, the choice of culture medium and the source and treatment of the follicular fluid itself.

Although follicular fluid alone exhibits a modest effect on oocyte maturation, the inhibitory activity can be profoundly increased by elevating cAMP. A low molecular weight fraction of porcine follicular fluid synergized dramatically with dbcAMP in both denuded and cumulus cell-enclosed oocytes to maintain meiotic arrest (Downs & Eppig, 1984). A similar interaction of follicular fluid was observed with forskolin in denuded oocytes and with FSH in cumulus cell-enclosed oocytes. Chari *et al.,* (1983) reported identical findings when human follicular fluid fractions were tested on rat oocyte maturation. The results raise the possibility that the level of cAMP within the oocyte or oocyte–cumulus cell complex at the time of isolation from the follicle influences the potency of follicular fluid, and perhaps other putative inhibitory factors, in suppressing GVB.

The source of inhibitor in follicular fluid has been shown to be the granulosa cells. Coculture of oocytes with granulosa cells results in suppressed meiotic maturation, and this effect is dependent upon the number of granulosa cells (Tsafriri & Channing, 1975; Sato & Ishibashi, 1977). Similarly, the addition of follicle walls to oocyte cultures prevents GVB (Tsafriri & Channing, 1975; Foote & Thibault, 1969; Leibfried & First, 1980). In addition, granulosa cell extracts and medium conditioned by granulosa cells exhibit inhibitory activity (Anderson, Stone & Channing, 1985; Sato & Koide, 1984; Tsafriri, Pomerantz & Channing, 1976*a*; Centola, Anderson & Channing, 1981), demonstrating that physical contact between germ and somatic cells is not required for this effect. Nevertheless, contact between somatic follicular components and the oocyte may facilitate transfer of inhibitory factors to the oocyte, perhaps via gap junctions, thereby maximizing the suppressive influence of this tissue *in vitro* (Foote & Thibault, 1969; Leibfried & First, 1989; Sato, Ishibashi & Iritani, 1982; Racowsky & Baldwin, 1989; Sirard & Bilodeau, 1990; Motlik, Nagai & Kikuchi, 1991). In fact, uncoupling the oocyte from somatic cell inhibitory input has been shown to induce meiotic maturation (Vilain, Moreau & Guerrier, 1980; Racowsky & Baldwin, 1989; Dekel & Piontkewitz, 1991; Cerada, Patrino & Wallace, 1993). That the inhibitory factor in follicular fluid was chemically similar to that in granulosa cell extracts and conditioned medium was demonstrated by Centola *et al.,* (1981).

Partial characterization of the porcine follicular fluid factor identified a small molecular weight (under 1000–2000 daltons), heat-stable peptide (Tsafriri *et al.,* 1976*a*). The inhibitory action of bovine follicular fluid, however, was heat-labile (Gwatkin & Anderson, 1976). The peptide nature of the inhibitor was based on sensitivity to trypsin treatment. Pomerantz and Billelo obtained several peaks of inhibitory activity (on pig oocytes) when a low molecular weight fraction of pig follicular fluid was chromatographed with QAE-Sephadex; purification was 80 000–150 000-fold (discussed in Tsafriri, 1988). A similar type of molecule can also be isolated from granulosa cells. Sato and colleagues have obtained an inhibitor from bovine granulosa cell extracts that appears to be a small (1450–3000 daltons) heat-stable polypeptide (Sato & Ishibashi, 1977; Sato & Koide, 1984). A specific peptide inhibitory molecule has not yet been identified.

The granulosa compartment is not necessarily the lone somatic source of inhibitory factor within the ovary. A recent study by Kotsuji *et al.,* (1994) has shown that when bovine cumulus cell-enclosed oocytes were cocultured with granulosa cells, little inhibitory action on spontaneous meiotic maturation was observed unless bovine thecal cells were also included in the cultures, and this effect was augmented with FSH. FSH was ineffective in the absence of thecal cells. Moreover, the inhibitory influence of thecal cells required the presence of granulosa tissue. Thus, the data indicate a co-operative interaction between granulosa and thecal cells that may be important physiologically in the mechanisms regulating bovine meiotic arrest (Kotsuji *et al.,* 1994).

Specific molecules found in follicular fluid that have been implicated in the control of meiotic maturation include steroid, fatty acids and purines. A possible role for steroids has recently been reviewed by Racowsky (1993). Estradiol and testosterone exert a negative effect on GVB while progesterone tends to provide a positive influence. Racowsky (1993) has proposed that shifts in the ratio of progesterone:oestradiol may be instrumental in modulating the oocyte's meiotic status. Homa and Brown (1992) have reported that a major fatty acid in bovine follicular fluid, linoleic acid, maintained bovine oocytes in meiotic arrest *in vitro*. The finding that the proportion of linoleic acid in follicular fluid declined with follicular development raised the possibility that this fatty acid serves as an important negative regulator of oocyte maturation in situ. Purines are a third type of specific molecule thought to be involved in meiotic control and will be the focus of the next section of this review.

Purines and meiotic arrest

Working with a low molecular weight fraction of porcine follicular fluid and a mouse oocyte maturation assay system, Downs & Eppig (1984) reported that the inhibitory component had a molecular weight less than 1000 daltons and was charcoal-extractable, but was resistant to heat treatment, acid hydrolysis, proteolysis and ether extraction. These data suggested the presence of a small, heat-stable hydrophobic molecule. Further characterization using ion exchange and high performance liquid chromatography identified not a protein, but hypoxanthine, as the principal inhibitory component (Downs, Coleman & Eppig, 1985). This purine base was found also in mouse follicular fluid, along with the nucleoside, adenosine, in millimolar concentrations (hypoxanthine: 2–4 mM; adenosine: 0.35–0.7 mM) (Eppig, Ward-Bailey & Coleman, 1985). These concentrations of purines are higher than those usually reported in biological fluids, but hypoxic conditions within the follicle due to its avascular nature may promote increased purine release into the follicular fluid. At these concentrations the two purines synergized to maintain nearly 100% of the cumulus cell-enclosed mouse oocytes in meiotic arrest in culture (Eppig *et al.*, 1985). The inhibitory effect of purines on spontaneous maturation *in vitro* has been confirmed in oocytes from mice, rats, cows, and monkeys (Downs, 1990*a*). Nevertheless, it should be cautioned that oocytes from different species may exhibit variable susceptibilities to putative inhibitory molecules such as hypoxanthine. Indeed, Racowsky (1993) found that maintaining meiotic arrest in hamster oocytes required significantly higher concentrations of this purine base than with mouse oocytes.

  In order for an inhibitory compound to quality as a physiological regulator of meiosis at least four criteria should be fulfilled: (1) the inhibitor should be present in the ovary; (2) the inhibitor should prevent spontaneous GVB *in vitro*; (3) gonadotropins should stimulate meiosis in the presence of the inhibitor; and (4) inhibition should be reversible/non-toxic. For hypoxanthine, the first two criteria have been met by data discussed above. Criteria (3) and (4) are supported by the following studies. Cumulus cell-enclosed oocytes maintained in meiotic arrest by hypoxanthine were stimulated to undergo GVB by addition of FSH to the culture medium (Downs, Daniel & Eppig, 1988). These results show the ability of gonadotropin to stimulate maturation but also indicate that purine inhibition is reversible. Further evidence for reversibility was provided by experiments in which cumulus cell-enclosed oocytes were maintained in meiotic arrest for 24 hours with hypoxanthine and adenosine followed by a 16 hour culture in inhibitor-free medium. Nearly 100% of the arrested oocytes resumed maturation, and, furthermore, the mature oocytes were successfully fertilized and demonstrated complete pre- and post-implantation development (Downs *et al.*, 1986*b*). Thus, not only are the effects reversible but no residual toxic effects on developmental capacity are evident. These data collectively support the idea that purines such as hypoxanthine and adenosine are physiologically important in the mechanisms controlling meiotic arrest *in vivo*.

Further corroborative data came from a study showing that hypoxanthine benefits the growth of granulosa cell-enclosed oocytes *in vitro* and keeps them in meiotic arrest after they have reached meiotic competence (Eppig & Downs, 1987). Perhaps more significantly, perturbants of purine metabolism, specifically inhibitors of inosine monophosphate dehydrogenase and *de novo* purine synthesis, stimulate GVB within ovarian follicles when administered by intraperitoneal injection to pregnant mare serum gonadotropin-primed mice (Downs & Eppig, 1987). This result demonstrated that interrupting normal purine metabolic pathways *in situ* upsets the intrafollicular control of meiotic arrest. Thus, once meiotic competence has been attained, these pathways contribute to the maintenance of meiotic arrest, preventing premature reinitiation of meiosis that would compromise developmental potential (Downs, 1994*b*).

The mechanisms of purine action on oocyte maturation

Follicular fluid is a complex mixture with numerous compounds that could potentially influence meiotic maturation in a negative capacity. It may therefore be short-sighted to assume that the inhibitory action is attributable to only one specific molecule or factor. A combined effect of several factors might be imposed upon the oocyte. The synergistic interaction of cAMP and follicular fluid is consistent with this idea. Furthermore, oocytes from different species could exhibit differential sensitivity to a particular follicular fluid component (e.g. Racowsky, 1993). Thus, it may be inappropriate to propose a general mechanism for meiotic arrest in mammalian oocytes based on experiments conducted with one species. Nevertheless, an understanding of how a particular molecule exerts its effects on the oocyte should lead to a better understanding of meiotic control mechanisms.

When hypoxanthine and adenosine were identified in mouse follicular fluid and were shown to interact in a synergistic manner to maintain meiotic arrest, it was proposed that this synergism was due to the interactive effects of adenosine-mediated cAMP generation and PDE inhibition by hypoxanthine (Eppig *et al.*, 1985). When low concentrations of PDE inhibitors like IBMX, dipyridamole and papaverine that have little inhibitory activity alone are combined with a low

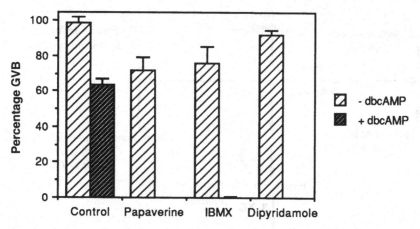

Fig. 2. Synergistic response of dbcAMP and phosphodiesterase inhibitors. Cumulus cell-enclosed oocytes were cultured 3 h in the presence or absence of 100 μM dbcAMP, plus or minus one of three inhibitors at a concentration of 5 μM. All three inhibitors synergized with dbcAMP to completely suppress oocyte maturation.

concentration of the cAMP analogue, dbcAMP, a similar inhibitory synergistic interaction results (Fig. 2). Thus, maintenance of elevated cAMP levels may be the primary mechanism responsible for purine-suppressed GVB. This relationship was demonstrated by the results of the following studies (Downs *et al.*, 1989): 1) hypoxanthine and adenosine alone each increased cAMP levels in cumulus cell-enclosed mouse oocytes, and cAMP increased even further when the two purine compounds were added together; higher cAMP levels were associated with a greater suppression of GVB. 2) Measurement of cAMP PDE activity revealed that guanosine, hypoxanthine and adenosine, in decreasing order of potency, prevented catabolism of cAMP. This agrees with their relative efficacy in suppressing spontaneous GVB. 3) Microinjection of an inhibitor of PKA into hypoxanthine-arrested, denuded oocytes induced GVB. In addition, like follicular fluid, hypoxanthine synergizes with dbcAMP or with agents that elevate cAMP, in maintaining meiotic arrest (Downs *et al.*, 1985).

Adenosine also potentiates the inhibitory action of FSH in cumulus cell-enclosed rat oocytes (Miller & Behrman, 1986) and the inhibitory action of forskolin in denuded mouse oocytes (Salustri *et al.*, 1988), perhaps by suppressing cAMP PDE activity. However, a more likely mechanism is through modulation of cAMP synthesis. Adenosine can be metabolized to ATP and therefore serve as a substrate for adenylate cyclase. This purine nucleoside has been shown to elevate ATP levels in oocyte–cumulus cell complexes (Billig & Magnusson, 1985). On the other hand, adenosine could activate adenylate cyclase by binding to receptors at the cell surface and amplify cAMP levels without acting as substrate.

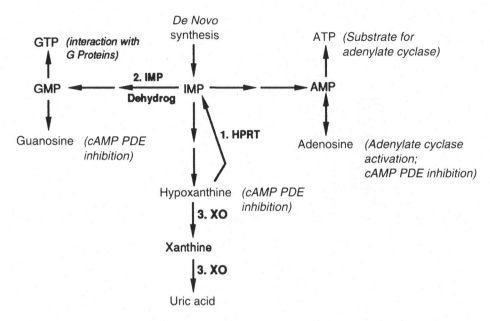

Fig. 3. Purine metabolic pathways. *De novo* synthesis produces inosine monophosphate (IMP), which serves as a central branchpoint for purine metabolism. IMP can be metabolized to adenyl compounds, guanyl compounds or hypoxanthine. Hypoxanthine phosphoribosyltransferase (HPRT; 1) catalyzes the salvage of hypoxanthine to IMP. IMP dehydrogenase (2) catalyzes the first step of a two-reaction pathway from IMP to GMP. Xanthine oxidase (3) metabolizes hypoxanthine to xanthine and uric acid. In parentheses are possible mechanisms whereby these purine compounds could influence oocyte maturation.

Evidence for this mode of action stems from the finding that poorly metabolized analogues of this nucleoside are as effective as the native compound in maintaining meiotic arrest (Downs, Coleman & Eppig, 1986*a*; Salustri *et al.*, 1988).

When a series of purines were tested for their inhibitory effect on meiotic maturation, guanyl compounds were found to be more potent than hypoxanthine (Downs *et al.*, 1985; Tornell *et al.*, 1990). Furthermore, when meiotic arrest was maintained *in vitro* with hypoxanthine, inhibitors of inosine monophosphate (IMP) dehydrogenase induced the resumption of maturation (Downs *et al.*, 1986*a*). This result fuelled the hypothesis that hypoxanthine was metabolized via hypoxanthine phosphoribosyltransferase (HPRT) to IMP and then to guanyl compounds, which act to maintain meiotic arrest (Fig. 3). However, experiments with HPRT inhibitors indicated that suppression of hypoxanthine salvage augments, rather than reverses, the inhibitory action of this purine base on meiotic maturation (Downs, 1993). An alternative route of hypoxanthine metabolism, that of conversion to uric acid via xanthine oxidase with concomitant generation of damaging free oxygen radicals, is also apparently not involved in mediating the meiotic arrest of hypoxanthine. Allopurinol, an inhibitor of xanthine oxidase, failed to induce GVB in hypoxanthine-arrested mouse oocytes and, in fact, augmented the inhibitory effect at high concentrations (Downs, 1993). This drug also proved to be inhibitory when microinjected into denuded mouse oocytes (Shim *et al.*, 1992). In addition, no evidence for metabolism of hypoxanthine via xanthine oxidase was obtained by high performance liquid chromatography when oocyte–cumulus cell complexes were cultured with radiolabelled hypoxanthine; rather, most of the hypoxanthine taken up was salvaged by HPRT and converted to guanyl and adenyl nucleotides (Downs, 1994*a, b*). Moreover, the addition of xanthine oxidase to culture medium relieved the meiotic arrest maintained by hypoxanthine (Downs, 1993), further supporting the conclusion that this enzyme is not responsible for the purine effect. It has been proposed that the negative action of hypoxanthine on GVB is due to an interaction between the suppression of cAMP phosphodiesterase by non-metabolized hypoxanthine and active purine metabolic pathways that lead to cAMP generation (Downs, 1993). Yet, the possibility that some metabolized hypoxanthine contributes to meiotic arrest cannot be discounted.

The suppressive effect of guanyl compounds, as discussed above, may be due to an inhibition of cAMP PDE. Alternatively, these compounds could be phosphorylated to GTP which then interacts with G-proteins, leading to activation of adenylate cyclase and generation of cAMP. Consistent with this latter idea, cholera toxin and microinjected GTPγS both exerted an inhibitory influence on oocyte maturation (Downs *et al.*, 1992). In addition, ADP-ribosylatable G-protein in mouse oocytes has been demonstrated (Allworth, Hildebrandt & Ziomek, 1990; Jones & Schultz, 1990). GTP could also act as a substrate for guanylate cyclase to increase cGMP levels. Cyclic GMP derivatives have been shown to block maturation in rat (Tornell, Brannstrom & Hillensjo, 1984; Tornell *et al.*, 1990) and hamster (Hubbard & Terranova, 1982) oocytes, but this cyclic nucleotide has little inhibitory effect in mouse oocytes (Downs *et al.*, 1988).

The resumption of meiotic maturation

Oocytes within healthy Graafian follicles do not resume meiotic maturation unless stimulated to do so by the pre-ovulatory gonadotropin surge. While the mechanism controlling this process *in situ* remains unknown, two models have arisen that offer an explanation of these events: 1) loss of inhibitory input and 2) positive stimulation.

Loss of inhibitory input and the paradox of cAMP

As discussed earlier, the syncytial nature of the ovarian follicle enables the direct transfer of small molecules and ions from the somatic compartment to the oocyte. One of the follicular responses to the pre-ovulatory gonadotropin surge is mucification and the expansion of the cumulus oophorus, with attendant loss of coupling and termination of the syncytial relationship. As a result, the oocyte can no longer receive direct regulatory signals via gap junctional channels. It has been proposed that this loss of intercellular communication serves as the trigger for resumption of meiotic maturation *in vivo* (Dekel & Beers, 1978, 1980). In this way, GVB would occur as a result of deprivation of somatic inhibitory input, much like removal of the oocyte from the follicle leads to spontaneous maturation. For this model to be valid, 1) the flow of inhibitory signal to the oocyte must be terminated as a result of the meiotic stimulus, and 2) coincidentally, metabolic coupling between the oocyte and follicle cells must be terminated in temporal agreement with the resumption of maturation. The problem in demonstrating the first criterion is identification of the inhibitory substance being transferred. In most studies the substance is assumed to be cAMP, but this fact has not been unequivocally established.

It is generally accepted that the actions of gonadotropins on cells result from binding to membrane receptors and transduction of the signal to adenylate cyclase, with subsequent elevation of intracellular cAMP levels. A similar mechanism functions in ovarian follicles in that gonadotropins generate increased cAMP in follicle cells that mediates a multitude of follicular responses, one of which is the resumption of meiosis (Lindner *et al.,* 1974). Yet, as discussed above, numerous studies have also demonstrated an inhibitory role for cAMP in oocyte maturation. Thus, this cyclic nucleotide has both inhibitory and stimulatory actions on meiotic maturation.

Following gonadotropin stimulation *in situ,* cAMP levels in mouse preovulatory follicles increase while cAMP in the oocyte declines prior to GVB (Schultz *et al.,* 1983*a*). A similar decrease precedes GVB in mouse (Schultz *et al.,* 1983*a*) and rat (Aberdam *et al.,* 1987) oocytes cultured *in vitro.* These results support the proposition that interruption of the transfer of follicle cell-derived cAMP to the oocyte is instrumental in the mechanism triggering GVB. However, in other species such as the sheep (Moor & Heslop, 1981), hamster (Racowsky, 1985*a*; Hubbard, 1986), rabbit (Yoshimura *et al.,* 1992*b*) and pig (Racowsky, 1985*b*; Mattioli *et al.,* 1994), a decline in oocyte cAMP from basal levels is not observed before resumption of meiosis. Therefore, nuclear maturation is not always associated with a decrease in cAMP.

How, then, can one reconcile the seemingly paradoxical actions of cAMP on oocyte maturation? As discussed by Dekel *et al.*, (1988), they may be due to the relative levels of the cAMP nucleotide the oocyte or follicle is exposed to and the temporal nature of this exposure. Treatment of cultured follicles with forskolin (Dekel & Sherizly, 1983; Ekholm *et al.*, 1984) or pulsing follicles with dbcAMP or IBMX (Tsafriri *et al.*, 1972; Ekholm & Ehren, 1978; Dekel *et al.*, 1988) stimulates GVB. Similarly, pulsing cumulus cell-enclosed mouse oocytes with a high concentration of cAMP analogue followed by culture in a lower, but normally inhibitory, concentration of the analogue, induces maturation (Downs *et al.*, 1988; Eppig, 1989). Identical treatment of denuded oocytes has no effect. However, evidence suggests that, if cAMP is maintained at a high level, follicular oocytes remain in the germinal vesicle stage (Tsafriri *et al.*, 1972; Hubbard, 1986; Hashimoto, Kishimoto & Nagahama, 1985; Ekholm *et al.*, 1984; Hosoi *et al.*, 1989). Moreover, treatment of follicles with agents that sustain elevated cAMP prevents gonadotropin-induced maturation (Hillensjo *et al.*, 1978; Hashimoto *et al.*, 1985; Dekel *et al.*, 1988). The evidence therefore indicates that, at least in species such as mice and rats where a role for cAMP in meiotic control is compelling, transient increases in cAMP within follicle cells promotes the resumption of oocyte maturation, and meiotic arrest is maintained as a result of persistently elevated cAMP in the oocyte (and follicle cells).

Temporary increases in cAMP within the oocyte itself may also play a role in the maturation response. In isolated rabbit follicles stimulated with human chorionic gonadotropin or forskolin (Yoshimura *et al.*, 1992*b*), a transient rise in oocyte cAMP levels was observed within 0.5 hours, but levels then decreased significantly by 4 hours, at which time GVB had been initiated. Under these conditions, about 60–75% of the oocytes had resumed meiosis after 6 hours when oocyte cAMP was either at, or well above, the basal level. These results suggest that a fall in cAMP may trigger the resumption in meiotic maturation even though oocyte cAMP does not necessarily fall below the level present at the germinal vesicle stage. This is consistent with the finding that, if isolated cumulus cell-enclosed rodent oocytes are maintained in meiotic arrest with cAMP analogues and stimulated with gonadotropin, GVB will occur despite the continued presence of analogue (Downs *et al.*, 1988; Dekel & Beers, 1978).

These data fail to consistently support the idea that gonadotropins provoke resumption of meiosis by terminating the transfer of cAMP to the oocyte. It is, of course, possible that the loss in transfer of a different low molecular weight molecule or ion may be important in the meiosis-inducing mechanism. As discussed above, dbcAMP maintains a higher frequency of cumulus cell-enclosed oocytes than denuded oocytes in meiotic arrest, suggesting that cumulus cells can be stimulated to produce a factor other than cAMP that acts on the oocyte in a meiosis-arresting capacity. But until such a putative factor is identified, its involvement in gap junction-mediated transfer between somatic and germ cell cannot be resolved.

A reduction in inhibitory input could also occur by increased metabolism of inhibitor to a form that does not suppress meiotic maturation or by removal of inhibitor from the cell by secretion. In the case of cAMP, increased PDE activity could conceivably lower its intracellular concentration below the inhibitory threshold despite continued influx from the follicular tissue. It does not appear that a lowering of follicular fluid purine concentration is involved in meiotic resumption, because a drop in hypoxanthine or adenosine in mouse follicular fluid did not occur *in situ* before the onset of GVB when primed mice were injected with an ovulatory dose of human chorionic gonadotropin (Eppig *et al.*, 1985).

Numerous studies have addressed the temporal relationship between breakdown of the germinal vesicle and oocyte-follicle cell metabolic coupling. When coupling in the oocyte–cumulus cell complex was measured using radioactive ligands such as uridine or choline (which are readily taken up by cumulus cells but not the denuded oocytes), no decrease in the coupling index was observed before the onset of gonadotropin-induced meiotic maturation *in vivo* or in cultured follicles of sheep (Moor *et al.*, 1981), mouse (Eppig, 1982; Salustri & Siracusa, 1983) or pig (Motlik, Fulka & Flechon, 1986). Furthermore, Freter and Schultz (1984) reported acceleration of meiotic maturation in LH-treated cumulus cell-enclosed mouse oocytes without a concomitant reduction in metabolic coupling. These authors proposed that increased metabolism of an inhibitor brought about the rapid maturation kinetics. However, decreases in metabolic and dye coupling were associated with GVB in hamster, rat and pig oocyte–cumulus cell complexes (Racowsky, 1984; Racowsky & Satterlie, 1985; Dekel *et al.*, 1988). In addition, GVB in rat complexes was associated with a decrease in cumulus cell gap junction fractional area (Larsen, Wert & Brunner, 1986). Nevertheless, these results do not demonstrate a causal role for uncoupling in the induction of GVB. For uncoupling to be the mechanism that triggers GVB, one might expect uncoupling to precede the onset of maturation by 30–45 minutes, because a similar period is required *in vitro* for rodent oocytes to become irreversibly committed when cultured in inhibitor-free medium. Results of a study in the hamster are consistent with this mechanism, as a decrease in granulosa cell gap junctional membrane was shown to occur during the irreversible commitment period (Racowsky *et al.*, 1989).

Another possibility is that the pre-ovulatory gonadotropin surge promotes the separation of the cumulus oophorus from the membrana granulosa and thereby isolates not only the oocyte but also the entire cumulus cell mass from inhibitory follicular input (see Fig. 4). Larsen, Wert & Brunner (1987) reported that

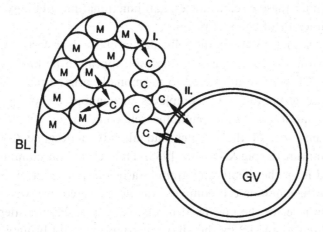

Fig. 4. Follicle diagram depicting possible sites of control of gap junctional inhibitor transfer. The entire follicle is a functional syncytium with component cells metabolically coupled by gap junctions. In scheme I, termination of inhibitor flow from the membrana granulosa cells (M) to the cumulus cells (C) reduces inhibitory input to the oocyte. In scheme II, direct communication from the cumulus cells to the oocyte is terminated, thereby eliminating the flow of inhibitor to the oocyte. BL, basal lamina. Note that the arrows are bidirectional and that regulatory signals could also travel from oocyte to follicle cells.

cumulus–cumulus gap junctions were down-regulated before cumulus–oocyte gap junctions in rats receiving an ovulatory injection of human chorionic gonadotropin (hCG). Further analysis revealed significant changes in gap junction particle packing patterns in cumulus cells that preceded GVB (Wert & Larsen, 1990). A similar study in hamsters (Racowsky *et al.*, 1989) showed that, at the cumulus–membrana boundary, a decrease in gap junction fractional area and particle density was associated with the oocyte's irreversible commitment to undergo GVB. Interestingly, in the follicles of superovulated pigs, the first evidence of mucification and, thus, disaggregation of adjacent follicle cells, was in the area where the stalk of the cumulus oophorus is connected to the follicle wall (Motlik, Fulka & Flechon, 1986). Thus, there is evidence to suggest that the integrity of gap junctions is altered prior to GVB, and this may influence their patency for the transfer of inhibitory factors. In an elegant series of experiments, Racowsky & Baldwin (1989) demonstrated that if hamster oocyte–cumulus cell complexes were microsurgically ablated from the membrana granulosa within intact follicles, meiotic arrest was abrogated. Re-establishment of gap junctions between the ablated complexes and the granulosa cells prevented the reinitiation of meiosis. Phillips & Dekel (1991) have suggested that the morphological integrity of the gap junctions may be maintained despite closure of the channel due to a gating mechanism. Under these circumstances, gap junctional morphology may not be an accurate indicator of channel patency.

If one assumes that cAMP is the follicular inhibitor transferred through gap junctions, then the above mechanism does not appear to be functioning in the mouse. When hCG was administered to hormonally primed mice, cAMP levels increased in oocyte–cumulus cell complexes throughout the period of meiosis re-initiation; in addition, oocyte–cumulus cell coupling was unaltered at 2 h post-hCG, when 79% of the oocytes had already undergone GVB or were committed to mature (Eppig & Downs, 1988). Thus, even if the cumulus oophorus were separated from the membrana granulosa before the onset of GVB, cAMP within the oocyte–cumulus cell complex was not lowered and was presumably available for transfer to the oocyte. It is, of course, possible that deprivation of a factor unrelated to cAMP by the above mechanism could bring about oocyte maturation.

Positive stimulation

Instead of depriving the oocyte of inhibitory substances originating in the follicle cells, gonadotropins could induce maturation by a mechanism that bypasses the meiosis-arresting pathway. This process would involve the production of a *positive* factor by the follicle cells that acts on the oocyte to trigger GVB despite the continued presence of inhibitor. This mechanism has a precedent in other well-characterized systems. For example, in the frog the follicle cell-derived stimulatory molecule is progesterone, while in starfish it is 1-methyladenine.

Evidence for such a mechanism has been accumulating in recent years. When cumulus cell-enclosed mouse oocytes are maintained in meiotic arrest *in vitro* they can be stimulated to undergo GVB by a variety of ligands, including gonadotropin, growth factors, lectins, cholera toxin, and phorbol esters (Fig. 5). In these instances, the frequency of maturation in ligand-treated cumulus cell-enclosed oocytes is greater than that in ligand-treated denuded oocytes. It has often been observed that the degree of inhibition *in vitro* by a particular inhibitory molecule is greater when the oocyte is enclosed by cumulus cells. Thus, denudation renders the resultant cumulus cell-free oocytes less susceptible to the inhibitory influence. The greater inhibition in cumulus cell-enclosed oocytes may result from uptake of the inhibitory substance by the cumulus cells and transfer to the oocyte or by metabolism of the substance by the cumulus cells to a form more inhibitory to the oocyte. If the stimulatory ligands were promoting maturation by simply uncoupling the oocyte from cumulus cell inhibitory input (i.e. by a sort of 'physiological denudation'), one would not expect the frequency of maturation to be different from that in similarly treated denuded oocytes. The

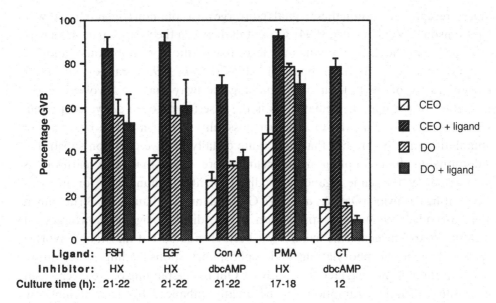

Fig. 5. The action of various ligands on meiotic maturation in denuded oocytes (DO) and cumulus cell-enclosed oocytes (CEO). Oocytes were maintained in meiotic arrest with hypoxanthine (HX) or dbcAMP and were treated with one of five stimulatory ligands: follicle-stimulating hormone (FSH), epidermal growth factor (EGF), concanavalin A (Con A), Phorbol 12-myristate 13-acetate (PMA) or cholera toxin (CT). Germinal vesicle breakdown was assessed after the designated culture period. In all instances, the percentage of GVB in ligand-treated CEO was significantly higher than the percentage of GVB in similarly treated DO. The inactive phorbol ester, phorbol 12-myristate 13-acetate 4-0-methyl ester, had no effect on oocyte maturation (data not presented). FSH and EGF data from Downs *et al.,* 1988; Con A data from Fagbohun and Downs, 1990; PMA data are unpublished; CT data from Downs *et al.,* 1992.

fact that a significantly greater number of cumulus cell-enclosed oocytes are stimulated to resume maturation suggests that the cumulus cells produce a positive factor in response to ligand treatment that bypasses the negative influence to bring about meiotic maturation. Also, since cAMP analogues and cAMP PDE inhibitors can act directly on the oocyte to maintain meiotic arrest, the positive action of stimulatory ligands on cumulus cell-enclosed oocytes maintained in meiotic arrest by such agents is direct evidence that GVB can be triggered despite the continued influence of the inhibitor (cf. Dekel & Beers, 1978; Downs *et al.,* 1988; Bilodeau *et al.,* 1993).

Different signal transduction cascades mediate the actions of these ligands on oocyte maturation, leading to activation of different protein kinases. Thus, PKA, protein kinase C or tyrosine-phosphorylated growth factor receptors can each generate a signal for meiotic maturation. Presumably at some point distal to kinase/receptor activation these signals converge on a common triggering pathway (cf. Johnson & Vaillancourt, 1994). Cross-talk between the various pathways may exist such that the activity of one may lead to activation or inhibition of another (e.g. Jalkanen *et al.*, 1987; Hubbard, 1994; Wu *et al.*, 1993; Graves *et al.*, 1993; Cohen, 1992), or more than one signalling pathway may be involved in the activation of a common mediator, as is the case for mitogen activated protein kinase (Anderson *et al.*, 1990). Another possibility is that multiple pathways of stimulation may be present that only quite distally involve common substrates. Additionally, dual coupling may occur, where more than one pathway is stimulated by the same ligand, providing potential redundancy for meiosis-stimulating pathways (Davis *et al.*, 1987; Gudermann, Birnbaumer & Birnbaumer, 1992; Berridge, 1993). How stimulation by the different ligands converges on meiotic control mechanisms has not yet been elucidated but inevitably involves specific protein phosphorylations and dephosphorylations leading to activation of maturation promoting factor (see below). Our understanding of the mechanism controlling meiotic resumption will be greatly enhanced by determining how these various signalling pathways interact in this capacity. The physiological relevance of gonadotropins in promoting the resumption of meiotic maturation has been well established (Lindner *et al.*, 1974), but the possible involvement of other non-gonadotropic ligands such as growth factors cannot be discounted.

Recent evidence indicates that a putative follicle cell-derived positive factor is transferred directly to the oocyte through gap junctions after stimulation of oocyte–cumulus cell complexes by one of these ligands. Alkanols, agents known to uncouple gap junctions, prevented the stimulation of GVB in cumulus cell-enclosed mouse oocytes by concanavalin A or FSH, and this response was associated with a decrease in the oocyte–cumulus cell metabolic coupling index (Fagbohun & Downs, 1991). Moreover, treatment with the weak base, methylamine, partially reversed the inhibition of metabolic coupling and increased the frequency of GVB in alkanol-treated complexes. Recent experiments using the uncoupling agent, glycerrhetinic acid, have also demonstrated suppression of FSH-induced maturation, thereby confirming these earlier results (Downs, unpublished observations). Alkanols have also been used to prevent hormone-stimulated meiotic maturation in frog (Patino & Purkiss, 1993) and pig (Coskun & Lin, 1994) oocytes. The most likely explanation for these data is that, as a result of hormone stimulation, stimulatory signals originating in the follicle cells are conveyed to the oocyte through the coupling pathway to trigger GVB.

Is calcium or a phosphoinositide metabolite the positive initiator of meiosis?

Phosphoinositides comprise an important second messenger system that responds to a variety of external signals. Phospholipase C, in response to a G-protein- or tyrosine-phosphorylation-mediated stimulus, hydrolyses phosphatidylinositol 4,5-bisphosphate to form inositol trisphosphate (IP_3), a Ca^{2+}-releasing ligand, and diacylglycerol, an activator of calcium-dependent protein kinase C (PKC) (Nishizuka, 1986; Berridge & Irvine, 1993). Both Ca^{2+} and PKC may be involved in the control of meiotic maturation.

Calcium has been shown to be vital for the mechanisms controlling cell cycle progression (Whitaker & Patel, 1990), and there has been a significant amount of research aimed at elucidating the potential role of calcium in the resumption of meiotic maturation in mammalian oocytes. A recent series of studies in frogs (Sandberg *et al.*, 1990, 1992) has shown that angiotensin II binding to follicle cells leads to phosphoinositide hydrolysis and an increase in intraoocytic calcium that is dependent on the heterologous gap junctional coupling pathway. It is not known whether the positive signal is calcium itself or some other factor that could traverse the gap junctions to influence calcium levels within the oocyte.

Consistent and direct evidence implicating calcium as a requisite mediator of meiotic resumption in mammals remains elusive. Intracellular calcium mobilization is required for nuclear envelope breakdown in mitotic cells (Silver, 1989; Kao *et al.*, 1990; Tombes *et al.*, 1992), and such calcium oscillations that occur during mouse spontaneous maturation are not causally associated with GVB (Carroll & Swann, 1992; Tombes *et al.*, 1992). An increase in intracellular calcium, however, has been reported to be required for the spontaneous maturation of mouse (DeFelici, Dolci & Siracusa, 1991) and pig (Kaufman & Homa, 1993) oocytes. The calcium requirement for maturation does not appear to be externally derived (DeFelici & Siracusa, 1982; Tsafriri & Bar-Ami, 1978; Leibfried & First, 1979; Kaufman & Homa, 1993), although the hamster is an exception (Racowsky, 1986), Calcium-deficient medium is detrimental to the maturation of denuded mouse oocytes (DeFelici & Siracusa, 1982), but this is thought to be an indirect effect due to maintenance of patent gap junctions between the oocyte and cumulus cell processes remaining in the zona pellucida, with resultant disruption of ionic balance within the oocyte (DeFelici, Dolci & Siracusa, 1989).

The phosphoinositide pathway is of prime importance in mobilizing Ca^{2+} within cells. IP_3 binds to receptor/channel complexes within the cell to release Ca^{2+} from internal stores (Ferris & Snyder, 1992; Berridge & Irvine, 1993), and elevating intraoocyte IP_3 levels in oocytes by microinjection, electroporation or photorelease elicits Ca^{2+} transients within the oocyte (Peres, Bertollini & Racca, 1991; Carroll & Swann, 1992; Rickords & White, 1993). Microinjection of IP_3 into bovine oocytes arrested with isobutyl methylxanthine elicited GVB (Homa, Webster & Russell, 1991), and similar treatment of mouse oocytes accelerated the kinetics of GVB (Pesty *et al.*, 1994), but in another report did not influence the resumption of meiosis (Paules *et al.*, 1991). IP_3, produced in the follicle cells in response to ligand stimulation, could enter the oocyte through the gap junctional coupling pathway to provoke calcium release from internal oocyte stores and trigger GVB (cf. Homa, Carroll & Swann, 1993).

PKC activators have differential effects on the oocyte depending on whether the oocyte is coupled to follicle cells. Phorbol esters cause meiotic arrest in denuded oocytes (Urner & Schorderet-Slatkine, 1984; Bornslaeger *et al.*, 1986; Homa, 1991; Lefevre *et al.*, 1992), but trigger GVB in cumulus cell-enclosed (Fig. 5; Lefevre *et al.*, 1988) or follicle-enclosed (Aberdam & Dekel, 1985; Yoshimura *et al.*, 1992a) oocytes. These opposing actions on the oocyte demonstrate the dramatic impact follicle cells have on the regulation of maturation and provide further compelling evidence for the generation of a meiosis-inducing signal within the follicle cells. Despite the positive action of PKC activators on GVB, studies in rabbits have failed to implicate PKC activity in mediating gonadotropin induction of meiotic resumption. Inhibitors of PKC such as staurosporine and calphostin C suppressed hCG-stimulated ovulation but were unable to prevent GVB (Kaufman *et al.*, 1992; Yoshimura *et al.*, 1992a).

Calcium ionophores, known to cause an increase in intracellular calcium, can stimulate the resumption of meiotic maturation in cultured rat follicles (Tsafriri & Bar-Ami, 1978) or reverse the meiotic arrest maintained by cAMP analogues in cumulus cell-enclosed mouse and hamster oocytes (Powers & Paleos, 1982; Racowsky, 1986). A direct, positive action on denuded hamster oocytes has also been reported (Racowsky, 1986). On the other hand, Bae and Channing (1985) reported that calcium ionophore inhibited the spontaneous maturation of rat oocytes. These data generally support a role for increased intracellular calcium in mediating the stimulatory role of gonadotropins on GVB. In the case of rat oocyte maturation, this calcium derives, at least in part, from external sources (Goron, Oron & Dekel, 1990).

Lithium is an agent that disrupts the phosphatidylinositol cycle by suppressing breakdown of inositol monophosphate (Hallcher & Sherman, 1980), thereby depleting inositol and interrupting phosphoinositide synthesis. Pesty *et al.* (1994) have shown that the spontaneous maturation of mouse oocytes was delayed by lithium treatment, and this effect was reversed by the addition of myo-inositol or microinjection of IP_3. In addition, both treatments accelerated the normal kinetics of spontaneous maturation (Pesty *et al.*, 1994). Lithium also blocked GVB in starfish oocytes (Picard & Doree, 1983; Pondaven & Meijer, 1986), but Gavin and Schorderet-Slatkine (1988) and Bagger *et al.* (1993) reported a positive action of this agent on mouse oocyte maturation.

Neomycin is a perturbant of phospholipase C that interferes with the hydrolysis of phosphatidylinositol 4,5-bisphosphate (Whitaker, 1989) and prevents the generation of IP_3 and diacylglycerol, the natural activator of protein kinase C. Neomycin has been shown to prevent GVB in spontaneously maturing bovine

(Homa, 1991) and porcine (Kaufman & Homa, 1993) oocytes. It also antagonizes progesterone-induced GVB in frog oocytes (Stith & Maller, 1987). It would be of interest to know whether this agent interferes with ligand-triggered GVB in mammalian oocytes.

While there is evidence that second messengers such as Ca^{2+}, IP_3 or diacylglycerol may be physiologically important in mediating the preovulatory resumption of meiotic maturation, the data are conflicting and incomplete. Of course, inconsistencies in the literature may be related to a number of variables, including 1) whether oocytes are cultured in the presence or absence of the cumulus oophorus; 2) whether maturation is spontaneous or ligand driven; 3) the species of mammal studied; and 4) composition of the culture medium used in the experiments. Additional factors, such as the method of zona pellucida removal prior to studying oocyte calcium fluxes, could influence the experimental outcome. Also, since cAMP is known to be an important second messenger involved in the regulation of meiotic maturation, it will be important to gain an understanding of the interaction between cyclic nucleotides and phosphoinositide metabolites as it relates to meiotic maturation. For example, Bornslaeger *et al.,* (1986) showed that mouse oocytes maintained in meiotic arrest with phorbol ester still exhibited a decrease in cAMP, thereby indicating an action downstream of where cAMP acts to suppress GVB. It will be interesting to determine whether these two transduction pathways are dependent upon one another or if they are redundant pathways that independently can bring about either meiotic arrest or breakdown of the germinal vesicle.

Energy substrates and oocyte maturation

When mouse oocytes are cultured in the denuded state, pyruvate, oxaloacetate or phosphoenolpyruvate alone will support spontaneous maturation, but glucose alone will not; however, when the cumulus oophorus is intact, glucose alone does support maturation (Biggers, Whittingham & Donahue, 1967). This difference is due to the ability of cumulus cells to metabolize glucose to pyruvate (Donahue & Stern 1968; Leese & Barton, 1985) that the oocyte can utilize (Biggers *et al.,* 1967; Eppig, 1976). Hence, the effect of glucose is indirect. The beneficial effect of pyruvate has been shown to be dependent upon oxygen (Haidri, Miller & Gwatkin, 1971; Zeilmaker *et al.,* 1972). It is therefore possible that oxidative metabolism of pyruvate provides conditions conducive to oocyte maturation that are not present in the absence of this energy source.

If oocytes are cultured in minimum essential medium containing millimolar amounts of pyruvate but no glucose, dbcAMP maintains denuded, but not cumulus cell-enclosed, oocytes in meiotic arrest (Fig. 6; Fagbohun & Downs,

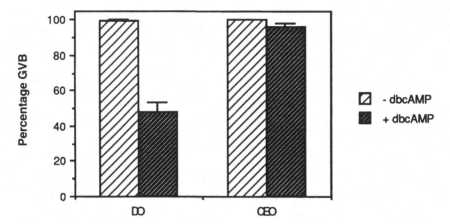

Fig. 6. Effect of pyruvate on dbcAMP-maintained meiotic arrest in denuded oocytes (DO) and cumulus cell-enclosed oocytes (CEO). Oocytes were cultured for 17–18 h in medium containing 0.23 mM pyruvate as the only energy source, in the presence or absence of 300 μM dbcAMP, and were then assessed for germinal vesicle breakdown.

1991). These results suggest that processing of pyruvate by the cumulus cells overcomes the meiosis-arresting action of dbcAMP on oocyte maturation. They also provide further support for a positive stimulus for oocyte maturation, since removal of the cumulus cells *decreased* the meiotic response of the oocyte in the presence of dbcAMP.

If small amounts of glucose are added to the above culture medium, a dramatic decrease in cumulus cell-enclosed oocyte maturation is observed, coincident with elevation of ATP levels, and these glucose effects are reversed by iodoacetate treatment (Downs & Mastropolo, 1994). External glucose has no effect on denuded oocyte maturation, thereby underscoring the importance of follicle cells in meiotic control. These data indicate that glycolytic hexose metabolism by the somatic tissue is important in generating ATP that can negatively influence meiotic progression (Downs & Mastropolo, 1994). This pathway may play an important role in meiotic control *in situ*, since high intrafollicular glucose concentrations and a relatively anaerobic environment at the site of the oocyte–cumulus cell complex (Gosden & Byatt-Smith, 1986) would promote glycolytic activity. The results of these studies also raise the possibility that ATP generated within the follicle cells can pass down a concentration gradient and enter the oocyte through the gap junctional coupling pathway to influence the latter's meiotic status (cf. Downs, 1995).

Experiments have shown that, when dbcAMP- or hypoxanthine-arrested, cumulus cell-enclosed mouse oocytes are stimulated to undergo GVB with FSH, the maximal meiotic response is dependent upon the presence of glucose

(Fagbohun & Downs, 1992; Downs & Mastropolo, 1994). Removal of glucose from the medium, replacing glucose with 2-deoxyglycose, or addition of phloretin, an inhibitor of facilitated glucose transport, resulted in a significant drop in the meiotic response to FSH (Fagbohun & Downs, 1992). The evidence suggests that uptake and metabolism of glucose by the cumulus cells mediates the stimulatory action of gonadotropin of oocyte maturation. Similar effects of gonadotropin on glucose metabolism in bovine oocyte–cumulus cell complexes have been reported (Zuelke & Brackett, 1992). It is therefore apparent that glucose can have both inhibitory and stimulatory actions on oocyte maturation depending on the culture conditions employed.

One possible interpretation of the above observations would be that increased glycolysis converts glucose to pyruvate that is made available to the oocyte in quantities large enough to overcome the meiotic block. Yet, it is not likely that the same metabolic pathway mediates both the inhibitory and stimulatory actions of glucose on oocyte maturation. Using lactate production as an indicator of glycolytic activity, we did not observe any causative relationship between lactate production and FSH-induced meiotic maturation. In addition, increasing pyruvate levels ten-fold failed to mimic the positive effect of FSH on GVB (Downs & Mastropolo, 1994). Furthermore, studies in the rat also provide evidence that this scheme is incorrect. Pyruvate added to culture medium does not stimulate GVB in isolated Graafian follicles (Lindner *et al.*, 1974), despite the fact that respiration is stimulated in isolated oocyte–cumulus cell complexes (Hillensjo, Hamberger & Ahren, 1975). In response to an ovulatory gonadotropin stimulus, the activities of hexokinase and phosphofructokinase, two rate-limiting enzymes of glycolysis, are stimulated within the rat oocyte (Tsutsumi *et al.*, 1992); nevertheless, glycolysis can be suppressed in cultured follicles without affecting meiotic maturation. If follicles are treated with gonadotropin, they respond with increased glucose uptake and glycolysis (Ahren, Hamberger & Rubinstein, 1969; Nilsson, 1974; Hillensjo, 1976; Tsafriri *et al.*, 1976*b*), and isolated granulosa cells also respond with increased lactate production (Hillier, Purohit & Reichert, 1985; Harlow *et al.*, 1987). When a low concentration of iodoacetate was added to medium, gonadotropin stimulation of lactate production was prevented in follicles but resumption of meiotic maturation was unaffected; at higher concentrations of the inhibitor, both activities were suppressed (Tsafriri *et al.*, 1976*b*). These data demonstrated that suppression of follicular glycolytic activity did not necessarily affect oocyte maturation.

However, the response of the entire follicle may not accurately reflect conditions within the microenvironment of the oocyte–cumulus cell complex; the limited contribution of the complex to the total response of the follicle may be obscured when the entire follicle is assayed. This is supported by the finding that oxygen consumption by isolated membrana granulosa cells increases in response to gonadotropin stimulation (Hamberger, 1968), yet oocyte–cumulus cell complexes exhibit a reduced respiratory rate under similar conditions (Hillensjo *et al.*, 1975; Dekel *et al.*, 1976; Billig & Magnusson, 1985). This change in metabolism by cumulus cells may reflect increased glycolysis, since cumulus cells exhibit increased lactate production in response to gonadotropin treatment *in vitro* (Billig, Hedrin & Magnusson, 1983). The inability of pyruvate to induce meiotic maturation in explanted follicles *in vitro* could reflect a limited accumulation of the carbohydrate in the microenvironment of the oocyte within the follicle or, alternatively, the presence of glucose produces a Crabtree effect, whereby utilization of the pyruvate is suppressed. On the other hand, it is possible that cumulus cell products of glucose-metabolizing pathways positively influence meiotic maturation via a respiration-independent mechanism. For example, faster, though less efficient, production of ATP via glycolysis may play a role in gonadotropin stimulation of maturation, or shunting glucose through alternative metabolic routes, such as through the pentose phosphate pathway, may be involved. Leese (1990) has suggested that a beneficial action of pyruvate could be through its known antioxidant properties (cf. Andrae, Singh & Ziegler-Skylakakis, 1985; O'Donnell-Tormey *et al.*, 1987).

RNA and protein synthesis

The addition of protein synthesis inhibitors to culture medium does not affect GVB in rodent oocytes, but does prevent the completion of maturation (i.e. progression to metaphase II) (Stern, Rayyis & Kennedy, 1972; Golbus & Stern, 1976; Wassarman, Josefowicz & Letourneau, 1976). Proteins important for maturation are present at the outset of culture in sufficient quantities for breakdown of the germinal vesicle but new protein synthesis is required for completion of nuclear maturation. In mammalian species demonstrating slower kinetics of GVB, protein synthesis inhibitors have a significant inhibitory effect on the resumption of maturation. GVB in oocytes from cows (Hunter & Moor, 1987), sheep (Moor & Crosby, 1986) and pigs (Fulka *et al.*, 1986) is suppressed in response to puromycin or cycloheximide. Since the time required for meiotic maturation is extended in these species, new protein synthesis is required for successful initiation of this nuclear maturation. In sheep oocytes, a protein associated with GVB fails to appear in the presence of cycloheximide coincident with suppression of maturation (Moore & Crosby, 1986).

After pig and sheep oocytes have been maintained in meiotic arrest with protein synthesis inhibitors and then washed free of the inhibitor and cultured in control medium, oocyte maturation proceeds with an accelerated kinetics when compared to freshly isolated oocytes. In the presence of inhibitor, the chromatin undergoes condensation despite the maintenance of an intact germinal vesicle. Thus, changes heralding the initiation of maturation take place but GVB is still blocked (Motlik, 1989). Both chromatin condensation and GVB can be prevented in spontaneously maturing pig oocytes by exposure to genistein, an inhibitor of protein phosphorylation (Jung *et al.,* 1993).

In rat oocytes treated with puromycin while maintained in meiotic arrest with dbcAMP, subsequent culture in dbcAMP-free medium containing puromycin prevented spontaneous maturation, and the efficacy of puromycin was dependent on the duration of the initial incubation period (Ekholm & Magnusson, 1979). This relationship has been confirmed in mouse oocytes as well (Downs, 1990*b*; Ecay & Powers, 1990). It has been concluded that the oocytes of rats and mice contain sufficient protein at the time of isolation to mediate GVB but that these proteins are short-lived and susceptible to degradation. Therefore, since the kinetics of rodent oocyte maturation are rapid (within 2-3 hours), GVB occurs before the protein involved is turned over.

Ligand-stimulated oocyte maturation is also sensitive to protein synthesis inhibitors. GVB is suppressed by inhibitors in cultured rat Graafian follicles stimulated with gonadotropin (Lindner *et al.,* 1974), in naturally cycling hamsters after subcutaneous injection of cycloheximide (Wang & Greenwald, 1987), and in FSH- or EGF-stimulated mouse cumulus cell-enclosed oocytes maintained in meiotic arrest *in vitro* (Downs, 1990*b*). It is not known whether the critical proteins are produced in the follicle cells, whether the cumulus cells direct protein synthesis within the oocyte, or whether a combination of these two mechanisms is involved.

To determine whether the protein synthesis required for GVB is dependent upon preexisting RNA transcripts, RNA synthesis inhibitors have been used. The spontaneous maturation of sheep, cow and rabbit oocytes is sensitive to transcription inhibitors (Osborn & Moor, 1983; Hunter & Moor, 1987; Motlik *et al.,* 1989; Farin & Yang, 1994), but not that of mouse or pig oocytes (Crozet & Szollosi, 1980; Motlik, 1989). Cumulus cells are apparently required for the inhibitory effect. This result suggest that RNA produced in the somatic cells participates in the control of meiotic maturation. Alternatively, the drug may not be readily taken up by the oocyte and, consequently, accumulation in the gamete may require the gap junctional pathway. Gonadotropin-stimulated oocyte maturation in rat follicles does not appear to be susceptible to inhibition of transcription (Tsafriri *et al.,* 1973); however, induction of maturation of porcine (Meinecke & Meinecke-Tillman, 1993) and mouse (Fig. 7) cumulus cell-enclosed oocytes by FSH or EGF is significantly suppressed by α-amanitin, and gonadotropin-stimulated maturation of bovine oocytes was suppressed by another inhibitor, 5,6-dichloro-1-β-D-ribofuranosylbenzimidazole (Farin & Yang, 1994). Again, somatic cell mediation is implicated, but the precise location of transcription is unresolved.

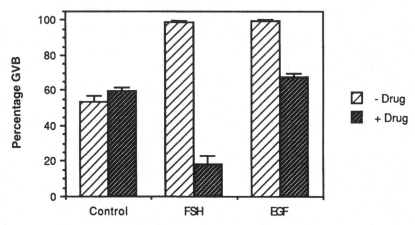

Fig. 7. Effect of a α-amanitin in ligand-induced meiotic maturation in cumulus-cell enclosed oocytes. CEO were maintained in meiotic arrest for 17–18 h with 4 mM hypoxanthine and were stimulated to resume maturation with 0.1 μg/ml follicle-stimulating hormone (FSH) or 0.1 ng/ml epidermal growth factor (EGF). α-Amanitin was added at a concentration of 10 μg/ml. The drug prevented ligand-induced maturation in a manner similar to that observed with protein synthesis inhibitors. The difference in degree of inhibition between the two ligand groups is likely due to the disparate effects of FSH and EGF on maturation kinetics (cf. Downs, 1990b.)

One protein that has been shown to be important in the control of meiotic maturation is the protooncogene product, c-*mos*. p39^{mos} is present in *Xenopus* oocytes only during progesterone-induced maturation (Sagata *et al.*, 1988). Injection of antisense oligonucleotides specific for p39^{mos} into immature frog oocytes prevented expression of the protein and suppressed hormone-dependent GVB; conversely, injection of synthetic c-*mos* RNA induced GVB in the absence of progesterone (Sagata *et al.*, 1988). p39^{mos} has also been detected in mouse oocytes, and injection of antisense oligonucleotides into these oocytes does not block the spontaneous resumption of maturation but does perturb later stages of meiosis (Paules *et al.*, 1989; O'Keefe *et al.*, 1989). This result is analogous to what occurs when spontaneously maturing mouse oocytes are treated with protein synthesis inhibitors and supports the idea that c-*mos* is important in the control of mammalian oocyte maturation. A role for c-*mos* in regulating GVB was suggested by the maintenance of meiotic arrest in mouse oocytes following treatment with c-*mos* antibody (Zhao *et al.*, 1990). However, this possibility was discounted by the recent study by Hashimoto *et al.* (1994), wherein oocytes from c-*mos*-deficient mice underwent GVB in culture. It seems that c-*mos* plays an important regulatory role later in mammalian oocyte maturation, maintaining the metaphase II arrest and preventing spontaneous parthenogenetic activation (Hashimoto *et al.*, 1994).

Maturation promoting factor

It has been known for many years that extracts of actively dividing somatic or germ cells, when microinjected into germinal vesicle-stage oocytes, will stimulate the resumption of meiotic maturation. This maturation, or M-phase, promoting factor (MPF) is highly conserved in eucaryotic cells and has been identified as a heterodimeric protein complex comprising a 34 kD homologue of the fission yeast *cdc*2 gene product (p34^{cdc2}) and cyclin, a 45 kD protein that is produced and degraded at specific times during the cell cycle. p34^{cdc2} functions as a kinase, and potential substrates include histone H1 and nuclear lamins. In fact, assessment of histone H1 kinase activity is routinely used as a measure of MPF activity. Activation of the p34^{cdc2} kinase is brought about by association with the cyclin regulatory subunit and dephosphorylation of p34 (Lewin, 1990). The activity of MPF is high as cells enter the M phase, in concert with increased cyclin synthesis; the degradation of cyclin leads to decreased MPF activity and an exit from M phase. If the translation of cyclin mRNA is prevented, oocytes will not resume maturation. In addition, if degradation of cyclin is prevented, the activity of MPF is maintained and the oocyte fails to exit metaphase II.

Although much of the work on MPF has been carried out with frog and starfish oocytes, evidence demonstrates that this complex functions in mammalian oocytes as well. Extracts of maturing mouse oocytes induced maturation when microinjected into immature starfish or frog oocytes (Kishimoto *et al.,* 1984; Sorensen, Cyert & Pedersen, 1985). Also, fusion of incompetent, immature mouse oocytes with maturing oocytes induced GVB (Balakier, 1978). These results indicate that oocytes having undergone GVB possess active MPF. This has been confirmed by Rime and Ozon (1990), who demonstrated histone H1 kinase activity in mouse oocytes coincident with entrance into M phase and has subsequently been demonstrated in porcine (Naito & Toyoda, 1991; Christmann, Jung & Moor, 1994), rabbit (Jelinkova *et al.,* 1994), and bovine (Kalous *et al.,* 1993) oocytes. The MPF activity fluctuates in concert with the cell cycle, peaking at each metaphase and reaching a nadir at the time of polar body extrusion (Hashimoto & Kishimoto, 1988). These latter authors report that the mouse MPF appears to be a *metaphase*-promoting factor.

That protein phosphorylation is important in the control of MPF in mammalian oocytes has been demonstrated by pharmacological modulation of the phosphorylated state of oocyte proteins. Spontaneous maturation of mouse (Rime *et al.,* 1989) and bovine (Fulka, Leibfried-Rutledge & First, 1991) oocytes can be blocked with 6-dimethylaminopurine, an inhibitor of phosphorylation. On the other hand, when mouse oocytes are maintained in meiotic arrest with dbcAMP, IBMX, or phorbol esters, the phosphatase inhibitor, okadaic acid, induces nuclear dissolution and chromosome condensation (Rime & Ozon, 1990; Alexandre *et al.*, 1991; Gavin, Tsukitani & Schorderet-Slatkine, 1991; Schwartz & Schultz, 1991). This agent also overcomes the block to GVB in bovine and porcine oocytes mediated by protein synthesis inhibitors (Kalous *et al.*, 1993) and elicits GVB in incompetent porcine oocytes (Christmann *et al.*, 1994). Decreases in phosphorylation forms of p34^{cdc2} were observed during the spontaneous maturation of mouse oocytes, and these changes were prevented by maintaining meiotic arrest with IBMX (Choi *et al.*, 1991). It was proposed that cAMP-dependent protein kinase prevents activation of MPF by maintaining p34^{cdc2} in the phosphorylated state. Moreover, okadaic acid treatment of IBMX-arrested oocytes induced the same maturation-associated changes in protein phosphorylation as was observed in oocytes maturing spontaneously in the absence of meiotic inhibitors (Schwartz & Schultz, 1991). Nevertheless, there is evidence that okadaic acid may induce GVB in mouse oocytes by means independent of PMF activation, as measured by histone H1 kinase activity (Gavin, Cavadore & Schorderet-Slatkine, 1994).

It is apparent that the control of the G2/M transition in mammalian oocytes by MPF parallels that in other eucaryotic cells. However, little is known concerning the mechanism(s) leading to this activation. While dephosphorylation of p34^{cdc2} is likely of central importance, other phosphorylations and dephosphorylations will no doubt prove important in both the positive and negative control of activation. Activators of protein kinases A and C maintain denuded oocytes in meiotic arrest, presumably through phosphorylation reactions that may or may not directly involve p34^{cdc2}. These same agents stimulate oocyte maturation in cumulus cell- or follicle-enclosed oocytes, and this action is mediated by the somatic compartment of the follicle. Thus, the somatic cell interactions are probably involved more proximally in the cascade of events leading to MPF activation and may involve different kinases and kinase substrates. It will be important to elucidate the intermediate events between hormonal stimulation of the follicle and generation of active MPF that will propel the prophase-arrested mammalian oocyte into M phase, including identification of substrates for the kinases and the cell type (somatic or germ) where this activity is manifested.

Concluding thoughts

The control of meiotic maturation involves a complex interplay between somatic and germ cells, with the participation of numerous metabolic pathways. Evidence has been presented that direct communication between the follicle cells and the oocyte facilitates the transfer of both inhibitory and stimulatory meiotic signals to the oocyte. The presence of cumulus cells that are metabolically coupled to the oocyte facilitates the acquisition by the oocyte of follicular fluid components, as well as direct contributions from the membrana granulosa, that serve to suppress the competent oocyte's inclination to undergo maturation. This same coupling pathway appears to convey positive meiotic signals to the oocyte that originate in the somatic compartment in response to ligand stimulation. Hence, the somatic cells are of vital importance in oocyte growth, maintenance of meiotic arrest, and in the induction of meiosis resumption.

Due to the importance of the somatic cell compartment, stripping the oocyte of its cumulus cell investment renders an artifactual condition, and although valuable information can be gleaned from experimentation with denuded oocytes, it is important to realize the caveat that the oocyte may not behave the same way physiologically as it would have if the cumulus oophorus remained intact. Furthermore, removing the oocyte from its inhibitory follicular environment and allowing it to resume nuclear maturation spontaneously may not duplicate physiological changes taking place in an oocyte that has been induced to resume maturation by ligand stimulation either *in situ* or within the follicle or oocyte–cumulus cell complex *in vitro*. This is an especially important consideration when examining different metabolic pathways involved in meiotic control. Completely different mechanisms or metabolic pathways could be functioning in the two types of maturation.

It has become increasingly apparent in recent years that oocytes from different mammalian species display disparate sensitivites to putative inhibitory agents and stimulatory ligands. It is therefore important to resist the temptation to make sweeping generalizations concerning meiotic control mechanisms based on data generated from a limited number of species. Nevertheless, it seems clear that, in most mammals, negative meiotic control within the follicle is mediated by the somatic compartment and is augmented by direct physical contact between the somatic and germ cells, and an increasing body of evidence is emerging that supports a positive stimulus for maturation at the time of the preovulatory gonadotropin surge. Future research will hopefully bring us closer to an understanding of the similarities as well as differences in meiotic control mechanisms within the different mammalian species.

References

Aberdam E, Dekel N. Activators of protein kinase C stimulate meiotic maturation of rat oocytes. *Biochem Biophys Res Commun* 1985; **132**: 570–4.

Aberdam E, Hanski E, Dekel N. Maintenance of meiotic arrest in isolated rat oocytes by the invasive adenylate cyclase of Bordetella Pertussis. *Biol Reprod* 1987; **36**: 530–5.

Ahren K, Hamberger L, Rubinstein L. Acute *in vivo* effects of gonadotrophins on the metabolism of the rat ovary. In: McKerns KW, ed. *The Gonads*. New York: Appleton-Centure-Crofts, 1969: 327–54.

Alexandre H, Van Cauwenberge A, Tsukitani Y, Mulnard J. Pleiotropic effect of okadaic acid on maturing mouse oocytes. *Development* 1991; **112**: 971–80.

Allworth AE, Hildebrandt JD, Ziomek CA. Changes in the amount of a pertussis toxin ribosylatable G-protein with egg maturation and early development in the mouse. *Dev Biol* 1990; **142**: 129–37.

Anderson NG, Maller JL, Tonks NK, Sturgill TW. Requirement for integration of signals from two distinct phosphorylation pathways for activation of MAP kinase. *Nature* 1990; **343**: 651–3.

Anderson LD, Stone SL, Channing CP. Influence of hormones on the inhibitory activity of oocyte maturation inhibitor present in conditioned media of porcine granulosa cells. *Gamete Res* 1985; **12**: 119–30.

Andrae U, Singh J, Ziegler-Skylakakis K. Pyruvate and related α-ketoacids protect mammalian cells in culture against hydrogen peroxide-induced cytotoxicity. *Toxicol Lett* 1985; **28**: 93–8.

Bae IH, Channing CP. Effect of calcium ion on the maturation of cumulus-enclosed pig follicular oocytes isolated from medium-sized follicles. *Biol Reprod* 1985; **33**: 79–87.

Bagger PW, Byskov AG, Christiansen MD, Bang L, Mortensen L. Lithium stimulates the first meiotic division in mouse oocytes. *Acta Obstet Gynecol Scand* 1993; **72**: 514–19.

Balakier H. Induction of maturation in small oocytes from sexually immature mice by fusion with meiotic or mitotic cells. *Exp Cell Res* 1978; **112**: 137–41.

Berridge MJ, Irvine RF. Inositol trisphosphates and calcium signaling. *Nature* 1993; **361**: 315–25.

Biggers JD, Whittingham DG, Donahue RP. The pattern of energy metabolism in the mouse oocyte and zygote. *Proc Natl Acad Sci USA* 1967; **58**: 560–7.

Billig H, Hedrin L, Magnusson C. Gonadotrophins stimulate lactate production by rat cumulus granulosa cells. *Acta Endocrinol* 1983; **103**: 562–6.

Billig H, Magnusson C. Gonadotrophin-induced inhibition of oxygen consumption in rat oocyte–cumulus complexes: relief by adenosine. *Biol Reprod* 1985; **33**: 890–8.

Bilodeau S, Fortier MA, Sirard MA. Effect of adenylate cyclase stimulation on meiotic resumption and cyclic AMP content of zona-free and cumulus-enclosed bovine oocytes *in vitro*. *J Reprod Fertil* 1993; **97**: 5–11.

Bornslaeger A, Poueymirou WT, Mattei P, Schultz RM. Effects of protein kinase C activators on germinal vesicle breakdown and polar body emission of mouse oocytes. *Exp Cell Res* 1986; **165**: 507–17.

Bornslaeger EA, Wilde MW, Schultz RM. Regulation of mouse oocyte maturation: involvement of cyclic AMP phosphodiesterase and calmodulin. *Dev Biol* 1984; **105**: 488–99.

Bornslaeger EA, Schultz RM. Adenylate cyclase activity in zona-free mouse oocytes *Exp Cell Res* 1985a; 156: 277–81.

Bornslaeger EA, Schultz RM. Regulation of mouse oocyte maturation: effect of elevating cumulus cell cAMP on oocyte levels. *Biol Reprod* 1985b; 33: 698–704.

Bornslaeger EA, Mattei P, Schultz RM. Involvement of cAMP-dependent protein kinase and protein phosphorylation in regulation of mouse oocyte maturation. *Biol Reprod* 1986; **114**: 453–62.

Canipari R, Palombi F, Riminucci M, Mangia F. Early programming of maturation competence in mouse oogenesis. *Dev Biol* 1984; **102**: 519–24.

Carroll J, Swann K. Spontaneous cytosolic calcium oscillations driven by inositol triphosphate occur during *in vitro* maturation of mouse oocytes. *J Biol Chem* 1992; **267**: 11196–210.

Carroll J, Whittingham DG, Wood MJ. Effect of dibutyryl cyclic adenosine monophosphate on granulosa cell proliferation, oocyte growth and meiotic maturation in isolated mouse primary ovarian follicles cultured in collagen gels. *J Reprod Fertil* 1991; **92**: 197–207.

Centola GM, Anderson LD, Channing CP. Oocyte maturation inhibitor (OMI) activity in protein granulosa cells. *Gamete Res* 1981; **4**: 451–61.

Chang MC. The maturation of rabbit oocytes in culture and their maturation, activation, fertilization and subsequent development in the fallopian tubes. *J Exp Zool* 1955; **128**: 379–99.

Channing CP, Liu CQ, Jones GS, Jones H. Decline of follicular oocyte maturation inhibitor coincident with maturation and achievement of fertilizability of oocytes recovered at midcycle of gonadotropin-treated women. *Proc Natl Acad Sci USA* 1983; **80**: 4184–8.

Chari S, Hillensjo T, Magnusson C, Sturm G, Daume E. *In vitro* inhibition of rat oocyte meiosis by human follicular fluid fractions. *Arch Gynecol* 1983; **233**: 155–64.

Chesnel JF, Wigglesworth K, Eppig JJ. Acquisition of meiotic competence by denuded mouse oocytes: participation of somatic cell product(s) and cAMP. *Dev Biol* 1994; **161**: 285–95.

Choi T, Ajoki F, Mori M, Yamashita M, Naganama Y, Kohmoto K. Activation of p34[cdc2] protein kinase activity in meiotic and mitotic cell cycles in mouse oocytes and embryos. *Development* 1991; **113**: 789–95.

Christmann L, Jung T, Moor RM. 1994. MPF components and meiotic competence in growing pig oocytes. *Molec Reprod Dev* 1994; **38**: 85–90.

Cohen P. Signal integration at the level of protein kinases, protein phosphatases and their substrates. *Trends Bioch Sci* 1992; **17**: 408–13.

Coskun S, Lin YC. Effects of transforming growth factors and activin-A on *in vitro* porcine oocyte maturation. *Molec Reprod Dev* 1994; **38**: 153–9.

Crozet N, Szollosi D. Effect of actinomycin D and α-amanitin on the nuclear ultrastructure of mouse oocytes. *Biol Cell* 1980; **38**: 163–70.

Davis JS, Weakland L, Farese RV, West LA. Luteinizing hormone increases inositol trisphosphate and cytosolic free Ca^{2+} in isolated bovine luteal cells. *J Biol Chem* 1987; **262**: 8515–21.

De Felici M, Dolci S, Siracusa G. Influence of cumulus cell processes on oolemma permeability and lethality of isolated mouse oocytes cultured in Ca^{2+} free medium. *Gamete Res* 1989; **23**: 245–53.

De Felici M, Dolci S, Siracusa G. An increase of intracellular free Ca^{2+} is essential for spontaneous meiotic resumption by mouse oocytes. *J Exp Zool* 1991; **260**: 401–5.

De Felici M, Siracusa G. Survival of isolated, fully grown mouse ovarian oocytes is strictly dependent upon external calcium. *Dev Biol* 1982; **92**: 539–43.

Dekel N, Beers WH. Rat oocyte maturation *in vitro*: relief of cyclic AMP inhibition by gonadotropins. *Proc Natl Acad Sci USA* 1978; **75**: 4369–73.

Dekel N, Beers WH. Development of the rat oocyte *in vitro*: inhibition and induction of maturation in the presence or absence of the cumulus oophorus. *Dev Biol* 1980; **75**: 247–54.

Dekel N, Hultborn R, Hillensjo T, Hamberger L, Kraicer P. Effect of luteinizing hormone on respiration of the preovulatory cumulus oophorus of the rat. *Endocrinology* 1976; **98**: 498–504.

Dekel N, Piontkewitz Y. Induction of maturation of rat oocytes by interruption of communication in the cumulus–oocyte complex. *Bulletin de l Association des Anatomistes*. 1991; **75**: 51–4.

Dekel N, Sherizly I. Induction of maturation in rat follicle-enclosed oocytes by forskolin. *FEBS Lett* 1983; **151**: 153–5.

Dekel N, Galiani D, Sherizly I. Dissociation between the inhibitory and the stimulatory action of cAMP on maturation of rat oocytes. *Molec Cell Endocrinol* 1988; **56**: 115–21.

Donahue RP, Stern S. Follicular cell support of oocyte maturation: production of pyruvate *in vitro*. *J Reprod Fert* 1968; 17: 395–98.

Downs SM. The maintenance of meiotic arrest in mammalian oocytes. In: Bavister BD, Cummins J, Roldman ERS, eds. *Fertilization in Mammals*. Norwell, MA: Serono Symposia, USA, 1990*a*: 5–16.

Downs SM. Protein synthesis inhibitors prevent both spontaneous and hormone-dependent maturation of isolated mouse oocytes. *Molec Reprod Dev* 1990*b*; **27**: 235–43.

Downs SM. Purine control of mouse oocyte maturation: evidence that nonmetabolized hypoxanthine maintains meiotic arrest. *Mol Reprod Dev* 1993; **35**: 82–94.

Downs SM. High performance liquid chromatography analysis of hypoxanthine metabolism in mouse oocyte–cumulus cell complexes: effects of purine metabolic perturbants. *Biol Reprod* 1994*a*; **50**: 1403–12.

Downs SM. Induction of meiotic maturation *in vivo* in the mouse by IMP dehydrogenase inhibitors: effects on the developmental capacity of ova. *Molec Reprod Dev* 1994*b*; **38**: 293–302.

Downs SM. The influence of glucose, cumulus cells, and metabolic coupling on ATP levels and meiotic control in the isolated mouse oocyte. *Dev Biol* 1995 (in press).

Downs SM, Eppig JJ. Cyclic adenosine monophosphate and ovarian follicular fluid act synergistically to inhibit mouse oocyte maturation. *Endocrinology* 1984; **114**: 418–27.

Downs SM, Coleman DL, Eppig JJ. Hypoxanthine is the principal inhibitor of murine oocyte maturation in a low molecular weight fraction of porcine follicular fluid. *Proc Natl Acad Sci USA* 1985; **82**: 454–8.

Downs SM, Coleman DL, Eppig JJ. Maintenance of murine oocyte meiotic arrest: uptake and metabolism of hypoxanthine and adenosine by cumulus cell-enclosed and denuded oocytes. *Dev Biol* 1986*a*; **117**: 174–83.

Downs SM, Mastropolo AM. The participation of energy substrates in the control of meiotic maturation in murine oocytes. *Dev Biol* 1994; **162**: 154–68.

Downs SM, Schroeder AC, Eppig JJ. The developmental capacity of mouse oocytes following maintenance of meiotic arrest *in vitro*. *Gamete Res* 1986*b*; **15**: 305–16.

Downs SM, Eppig JJ. Induction of mouse oocyte maturation *in vivo* by perturbants of purine metabolism. *Biol Reprod* 1987; **36**: 431–7.

Downs SM, Daniel SAJ, Eppig JJ. Induction of maturation in cumulus cell-enclosed mouse oocytes by follicle stimulation hormone and epidermal growth factor: evidence for a positive stimulus of somatic cell origin. *J Exp Zool* 1988; **245**: 86–96.

Downs SM, Daniel S, Bornslaeger EA, Hoppe PC, Eppig JJ. Maintenance of meiotic arrest in mouse oocytes by purines: modulation of cAMP levels and cAMP phosphodiesterase activity. *Gamete Res* 1989; **23**: 323–34.

Downs SM, Buccione R, Eppig JJ. Modulation of meiotic arrest in mouse oocytes by guanyl nucleotides and modifiers of G-proteins. *J Exp Zool* 1992; **262**: 391–404.

Ecay TW, Powers RD. Differential effects of testosterone and dibutyryl cyclic AMP on the meiotic maturation of mouse oocytes. *in vitro. J Exp Zool* 1990; **253**: 88–98.

Ekholm C, Magnusson C. Rat oocyte maturation: effects of protein synthesis inhibitors. *Biol Reprod* 1979; **21**: 1287–93.

Ekholm C, Hillensjo T, Magnusson C, Rosberg S. Stimulation and inhibition of rat oocyte meiosis by forskolin. *Biol Reprod* 1984; **30**: 537–43.

Eppig JJ. Analysis of mouse oogenesis *in vitro*. oocyte isolation and the utilization of exogenous energy sources by growing oocytes. *J Exp Zool* 1976; **198**: 375–82.

Eppig JJ. The relationship between cumulus cell–oocyte coupling, oocyte meiotic maturation, and cumulus expansion. *Dev Biol* 1982; **89**: 268–72.

Eppig JJ. The participation of cyclic adenosine monophosphate (cAMP) in the regulation of meiotic maturation of oocytes in the laboratory mouse. *J Reprod Fertil Suppl* 1989; **38**: 3–8.

Eppig JJ, Downs SM. Chemical signals that regulate mammalian oocyte maturation. *Biol Reprod* 1984; **30**: 1–11.

Eppig JJ, Ward-Bailey PF, Coleman DL. Hypoxanthine and adenosine in murine ovarian follicular fluid: concentrations and activity in maintaining oocyte meiotic arrest. *Biol Reprod* 1985; **33**: 1041–49.

Eppig JJ, Downs SM. The effect of hypoxanthine on mouse oocyte growth and development *in vitro*: maintenance of meiotic arrest and gonadotropin-induced oocyte maturation. *Dev Biol* 1987; **119**: 313–21.

Eppig JJ, Downs SM. Gonadotropin-induced murine oocyte maturation *in vivo* is not associated with decreased cyclic adenosine monophosphate in the oocyte–cumulus cell complex. *Gamete Res* 1988; **20**: 125–31.

Fagbohun CF, Downs SM. Maturation of the mouse oocyte–cumulus cell complex: stimulation by lectins. *Biol Reprod* 1990; **42**: 412–23.

Fagbohun CF, Downs SM. Metabolic coupling and ligand-stimulated meiotic maturation in the mouse oocyte–cumulus cell complex. *Biol Reprod* 1991; **45**: 851–9.

Fagbohun CF, Downs SM. Requirement for glucose in ligand-stimulated meiotic maturation of cumulus cell-enclosed mouse oocytes. *J Reprod Fert* 1992; **96**: 681–97.

Farin CE, Yang L. Inhibition of germinal vesicle breakdown in bovine oocytes by 5,6-dichloro-1-β-D-ribofuranosylbenzimidazole (DRB). *Molec Reprod Dev* 1994; **37**: 284–92.

Ferris CD, Snyder SH. Inositol phosphate receptors and calcium disposition in the brain. *J Neurosci* 1992; **12**: 1567–74.

Fleming AD, Khalil W, Armstrong DT. Porcine follicular fluid does not inhibit maturation of rat oocytes *in vitro. J Reprod Fert* 1983; **69**: 665–70.

Foote WD, Thibault C. Recherches experimentales sur la maturation *in vitro* des ovocytes de truie et de veau. *Ann Biol Anim Biochim Biophys* 1969; **9**: 329–49.

Freter RR, Schultz RM. Mechanism of gonadotropin regulation of mouse oocyte maturation. *J Cell Biol* 1984; **98**: 1119–28.

Fulka J Jr, Leibfried-Rutledge ML, First NL. Effect of 6-dimethylaminopurine on germinal vesicle breakdown of bovine oocytes. *Molec Reprod Dev* 1991; **29**: 379–84.

Fulka J Jr, Motlik J, Fulka J, Jilek F. Effect of cycloheximide on nuclear maturation of pig and mouse oocytes. *J Reprod Fert* 1986; **77**: 281–5.

Gavin A-C, Cavadore J-C, Schorderet-Slatkine S. Histone H1 kinase activity, germinal vesicle breakdown and M-phase entry in mouse oocytes. *J Cell Sci* 1994; **107**: 275–83.

Gavin A-C, Schorderet-Slatkine S. The interaction of lithium with forskolin-inhibited meiotic maturation of denuded mouse oocytes. *Exp Cell Res* 1988; **179**: 298–302.

Gavin A-C, Tsukitani Y, Schorderet-Slatkine S. Induction of M-phase entry of prophase-blocked mouse oocytes through microinjection of okadaic acid, a specific phosphatase inhibitor. *Exp Cell Res* 1991; **192**: 75–81.

Golbus MS, Stein MP. Qualitative patterns of protein synthesis in the mouse oocyte. *J Exp Zool* 1976; **198**: 337–42.

Goron S, Oron Y, Dekel N. Rat oocyte maturation: role of calcium in hormone action. *Molec Cell Endocrinol* 1990; **72**: 131–8.

Gosden RG, Byatt-Smith JG. Oxygen concentration gradient across the ovarian follicular epithelium: model, predictions and implications. *Human Reprod* 1986; **1**: 65–8.

Graves LE, Bornfeldt KE, Raines EW, Potts BC, MacDonald SG, Ross R, Krebs EG. Protein kinase A antagonizes platelet-derived growth factor-induced signaling by mitogen-activated protein kinase in human arterial smooth muscle cells. *Proc Natl Acad Sci USA* 1993; **90**: 10300–4.

Gudermann T, Birnbaumer M, Birnbaumer L. Evidence for dual coupling of the murine luteinizing hormone receptor to adenyl cyclase and phosphoinositide breakdown and Ca^{2+} mobilization. *J Biol Chem* 1992; **267**: 4479–88.

Gwatkin RBL, Anderson OF. Hamster oocyte maturation *in vitro*: inhibition by follicular components. *Life Sci* 1976; **19**: 527–36.

Haidri AA, Miller IM, Gwatkin RBL. Culture of mouse oocytes *in vitro*, using a system without oil or protein. *J Reprod Fert* 1971; **26**: 409–11.

Hallcher LM, Sherman WR. The effects of lithium ion and other agents on the activity of *myo*-inositol-1-phosphatase from bovine brain. *J Biol Chem* 1980; **255**: 10896–901.

Harlow CR, Winston RML, Margara RA, Hillier SG. Gonadotrophic control of human granulosa cell glycolysis. *Human Reprod* 1987; **2**: 649–53.

Hashimoto H, Kishimoto T. Regulation of meiotic metaphase by a cytoplasmic maturation-promoting factor during mouse oocyte maturation. *Dev Biol* 1988; **126**: 242–52.

Hashimoto N, Kishimoto T, Nagahama Y. Induction and inhibition of meiotic maturation in follicle-enclosed mouse oocytes by forskolin. *Dev Growth Differentiation* 1985; **27**: 709–16.

Hashimoto N, Watanabe N, Furuta Y, Tamemoto H, Sagata N, Yokoyama M, Okazaki K, Nagayoshi M, Takeda N, Ikawa Y, Alzawa S. Parthenogenetic activation of oocytes in c-*mos*-deficient mice. *Nature* 1994; **370**: 68–71.

Hillensjo T, Hamberger L, Ahren K. Respiratory activity of oocytes isolated from ovarian follicles of the rat. *Acta Endocrinol* 1975; **78**: 751–9.

Hillensjo T. oocyte maturation and glycolysis in isolated pre-ovulatory follicles of PMS-injected immature rats. *Acta Endocrinol* 1976; **82**: 809–30.

Hillensjo T, Ekholm C, Ahren K. Role of cyclic AMP in oocyte maturation and glycolysis in the pre-ovulatory rat follicle. *Acta Endocrinol* 1978; **87**: 377–88.

Hillier JSG, Purohit A, Reichert LE. Control of granulosa cell lactate production by FSH and androgen. *Endocrinology* 1985; **116**: 1163–7.

Homa ST. Effects of cyclic AMP on the spontaneous meiotic maturation of cumulus-free bovine oocytes cultured in chemically defined medium. *J Exp Zool* 1988; **248**: 222–31.

Homa ST. Neomycin, an inhibitor of phosphoinositide hydrolysis, inhibits the resumption of bovine oocyte spontaneous meiotic maturation. *J Exp Zool* 1991; **258**: 95–103.

Homa ST, Brown CA. Changes in linoleic acid during follicular development and inhibition of spontaneous breakdown of germinal vesicles in cumulus-free bovine oocytes. *J Reprod Fertil* 1992; **94**: 153–60.

Homa ST, Carroll J, Swann K. The role of calcium in mammalian oocyte maturation and egg activation. *Human Reprod* 1993; **8**: 1274–81.

Hosoi Y, Yoshimura Y, Atlas SJ, Adachi T, Wallach EE. Effects of dibutyryl cyclic AMP on oocyte maturation and ovulation in the perfused rabbit ovary. *J Reprod Fertil* 1989; **85**: 405–11.

Hubbard CJ. EGF modulates phosphoinositide levels in ovarian granulosa cells stimulated by luteinizing hormone. *J Cell Physiol* 1994; **160**: 227–32.

Hubbard CJ, Terranova PF. Inhibitory action of cyclic guanosine 5'-phosphoric acid (GMP) on oocyte maturation: dependence on an intact cumulus. *Biol Reprod* 1982; **26**: 628–32.

Hubbard CJ. Cyclic AMP changes in the component cells of Graafian follicles: possible influences on maturation in the follicle-enclosed oocytes of hamsters. *Dev Biol* 1986; **118**: 343–51.

Hunter AG, Moor RM. Stage-dependent effects of inhibiting ribonucleic acids and protein synthesis on meiotic maturation of bovine oocytes *in vitro*. *J Dairy Sci* 1987; **70**: 1646–51.

Jagiello G, Ducayen MB, Goonan WD. A note on the inhibition of *in vitro* meiotic maturation of mammalian oocytes by dibutyryl cyclic AMP. *J Exp Zool* 1981; **218**: 309–11.

Jalkanen J, Ritvos O, Huhtaniema I, Stenman U-H, Laatikainen T, Ranta T. Phorbol ester stimulates human granulosa-luteal cell cyclic adenosine 3',5'-monophosphate and progesterone production. *Mol Cell Endocrinol* 1987; **51**: 273–6.

Jelinkova L, Kubelka M, Motlik J, Guerrier P. Chromatin condensation and histone H1a kinase activity during growth and maturation of rabbit oocytes. *Molec Reprod Dev* 1994 **37**: 210–15.

Johnson GL, Vaillancourt RR. Sequential protein kinase reactions controlling cell growth and differentiation. *Curr Op Cell Biol* 1994; **6**: 230–8.

Jones J, Schultz RM. Pertussis toxin-catalyzed ADP-ribosylation of a G protein in mouse oocytes, eggs and preimplantation embryos: developmental changes and possible functional roles. *Dev Biol* 1990; **139**: 250–62.

Jung T, Fulka Jr J, Lee C, Moor RM. Effects of the protein phosphorylation inhibitor genistein on maturation of pig oocytes *in vitro*. *J Reprod Fertil* 1993; **98**: 529–35.

Kalous J, Kubelka M, Rimkevicova Z, Guerrier P, Motlik J. Okadaic acid accelerates germinal vesicle breakdown (GVBD) and overcomes cycloheximide and 6-dimethylaminopurine block in cattle and pig oocytes. *Dev Biol* 1993; **157**: 448–54.

Kao JP, Alderton JM, Tsien RY, Steinhardt RA. Active involvement of Ca^{2+} in mitotic progression of Swiss 3T3 fibroblasts. *J Cell Biol* 1990; **111**: 183–96.

Kaufman G, Dharmarajan AM, Takehara Y, Cropp CS, Wallach EE. The role of protein kinase-C in gonadotropin-induced ovulation in the *in vitro* perfused rabbit ovary. *Endocrinology* 1992; **131**: 1804–9.

Kaufman ML, Homa ST. Defining a role for calcium in the resumption and progression of meiosis in the pig oocyte. *J Exp Zool* 1993; **265**: 69–76.

Kishimoto T, Yamazaki K, Kato Y, Koide SS, Kanatani H. Induction of starfish oocyte maturation by maturation-promoting factor of mouse and surf clam oocytes. *J Exp Zool* 1984; **231**: 293–5.

Kuyt JRM, Kruip TAM, DeJong-Brink M. Cytochemical localization of adenylate cyclase in bovine cumulus–oocyte complexes. *Exp Cell Res* 1988; **174**: 139–45.

Larsen WJ, Wert S, Brunner GD. A dramatic loss of cumulus cell gap junctions is correlated with germinal vesicle breakdown in rat oocytes. *Dev Biol* 1986; **113**: 517–21.

Larsen WJ, Wert S, Brunner GD. Differential modulation of rat follicle cell gap junction populations at ovulation. *Dev Biol* 1987; **122**: 61–71.

Larsen WJ, Wert S. Roles of cell junctions in gametogenesis and in early embryonic development. *Tissue & Cell* 1988; **20**: 809–48.

Leese HJ. Physiology of the fallopian tube: the provision of nutrients for oocytes and early embryos. In: Evers JHL, Heinemann MJ, eds. *Ovulation to Implantation*. New York, Elsevier Science Pub., 1990: 121–5.

Leese HJ, Barton AM. Production of pyruvate by isolated mouse cumulus cells. *J Exp Zool* 1985; **234**: 231–6.

Lefevre B, Gongeon A, Peronny H, Testart J. A gonadotropin-releasing hormone agonist and an activator of protein kinase C improve *in vitro* maturation in *Macaco fascicularis*. *Gamete Res* 1988; **21**: 193–7.

Lefevre B, Pesty A, Koziak K, Testart J. Protein kinase C modulators influence meiosis kinetics but not fertilizability of mouse oocytes. *J Exp Zool* 1992; **264**: 206–13.

Leibfried L, First NL. Effects of divalent cations on *in vitro* maturation of bovine oocytes. *J Exp Zool* 1979; **210**: 575–80.

Leibfried L, First NL. Follicular control of meiosis in the porcine oocyte. *Biol Reprod* 1980; **23**: 705–9.

Lewin B. Driving the cell cycle: M phase kinase, its partners and substrates. *Cell* 1990; **61**: 743–52.

Lindner HR, Tsafriri A, Lieberman ME *et al.* Gonadotropin action on cultured Graafian follicles: induction of maturation division of the mammalian oocyte and differentiation of the luteal cell. *Rec Prog Horm Res* 1974; **30**: 79–127.

Mattioli M, Galeati G, Barboni B, Seren E. Concentration of cyclic AMP during the maturation of pig oocytes *in vivo* and *in vitro*. *J Reprod Fertil* 1994; **100**: 403–9.

Meinecke B, Meinecke-Tillman. Effects of α-amanitin on nuclear maturation of porcine oocytes *in vitro*. *J Reprod Fertil* 1993; **98**: 195–201.

Miller JGO, Behrman HR. Oocyte maturation is inhibited by adenosine in the presence of follicle-stimulating hormone. *Biol Reprod* 1986; **35**: 833–7.

Moor RM, Heslop JP. Cyclic AMP in mammalian follicle cells and oocytes during maturation. *J Exp Zool* 1981; **216**: 205–9.

Moor RM, Osborn JC, Cran DG, Walters DE. Selective effect of gonadotropins on cell coupling, nuclear maturation, and protein synthesis in mammalian oocytes. *J Embryol Exp Morphol* 1981; **61**: 347–65.

Moor RM, Crosby IM. Protein requirements for germinal vesicle breakdown in ovine oocytes. *J Embryol Exp Morphol* 1986; **94**: 207–20.

Motlik J. Cytoplasmic aspects of oocyte growth and maturation in mammals. *J Reprod Fert* 1989; **Suppl 38**: 17–25.

Motlik J, Fulka J, Flechon JE. Changes in intercellular coupling between pig oocytes and cumulus cells during maturation *in vivo* and *in vitro*. *J Reprod Fert* 1986; **76**: 31–7.

Motlik J, Fulka J Jr, Prochazka R, Rimkevicova Z, Kubelka M, Fulka J. RNA and protein synthesis requirement for the resumption of meiosis in rabbit oocytes: the role of cumulus cells. *Reprod Nutr Dev* 1989; **29**: 601–9.

Motlik J, Nagai T, Kikuchi K. Resumption of meiosis in pig oocytes cultured with cumulus and parietal cells: the effect of protein synthesis inhibition. *J Exp Zool* 1991; **259**: 386–91.

Naito K, Toyoda Y. Fluctuation of histone H1 kinase activity during meiotic maturation in porcine oocytes. *J Reprod Fertil* 1991; **93**: 467–73.

Nilsson L. Acute effects of gonadotrophins and prostaglandins on the metabolism of isolated ovarian follicles from PMSG-treated immature rats. *Acta Endocrinol* 1974; **77**: 540–58.

Nishizuka Y. Studies and perspectives of protein kinase C. *Science* 1986; **233**: 305–12.

O'Donnell-Tormey J, Nathan CF, Lanks K, DeBoer CJ, De La Harpe J. Secretion of pyruvate: an antioxidant defence of mammalian cells. *J Exp Med* 1987; **165**: 500–14.

O'Keefe SJ, Wolfes H, Kiessling AA, Cooper GM. Microinjection of antisense *c-mos* oligonucleotides prevents meiosis II in the maturing mouse egg. *Proc Natl Acad Sci USA* 1989; **86**: 7038–42.

Olsiewski PJ, Beers WH. cAMP synthesis in the rat oocyte. *Dev Biol* 1983; **100**: 287–93.

Osborn JC, Moor RM. Time-dependent effects of α-amanitin on nuclear maturation and protein synthesis in mammalian oocytes. *J Embryol Exp Morphol* 1983; **73**: 317–38.

Patino R, Purkiss RT. Inhibitory effects of *n*-alkanols on the hormonal induction of maturation in follicle-enclosed *Xenopus* oocytes: implications for gap junctional transport of maturation-inducing steroid. *Gen Comp Endocrinol* 1993; **91**: 189–98.

Paules RS, Buccione R, Moschel RC, Vande Woude GF, Eppig JJ. Mouse Mos protooncogene product is present and functions during oogenesis. *Proc Natl Acad Sci USA* 1989; **86**: 5395–9.

Peres A, Bertollini L, Racca C. Characterization of Ca^{2+} transients induced by intracellular photorelease of $InsP_3$ in mouse oocytes. *Cell Calcium* 1991; **12**: 457–65.

Pesty A, Lefevre B, Kubiak J, Geraud G, Tesarik J, Maro B. Mouse oocyte maturation is affected by lithium via the polyphosphoinositide metabolism and the microtubule network. *Molec Reprod Dev* 1994; **38**: 187–99.

Phillips DM, Dekel N. Maturation of the rat cumulus–oocyte complex: structure and function. *Molec Reprod Dev* 1991; **28**: 297–306.

Picard A, Doree M. Lithium inhibits amplification or action of the maturation-promoting factor (MPF) in meiotic maturation of starfish oocytes. *Exp Cell Res* 1983; **147**: 41–50.

Pondaven P, Meijer L. Protein phosphorylation and oocyte maturation. I. induction of starfish oocyte maturation by intracellular microinjection of a phosphatase inhibitor, alphanaphthylphosphate. *Exp Cell Res* 1986; **163**: 477–88.

Powers RD, Paleos GA. Combined effects of calcium and dibutyryl cyclic-AMP on germinal vesicle breakdown in the mouse oocyte. *J Reprod Fertil* 1982; **66**: 1–8.

Racowsky C. Effect of forskolin on the spontaneous maturation and cyclic AMP content of hamster oocyte–cumulus complexes. *J Exp Zool* 1985*a*; 234: 87–96.

Racowsky C. Effect of forskolin on maintenance of meiotic arrest and stimulation of cumulus expansion, progesterone and cyclic AMP production by pig oocyte–cumulus complexes. *J Reprod Fert* 1985*b*; **74**: 9–21.

Racowsky C. The releasing action of calcium upon cyclic AMP-dependent meiotic arrest in hamster oocytes. *J Exp Zool* 1986; **239**: 263–75.

Racowsky C. Follicular control of meiotic maturation in mammalian oocytes. In: Bavister BD, ed. *Preimplantation Embryo Development*. New York, Springer-Verlag, 1993: 22–37.

Racowsky C, Satterlie RA. Metabolic, fluorescent dye and electrical coupling between hamster oocytes and cumulus cells during meiotic maturation *in vivo* and *in vitro*. *Dev Biol* 1985; **108**: 191–202.

Racowsky C, Baldwin KV. *In vitro* and *in vivo* studies reveal that hamster oocyte meiotic arrest is maintained only transiently by follicular fluid, but persistently by membrana/cumulus granulosa cell contact. *Dev Biol* 1989; **134**: 297–306.

Racowsky C, Baldwin KV, Larabell CA, DeMarais AA, Kazilek CJ. Down-regulation of membrana granulosa cell gap junctions is correlated with irreversible commitment to resume meiosis in golden Syrian hamster oocytes. *Eur J Cell Biol* 1989; **49**: 244–51.

Rickords LF, White LF. Electroporation of inositol 1,4,5-triphosphate induces repetitive calcium oscillations in murine oocytes. *J Exp Zool* 1993; **265**: 178–84.

Rime H, Neant I, Guerrier P, Ozon R. 6-Dimethylaminopurine (6-DMAP), a reversible inhibitor of the transition to metaphase during the first meiotic division of the mouse oocyte. *Dev Biol* 1989; **133**: 169–79.

Rime H, Ozon R. Protein phosphatases are involved in the *in vivo* activation of histone H1a kinase in mouse oocyte. *Dev Biol* 1990; **141**: 115–22.

Sagata, N, Oskarsson M, Copeland T, Brumbaugh J, Vande Woude GF. Function of c-mos proto-oncogene product in meiotic maturation in Xenopus oocytes. *Nature* 1988; **335**: 519–25.

Salustri A, Siracusa G. Metabolic coupling, cumulus expansion and meiotic resumption in mouse cumuli oophori cultured *in vitro* in the presence of FSH or dbcAMP, or stimulated *in vivo* by hCG. *J Reprod Fert* 1983; **68**: 335–41.

Salustri A, Petrungaro S, DeFelici M, Conti M, Siracusa G. Effect of follicle-stimulating hormone on cyclic adenosine monophosphate level and on meiotic maturation in mouse cumulus cell-enclosed oocytes cultured *in vitro*. *Biol Reprod* 1985; **33**: 797–802.

Salustri A, Petrungaro S, Conti M, Siracusa G. Adenosine potentiates forskolin-induced delay of meiotic resumption by mouse denuded oocytes: evidence for an oocyte surface site of adenosine action. *Gamete Res* 1988; **21**: 157–68.

Sandberg K, Bor M, Ji H, Markwick AJ, Millan MA, Catt KJ. Angiotensin II-induced calcium mobilization in oocytes by signal transfer through gap junctions. *Science* 1990; **249**: 298–301.

Sandberg K, Ji H, Iida T, Catt KJ. Intercellular communication between follicular angiotensin receptors and *Xenopus laevis* oocytes: mediation by an inositol 1,4,5-trisphosphate-dependent mechanism. *J Cell Biol* 1992; **117**: 157–67.

Sato E, Ishibashi T, Iritani A. Meiotic arresting substance separated from porcine granulosa cells and hypothetical arresting mechanism of meiosis. In: Channing CP, Segal SJ, eds. *Intraovarian Control Mechanisms*. New York: Plenum Publ Corp 1982: 161–73.

Sato E, Koide SS. A factor from bovine granulosa cells preventing oocyte maturation. *Differentiation* 1984; **26**: 59–62.

Sato E, Ishibashi T. Meiotic arresting action of the substance obtained from the cell surface of porcine granulosa cells. *Jpn J Zootech Sci* 1977; **48**: 22–6.

Schultz RM. Molecular aspects of mammalian oocyte growth and maturation. In: Rossant J, Pederson RA, eds. *Experimental Approaches to Mammalian Embryonic Development*. Cambridge: Cambridge University Press, 1986: 195–237.

Schultz RM, Montgomery RR, Belanoff JR. Regulation of mouse oocyte maturation: implication of a decrease in oocyte cAMP and protein dephosphorylation in commitment to resume meiosis. *Dev Biol* 1983a; **97**: 264–73.

Schultz RM, Montgomery RR, Ward-Bailey PF, Eppig JJ. Regulation of oocyte maturation in the mouse: possible roles of intercellular communication, cAMP, and testosterone. *Dev Biol* 1983*b*; **95**: 294–304.

Schwartz DA, Schultz RM. Stimulatory effect of okadaic acid, an inhibitor of protein phosphatases, on nuclear envelope breakdown and protein phosphorylation in mouse oocytes and one-cell embryos. *Dev Biol* 1991; **145**: 119–27.

Sherizly I, Galiani D, Dekel N. Regulation of oocyte maturation: communication in the rat cumulus–oocyte complex. *Human Reprod* 1988; **3**: 761–6.

Shim C, Lee DK, Lee CC, Cho WK, Kim K. Inhibitory effect of purines in meiotic maturation of denuded mouse oocytes. *Molec Reprod Dev* 1992; **31**: 280–6.

Silver RB. Nuclear envelope breakdown and mitosis in sand dollar embryos is inhibited by microinjection of calcium buffers in a calcium-reversible fashion, and by antagonists of intracellular Ca^{2+} channels. *Dev Biol* 1989; **131**: 11–26.

Sirard MA. Temporary inhibition of *in vitro* meiotic resumption by adenylate cyclase stimulation in immature bovine oocytes. *Theriogenology* 1990; **33**: 757–67.

Sirard MA, Bilodeau S. Effects of granulosa cell co-culture on *in vitro* meiotic resumption of bovine oocytes. *J Reprod Fertil* 1990; **89**: 459–65.

Sirard MA, First NL. *In vitro* inhibition of oocyte nuclear maturation in the bovine. *Biol Reprod* 1988; **39**: 229–34.

Sorensen RA, Cyert MS, Pedersen RA. Active maturation-promoting factor is present in mature mouse oocytes. *J Cell Biol* 1985; **100**: 1637–40.

–7Stern S, Rayyis A, Kennedy JF. Incorporation of amino acids during maturation *in vitro* by the mouse oocyte: effect of puromycin on protein synthesis. *Biol Reprod* 1972; **7**: 341–6.

Stith BJ, Maller JL. Induction of meiotic maturation in *Xenopus* oocytes by 12-*o*-tetradecanoylphorbol 13-acetate. *Exp Cell Res* 1987; **169**: 514–23.

Tombes RM, Simerly C, Borisy G, Schatten G. Meiosis, egg activation, and nuclear envelope breakdown are differentially reliant on Ca^{2+}, whereas germinal vesicle breakdown is Ca^{2+}-independent in the mouse oocyte. *J Cell Biol* 1992; **117**: 799–811.

Tornell J, Brannstrom M, Hillensjo T. Different effects of cyclic nucleotide derivatives upon the rat oocyte–cumulus complex *in vitro*. *Acta Physiol Scand* 1984; **122**: 507–13.

Tornell J, Brannstrom M, Magnusson C, Billig H. Effects of follicle stimulating hormone and purines on rat oocyte maturation. *Molec Reprod Dev* 1990; **27**: 254–60.

Tsafriri A. Local nonsteroidal regulators of ovarian function. In: Knobil E, Neill J *et al* eds. *The Physiology of Reproduction*. New York, Raven Press Ltd., 1988: 527–65.

Tsafriri A, Bar-Ami S. Role of divalent cations in the resumption of meiosis of rat oocytes. *J Exp Zool* 1978; **205**: 293–300.

Tsafriri A, Lindner HR, Zor U, Lamprecht SA. *In vitro* induction of meiotic division in follicle-enclosed rat oocytes by LH, cyclic AMP and prostaglandin E2. *J Reprod Fert* 1972; **31**: 39–50.

Tsafriri A, Lieberman ME, Barnea A, Bauminger S, Lindner HR. Induction by luteinizing hormone of ovum maturation and of steroidogenesis in isolated Graafian follicles of the rat: role of RNA and protein synthesis. *Endocrinology* 1973; **93**: 1378–86.

Tsafriri A, Channing CP. An inhibitory influence of granulosa cells and follicular fluid upon porcine oocyte meiosis *in vitro*. *Endocrinology* 1975; **96**: 922–7.

Tsafriri A, Pomerantz SH, Channing CP. Inhibition of oocyte maturation by porcine follicular fluid: partial characterization of the inhibitor. *Biol Reprod* 1976*a*; **14**: 511–16.

Tsafriri A, Lieberman ME, Ahren K, Lindner HR. Dissociation between LH-induced aerobic glycolysis and oocyte maturation in cultured Graafian follicles of the rat. *Acta Endocrinol* 1976*b*; **81**: 362–6.

Tsafriri A, Dekel N, Bar-Ami S. The role of oocyte maturation inhibitor in follicular regulation of oocyte maturation. *J Reprod Fert* 1982; **64**: 541–51.

Tsutsumi O, Satoh K, Taketani Y, Kato T. Determination of enzyme activities of energy metabolism in the maturing rat oocyte. *Molec Reprod Dev* 1992; **33**: 333–7.

Urner F, Herrmann WL, Baulier EE, Schorderet-Slatkine S. Inhibition of denuded mouse oocyte meiotic maturation by forskolin, an activator of adenylate cyclase. *Endocrinology* 1983; **113**: 1170–2.

Urner F, Schorderet-Slatkine S. Inhibition of denuded mouse oocyte meiotic maturation by tumor-promoting phorbol esters and its reversal by retinoids. *Exp Cell Res* 1984; **154**: 600–5.

Vilain JP, Moreau M, Guerrier P. Uncoupling of oocyte–follicle cells triggers re-initiation of meiosis in amphibian oocytes. *Dev Growth Differ* 1980; **22**: 687–91.

Vivarelli E, Conti M, DeFelici M, Siracusa G. Meiotic resumption and intracellular cAMP levels in mouse oocytes treated with compounds which act on cAMP metabolism. *Cell Differentiation* 1983; **12**: 271–6.

Wang S-C, Greenwald GS. Effects of cycloheximide during the periovulatory period on ovarian follicular FSH, hCG, and prolactin receptors and on follicular maturation in the hamster. *Proc Soc Exp Biol Med* 1987; **185**: 55–61.

Wassarman PM, Josefowicz WJ, Letourneau GE. Meiotic maturation of mouse oocytes *in vitro*: inhibition of maturation at specific stages of nuclear progression. *J Cell Sci* 1976; **22**: 531–45.

Wert SE, Larsen WJ. Preendocytotic alterations in cumulus cell gap junctions precede meiotic resumption in the rat cumulus–oocyte complex. *Tissue & Cell* 1990; **22**: 827–51.

Whitaker M. Phosphoinositide second messengers in eggs and oocytes. In: Michell RH, Drummond AH, Downes CP, eds. *Inositol Lipids in Cell Signalling*. New York: Academic Press, 1989: 459–83.

Whitaker M, Patel R. Calcium and cell cycle control. *Development* 1990; **108**: 525–42.

Wu J, Dent P, Jelinek T, Wolfman A, Weber MJ, Sturgill TW. Inhibition of the EGF-activated MAP kinase signaling pathway by adenosine 3,5-monophosphate. *Science* 1993; **262**: 1065–9.

Yoshimura Y, Nakamura Y, Ando M, Jinno M, Nanno T, Oda T, Koyama N, Shiokawa S. Protein kinase C mediates gonadotropin-releasing hormone agonist-induced meiotic maturation of follicle-enclosed rabbit oocytes. *Biol Reprod* 1992*a*; **47**: 118–25.

Yoshimura Y, Nakamura Y, Oda T, Ando M, Ubukata Y, Karube M, Koyama N, Yamada H. Induction of meiotic maturation of follicle-enclosed oocytes of rabbits by a transient increase followed by an abrupt decrease in cyclic AMP concentration. *J Reprod Fertil* 1992*b*; **95**: 803–12.

Zeilmaker GH, Hulsmann WC, Wensinck F, Verhamme C. Oxygen-triggered mouse oocyte maturation *in vitro* and lactate utilization by mouse oocytes and zygotes. *J Reprod Fert* 1972; **29**: 151–2.

Zhao H, Batten B, Singh B, Arlinghaus RB. Requirement of the *c-mos* protein kinase for murine meiotic maturation. *Oncogene* 1990; **5**: 1727–30.

Zuelke KA, Brackett BG. Effects of luteinizing hormone on glucose metabolism in cumulus-enclosed bovine oocytes matured *in vitro*. *Endocrinology* 1992; **131**: 2690–6.

8

Ovulation 3: Endocrinology of ovulation

W. L. LEDGER AND D. T. BAIRD

Introduction

Mammalian fertilization is the result of a single sperm cell penetrating the barriers surrounding the oocyte, allowing the male and female gametes to fuse. The 'successful' gametes, both male and female, each arise from amongst millions of potential candidates for fertilization, but the means by which they arrive at the point of fertilization differs markedly between the sexes. Sperm cells are synthesized continuously within the testis, providing a steady state in turnover of male gametes. In contrast, formation of the total lifetime pool of primordial follicles containing the oocytes is completed within the seventh month of fetal life and no new female gametes are produced thereafter (Block, 1951). Of the several millions of oocytes present within the ovary in late fetal life, at most only about 500 will ever ovulate and hence be exposed to the possibility of fertilization. This chapter will review our patchy knowledge of the endocrine processes by which these few follicles are induced to grow and develop to contain a mature oocyte by the time of ovulation.

Early follicular phase

The oocyte lies within its primordial follicle in a resting state, with its chromosomal development arrested at the diplotene stage of the first meiotic division (Baker, 1982). The process by which follicles leave this resting state and resume development is independent of gonadotrophin stimulation and occurs continuously throughout childhood and the reproductive years until menopause is reached. Although the origin of the dominant follicle of the month is commonly termed 'selection', there is no evidence to suggest that it is anything other than a random process. One hypothesis devised to explain the process by which a single follicle is induced to mature out of the high number available holds that there is a constant level of activity within the ovary with individual primordial follicles acquiring the ability to mature at different times during the reproductive life of the organism. A 'gate' mechanism may then operate, with the gate remaining open for a brief period in the early follicular phase of the cycle under the influence of the elevated levels of FSH seen at this time (Baird, 1987). Only those follicles which have acquired the 'ability to mature' at the correct time can escape to form a cohort of potential dominant follicles. Those follicles which, by chance, acquire the 'ability to mature' at other times in the cycle encounter low levels of FSH which keep the gate closed, leading to the follicles failing to grow with subsequent progression to atresia. This process would account for the apparently constant rate of attrition in the numbers of primary follicles within the ovary.

Nothing is known of the factors which regulate the rate of turnover of primordial follicles, although an increase in our level of understanding of this process may hold important clues to the aetiology of premature menopause and certain types of infertility. The process is apparently independent of endocrine changes such as alterations in the circulating levels of gonadotrophins and sex steroids. This independence is most clearly demonstrable in two groups of patients. Those with olfactogenital dysplasia (Kallman's syndrome) have congenital deficiency of gonadotrophin secretion and are hypogonadotrophic and hypo-oestrogenic. However, development of primary follicles seems to continue unabated in these patients despite their severely hypogonadotrophic state (Gauthier, 1960). In contrast, approximately 30% of patients with premature ovarian failure (premature menopause) have numerous ovarian follicles on ovarian biopsy but exhibit post-menopausal levels of gonadotrophins in the circulation, are hypo-oestrogenic and acyclic (Russell *et al.*, 1982; Friedman, Barrows & Moon, 1983). However, suppression of their grossly elevated levels of circulating gonadotrophins using a long-acting analogue of GnRH did not restore the ability to ovulate, again demonstrating the gonadotrophin-independent nature of the earliest stages of folliculogenesis (Ledger *et al.*, 1989).

Mid-follicular phase

The gate theory of follicle selection suggests that the gate is opened by the elevated levels of FSH seen during the early part of the menstrual cycle (Baird, 1983). Such follicles as are ready to respond to FSH are then recruited into a roughly synchronous cohort of primary follicles, all of which are potentially ready to form the final dominant follicle (de Zerega & Hodgen, 1981). The size of this cohort is dependent upon the gonadotrophin-independent rate of intra-ovarian primordial follicle turnover and the period of time over which the FSH level remains elevated. This latter variable has been utilized clinically to induce multiple follicular development using anti-oestrogens or exogenous injection of FSH to prolong the period over which follicles can be recruited to join the developing cohort.

The early follicular phase ends with the emergence of a single dominant follicle from the recruited cohort. Although this is termed 'follicle selection', this term implies the existence of a non-random element in the mechanism by which one follicle comes to maturity and suppresses the growth and development of the remainder of the cohort. Again, there is no evidence that this is anything other than a random process which is probably largely governed by the individual stage of development of each individual follicle at the time of initial entry into the cohort. 'Selection' of the dominant follicle occurs as the circulating level of FSH falls under the influence of the increasing amounts of oestrogen secreted into the circulation by the dominant follicle. Once a dominant follicle has emerged, the remainder of the cohort shrink and become atretic. 'Dominance' must be a true endocrine phenomenon since the contra-lateral ovary is induced to remain quiescent throughout the succeeding events of the cycle. The choice of which ovary will be the source of the dominant follicle of the month has been shown by ultrasound studies of developing follicles to be a random process (Sallam, Whitehead & Collins, 1983) and unilateral ovariectomy results only in incessant ovulation from the remaining ovary, indicating that the mechanism of selection of the site of the dominant follicle of the month resides within the ovaries themselves rather than being under central control.

The degree to which the dominant follicle controls the events of the follicular phase of the cycle is demonstrated by experiments in which the dominant follicle is surgically ablated (Nilsson, Wikland & Hamberger, 1982). This results in postponement of ovulation for approximately 14 days, the length of one follicular phase, indicating that the dominant follicle has suppressed the development of the other members of its cohort to such an extent as to make it impossible for one of them to resume maturation and replace the erstwhile dominant follicle after its destruction. Ablation of the dominant follicle seems to result instead in the resumption of the whole process of cohort recruitment and 'follicle selection'.

As the follicle grows and develops, its antrum enlarges and the granulosa and theca interna layers become distinguishable. The granulosa cells secrete increasing amounts of oestradiol into the circulation. The rising levels of oestradiol seen during the mid-follicular phase of the cycle impose numerous endocrine changes, including the crucial actions on endometrial proliferation and priming of the hypothalamus and pituitary in preparation for the mid-cycle gonadotrophin surge. The dominant follicle is thus responsible for the synchronized preparation of the reproductive tract for ovulation, fertilization and implantation.

Regulation of the gonadotrophin surge

The dramatic sequence of events which result in ovulation represents one of the few biological examples of a positive feedback cascade. Information from the ovary and the central nervous system is integrated at the level of the anterior pituitary gland to trigger a massive release of LH, the ovulatory hormone (Knobil *et al.*, 1980). The central position of the LH surge in the control of ovulation is seen throughout the animal kingdom, both in species which ovulate as reflex to mating and to those which ovulate spontaneously, both seasonal breeders and those with oestrous or menstrual cycles. Three physiological processes are initiated within the follicle around the time of the LH surge. First, meiosis I resumes and oocyte maturation occurs with transition from prophase I through metaphase I to extrusion of the first polar body at metaphase II. Nuclear maturation is synchronized with maturation of the cytoplasm and zona pellucida, rendering the oocyte capable of fertilization. Second, luteinization begins as the follicular granulosa cells switch to synthesis and secretion of progesterone rather than oestradiol. Initiation of luteinization may occur independently of the changes in LH pulse frequency and amplitude, possibly under regulation by an intra-ovarian paracrine mechanism. The possible significance of the preovular rise in circulating levels of progesterone is discussed below. Third in this sequence of events is ovulation itself. The breakdown of the ovarian epithelial surface at ovulation may represent a process of programmed cell death (apoptosis), possibly induced by local synthesis of prostaglandins (Ackerman & Murdoch, 1993). The gonadotrophin surge is also associated with an increase in the amount of plasminogen activator in follicular fluid and granulosa cells (Strickland & Beer, 1987; Deutinger *et al.*, 1988) with eventual enzymic breakdown of the follicle wall with subsequent release of the follicular fluid and oocyte–cumulus complex.

Data concerning the mechanism regulating the gonadotrophin surge have been derived from rodents, ungulates and primates. It is apparent that the LH surge is initiated by positive feedback from rising levels of oestrogen secreted from the maturing follicle acting on the hypothalamus and pituitary. In rats, the amount of LHRH released into the portal vessels increases in the afternoon of pro-oestrous (Sarkar *et al.*, 1976). The development of push-pull perfusion of the rat anterior pituitary by Levine and Ramirez (1980) allowed measurement of LHRH in conscious freely moving animals. Using this method it soon became apparent that the LHRH pulse frequency does not increase dramaticaly during the initiation of the LH surge. Subsequent work showed that the increase in LHRH release from the hypothalamus in response to rising levels of oestradiol is mainly the result of an increase in pulse amplitude (Levine & Ramirez, 1982; Park & Ramirez, 1989). Further data from studies on the rat and sheep suggested that concentrations of oestradiol acted synergistically in late pro-oestrus at the level of the pituitary, increasing both the number of receptors for GnRH (Menon, Pregel & Katta, 1985; Gregg, Allen & Nett, 1990) and the responsiveness of the gonadotrophs to GnRH (Fink, 1979), at least partially by increasing intracellular synthesis of LH (Naftolin, Brown-Grant & Corker, 1972). GnRH receptor complexes act on pituitary gonadotrophs via a G-protein coupled activation of phospholipase C. This generates both inositol 1,4,5,-triphosphate, mobilizing intracellular calcium, and diacylglycerol which activates protein kinase C. It has been suggested that oestradiol can modulate both the calcium and protein kinase C-mediated signalling systems (McArdle *et al.*, 1992), increasing the post-receptor sensitivity of the gonadotroph cells to GnRH. From the above mentioned studies, it is apparent that the positive feedback effects of oestradiol on the hypothalamo-pituitary axis before the LH surge are mediated by a variety of means which combine to produce the dramatic, abrupt increase in peripheral levels of LH seen at the time of the surge. Although the LH surge itself is the most obvious marker that ovulation is imminent, it can only occur if follicular maturation proceeds normally. While it is clear that positive feedback of oestradiol initiates the LH surge, other endocrine signals have been implicated in the regulation of ovulation.

Role of progesterone in mediating the LH surge

Although an increase in circulating levels of gonadotrophins, both LH and FSH, can be induced in suitable subjects by administration of oestrogen alone. (Monroe, Jaffe & Midgley, 1972; Liu & Yen, 1983) there is evidence that progesterone may also participate in the events leading to the onset of the gonadotrophin surge in normally cycling women. In most studies, peripheral levels of progesterone begin to rise some hours before the onset of the surge (Pauerstein *et al.*, 1978; Hoff, Quigley & Yen, 1983) and administration of progesterone after oestrogen priming will advance the time of the surge and amplify its magnitude and duration (Aono *et al.*, 1976; Permezel *et al.*, 1989). It therefore seems likely that progesterone may also participate in the initiation of the mid-cycle surge. The recent introduction of effective progesterone antagonists has provided a novel method of evaluating the role of progesterone in the late follicular phase of the menstrual cycle. We have shown that very low doses of mifepristone (2 mg/day) will attenuate the LH surge without reducing the pre-ovulatory rise of oestradiol (Ledger *et al.*, 1992) (Fig. 1), thereby effectively dissociating the positive feedback effects of oestrogen and progesterone on the hypothalamus and pituitary. Treatment with even lower doses of mifepristone (1 mg/day) during the late follicular phase will retard the onset of the LH surge (Batista *et al.*, 1992*a*,*b*). This effect was reversible by

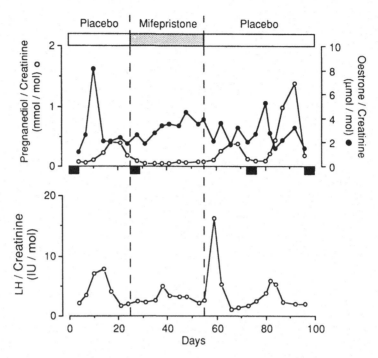

Fig. 1. Concentrations of urinary oestrone glucuronide, pregnanediol glucuronide and luteinizing hormone (LH) in placebo, treatment and washout cycles in one subject taking 2 mg mifepristone. Filled bars represent menses. (From Ledger *et al.*, 1992.)

concurrent treatment with progesterone. These experiments suggest that the pre-ovulatory rise in progesterone participates in the development of an adequate LH surge, as in the monkey (Collins & Hodgen, 1986).

The site of action of progesterone on the hypothalamo-pituitary axis is not known. Treatment of women with mifepristone, albeit at doses (10–100 mg/day) which might exert direct antifolliculotrophic effects (Croxatto *et al.*, 1993) significantly reduced plasma LH concentrations, but by altering pulse amplitude rather than pulse frequency (Permezel *et al.*, 1989). This reduction could occur either through a direct effect on the pituitary, reducing the response to each pulse of GnRH, or by reducing the amplitude of pulses released from the hypothalamus.

Low dose mifepristone has dose-dependent effects on both the follicle and endometrium, in addition to the pituitary and hypothalamus (Croxatto *et al.*, 1993). Doses of 5 or 10 mg/day arrest oestradiol synthesis and/or secretion by the dominant follicle and inhibit ovulation by preventing the pre-ovular oestradiol surge. Doses of 1 mg/day allow breakthrough ovulation and luteinisation but interfere with endometrial maturation (Batista *et al.*, 1992). Use of the 2 mg/day dose (Ledger *et al.*, 1992) appears to have unmasked the contribution made by rising pre-ovular levels of progesterone to the initiation of the LH surge by allowing follicle growth and secretion of amounts of oestradiol which would normally be sufficient to activate the positive feedback mechanism triggering the LH surge. The fact that the positive feedback mechanism failed in patients treated with this dose suggests that this is due to abolition of the synergistic effect of progesterone.

Role of inhibin

The glycoprotein hormone, inhibin, is secreted by the corpus luteum and circulating levels rise during the luteal phase of the human cycle (McLachlan *et al.*, 1987*a,b*). Inhibin is believed to participate in the regulation of FSH secretion by the pituitary (Franchimont *et al.*, 1979) and to act within the ovary as a paracrine regulator (Ying, 1988). Despite early evidence suggesting a rise in inhibin during the follicular phase of the human cycle, concomitant with the fall in FSH before ovulation, it is now clear that inhibin levels remain low prior to ovulation (Reddi *et al.*, 1990). Measurement of inhibin in blood drawn from the ovarian veins in the late follicular phase of the cycle indicates that inhibin is secreted from both ovaries in similar amounts, excluding the dominant follicle as the major source (Illingworth *et al.*, 1991). It does not therefore seem likely that inhibin participates in the mechanism of communication between the dominant follicle and the hypothalamo-pituitary axis at the time of the LH surge. However, frequent measurement of peripheral levels of inhibin in the peri-ovulatory period in women have revealed a peri-ovular rise in circulating inhibin levels in the peripheral circulation (McLachlan *et al.*, 1990). In this study, samples of blood collected every three hours showed that inhibin levels begin to rise at the time of onset of the LH surge and that this rise in inhibin is sustained until approximately 36 hours after the peak of the LH surge and approximately 17 hours after the disappearance of the dominant follicle as observed by serial ultrasound examinations. However, the samples in this study were grouped relative to the peak level of LH rather than the onset of the surge.

In an attempt to clarify the relationship between gonadotrophins, sex steroids and inhibin in the human midcycle we have recently completed a study which combined a regime of three-hourly blood sampling with frequent transvaginal ultrasound to identify the time of follicular rupture (Ledger, Thong and Baird, unpublished data). In this study, six regularly cycling volunteers were monitored using daily urinary LH estimation over at least three cycles to identify the day of onset of the LH surge. They were then admitted to the research unit at least 48 hours prior to the expected time of onset of the surge in the following cycle.

Blood samples were taken for assay for LH, FSH, progesterone, oestradiol and immunoactive inhibin (Robertson *et al.*, 1988). Six hourly transvaginal ultrasound, using a 7.5 mHz transducer was performed to provide serial estimation of follicle size. The time of onset of the LH surge was defined as the sampling time at which the concentration of LH increased by at least 100% over the preceding level and which was then followed by a sustained increase in LH levels (Djahanbakhch *et al.*, 1981).

When data were normalized to the time of onset of the LH surge, it became clear that there were detectable increases in circulating levels of both progesterone and immunoactive inhibin at the time of the onset of LH surge (Fig. 2). However, scrutiny of results from individual women revealed that a clear-cut rise in progesterone concentration occurred before the onset of the LH surge in only three out of the six cases. There was similar variation in levels of immunoactive inhibin, with no change being seen in four out of six cases until at least three hours after the onset of the LH surge. It is noteworthy that similar variation between individuals in circulating concentrations of inhibin around the time of the LH surge has been observed in the autotransplanted ewe (Campbell *et al.*, 1990). Taken together with the evidence of secretion of inhibin in the late follicular phase by non-dominant follicles (Illingworth *et al.*, 1991), it seems unlikely that this peptide plays a major endocrine role in the initiation of the LH surge or in control of ovulation. The part played by progesterone at mid-cycle is more clearly defined. Observations of the temporal relationships between oestradiol, progesterone and gonadotrophins, and the results of studies using progesterone antagonists, support the hypothesis that a pre-ovulatory rise in progesterone participates in the positive feedback mechanism at the level of the hypothalamus or pituitary, at least in some women. Further studies of the effects of progesterone antagonism on gonadotrophin pulsatility and the effects of increasing circulating levels of oestrogen at the time of the pre-ovular surge by exogenous treatment to overcome the block to positive feedback exerted by mifepristone remain to be performed.

Opioid peptides

The availability of the opioid μ-receptor antagonists naloxone and naltrexone has allowed detailed pharmacological manipulation of the opioid input to the hypothalamic pulse generator in both animals and humans. The opioid pathway can also be stimulated by agonists such as morphine and β-endorphin. Opioids appear to inhibit gonadotrophin secretion by the hypothalamus, most markedly in the late follicular and luteal phases of the human cycle (Rossmanith *et al.*, 1989). The inhibitory effect of opioids is not readily apparent during the early follicular phase, suggesting that the exertion of endorphin tone is dependent upon

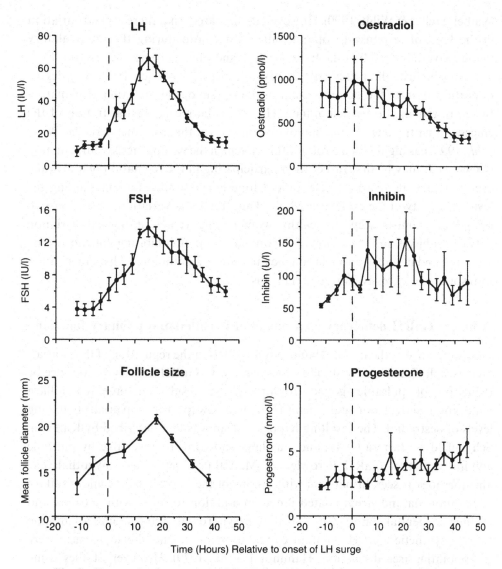

Fig. 2. Changes in the concentration of LH, FSH, oestradiol, progesterone and inhibin in samples of blood collected at 3-hourly intervals around ovulation. The samples have been grouped around the onset of the LH surge as indicated by the dotted line. (Ledger, Thong & Baird, unpublished data.)

the presence of relatively high background levels of ovarian steroids. However, the sleep-specific suppression of gonadotrophin secretion that occurs in the early follicle phase is opioid mediated (Rossmanith & Yen, 1987). Alteration of opioid tone by sex steroids has been implicated as a mechanism by which hypothalamic GnRH secretion might be regulated by the developing follicle (Leyendecker,

Waibel-Treber & Wildt, 1990). However, it is apparent that there is great variation in the level of response to opioid antagonism, both during the pre-ovulatory phase (Rossmanith, Mortola & Yen, 1988) and after chronic administration of antagonists throughout the cycle (Bryzski, Viniegra & Archer, 1992). The degree of participation of the opioid system in the physiological initiation of ovulation therefore remains to be determined. However, the recent demonstration of the efficacy of naltrexone in inducing ovulation in hypothalmic amenorrhoea (Wildt *et al.*, 1993) has highlighted a role for this system in the pathogenesis of anovulation (see later). It may be that rather than participating in the regulation of individual events within the ovarian cycle, opioid tone is responsible for maintaining the level of activity of the cycle as a whole. Thus, the large variations in response to opioid antagonists seen in healthy women may represent normal variation between subjects and the action of the opioid system in inhibiting gonadotrophin secretion and inducing anovulation may be seen as a pathological hyperactivation in response to excessive stress, weight loss, etc.

Clinical GnRH deficiency as a model of hypothalamo-pituitary function

The dominance of the hypothalamo-pituitary axis in the regulation of the ovarian cycle is well illustrated by studies on patients with GnRH deficiency. Absence or reduction of pulsatile gonadotrophin release results in impaired follicle maturation, anovulation and amenorrhoea with low (post-menopausal) circulating levels of oestradiol. The resulting hypogonadism was first described by Kallman, Schoenfeld & Barrera (1944) and was later shown to be reversible by pulsatile administration of GnRH (Crowley & McArthur, 1980). Such 'hypothalamic' amenorrhoea is seen in patients with lesions of the hypothalamus and pituitary stalk, anorexia and stress related illness in addition to those with anosmia and midline congenital abnormalities (Kallman Syndrome). Initial studies attempting to use synthetic GnRH to induce ovulation in amenorrhoeic women were disappointing (see discussion, Hammond *et al.*, 1979). However, studies using GnRH-deficient monkeys with lesions in the arcuate nucleus (Knobil, 1980) had already demonstrated that continuous treatment with long-acting GnRH agonists induced desensitisation of gonadotrophin secretion whereas pulsatile administration of GnRH resulted in physiological levels and patterns of gonadotrophins and sex steroids. Once the necessity for pulsatile administration of GnRH was understood, the success of treatment with GnRH, seen both in terms of ovulation and pregnancy, improved. Thus studies on patients exhibiting total absence of GnRH pulses demonstrated that doses of GnRH of 1.25–1.5 μg/pulse delivered intravenously every 60–90 minutes would induce ovulation and reconstitute normal menstrual cyclicity and fertility (Leyendecker, Wildt & Hansmann, 1980).

Refinement of the technology involved in administering subcutaneous or intravenous GnRH in a pulsatile manner through a small infusion pump has allowed successful use of this treatment modality in large numbers of patients with hypothalamic amenorrhoea. Use of pulsatile GnRH to induce ovulation avoids the high incidence of multiple pregnancy seen after treatment by daily injection of human menopausal gonadotrophin since restoration of GnRH pulsatility mimics the physiology of the normal cycle with preservation of the negative feedback effect of rising level of oestradiol on FSH secretion, reducing the chance of multi-follicular development to near normal (Leyendecker, Wildt & Hansmann, 1980). The positive feedback effect of oestradiol on the hypothalamus and pituitary is also preserved, with most GnRH induced cycles exhibiting a spontaneous LH surge and ovulation without the necessity for injection of human chorionic gonadotrophin. The low risk of multiple pregnancy and likelihood of spontaneous ovulation reduce the need for monitoring of GnRH induced cycles when compared to human menopausal gonadotrophin treatment. This has obvious benefits for the patient undergoing treatment and also results in significant cost saving (Baird, Ledger & Glasier, 1990).

Treatment of 'hypothalamic' amenorrhoea with pulsed GnRH has its drawbacks, however, The patient is required to wear a portable pump continuously often for many days with some disruption of lifestyle. More importantly, maintaining prolonged intravenous access carries a small but significant risk of sepsis. Subcutaneous injection of GnRH seems less effective than the intravenous route (Homburg *et al.*, 1989). Just as the understanding of the physiology of the regulation of the pituitary gonadotroph led to the clinical use of pulsed GnRH therapy, basic studies of the effects of opioids on the hypothalamic pulse generator have led directly to trials of drugs designed to modify GnRH secretion by acting on the hypothalamic opioid receptor. This approach offers a new alternative to GnRH pulse therapy, avoiding the above mentioned disadvantages, Opioid peptides are known to have profound effects on the hypothalamus in animals and humans, inhibiting pulsatile gonadotrophin secretion (Kesner *et al.*, 1986; Wildt *et al.*, 1993). Initial studies in which normal menstrual cycles were restored in women suffering from severe secondary hypothalamic amenorrhoea using the specific opiate μ-receptor antagonist naltrexone (Wildt & Leyendecker, 1987), have now been followed by a clinical trial of the drug in a large group of women with primary and secondary amenorrhoea (Wildt *et al.*, 1993). 16 women were able to conceive and a further 33 women experienced endocrinologically normal menstrual cycles in the study group of 66 patients. Naltrexone was more effective in cases of secondary amenorrhoea and the identification of a group of non-responders to the drug suggests the existence of opioid independent mechanisms of suppression of gonadotrophin secretion. However, opioid antagonism appears to offer a high pregnancy rate with few side effects and a convenient daily oral treatment regime for infertile women with secondary hypothalamic amenorrhoea.

Effect of ageing on ovulation

There is little doubt that fertility declines with age, even before ovulation ceases at the menopause. In classic studies of the Hutterite sect in North America, who condemn contraception and who are amongst the most fertile groups in the Western world, Tietze (1957) demonstrated the decline of fecundity with age. In his population study, the average age of women entering their last pregnancy was 40.9 years, some ten years before the menopause. More recently, the advent of assisted conception using *in vitro* fertilization and associated technologies has permitted detailed assessment of the effects of age on fertility by excluding such variables as frequency of intercourse and sperm quality. The prognosis for the success of *in vitro* fertilization in women over 40 years of age is poor, even in those with regular menstrual cycles (Romeu *et al.*, 1986). This decline in fertility is correlated with a rise in the basal level of FSH (Pearlstone *et al.*, 1992), with basal levels of FSH in excess of 25 IU/L being associated with a very poor prognosis. The relative contributions of the decline in quality of the oocyte and endometrium with age in IVF cycles have been elegantly demonstrated in studies using oocytes donated by young women to older infertile couples (Sauer, Paulson & Lobo, 1990; Navot *et al.*, 1991). It is clear from such work that oocyte age is the most important determinant of outcome in the donor cycle, identifying the oocyte as the major cause of the decline in fertility in older women (Navot *et al.*, 1991).

The rise of FSH with age is the first detectable endocrine marker of the onset of the peri-menopause. The FSH rise commonly occurs while menstrual cyclicity is retained (Lee *et al.*, 1988) and occurs independently of a rise in LH. This dissociation of FSH and LH has been attributed to an effect of the decline in the amount of inhibin released from follicles with ageing (Van Look *et al.*, 1977). Thus, although follicular phase levels of oestradiol do not differ between groups of regularly cycling women aged 20–29 and 40–44, FSH levels were higher and immunoactive inhibin levels lower in the older women (MacNaughton *et al.*, 1992). The fall in circulating levels of inhibin with age might reflect a combination of the diminution in the number of primordial follicles in the ovaries and a reduction in the ability of the granulosa cells to synthesize inhibin and possibly other peptides. The combination of normal follicular phase levels of oestradiol and reduced levels of immunoactive inhibin was identified by Buckler *et al.* (1991) in a group of regularly cycling infertile women with incipient ovarian failure, shown by persistently elevated levels of FSH. Although the steroidogenic capacity of the granulosa cells in this group was clearly not impaired, the ability to synthesize inhibin was again presumably reduced. Given the well-known effects of ageing on the incidence of chromosomal abnormalities in oocytes (see Angell *et al.*, 1988), it is attractive to hypothesize that the fall in inhibin secretion and concomitant rise in FSH secretion with disruption of the normal mechanism of successful folliculogenesis and ovulation represents a mechanism for reducing fertility at a time when the risks of miscarriage and fetal malformation due to oocyte abnormalities are increasing.

References

Ackerman RC, Murdoch WJ. Prostaglandin-induced apoptosis of ovarian surface epithelial cells. *Prostaglandins* 1993; **45**: 475–85

Angell RR, Hillier SG, West JD, Glasier AF, Rodger MW, Baird DT. Chromosome anomalies in early human embryos. *J Reprod Fertil Suppl.* 1988; **36**: 73–81.

Anonymous. Declining fertility: egg or uterus? *Lancet* 1991; **338**: 285–6 (Editorial).

Aono T, Miyake A, Kinugasa, TY, Kurachi, K. Progesterone advancement of oestrogen-induced luteinizing hormone release during the mid-follicular phase in normal cyclic women. *J Endocrinol* 1976; **71**: 451–2.

Baird DT. Factors regulating the growth of the pre-ovulatory follicle in the sheep and the human. *J Reprod Fertil* 1983; **69**: 343–52.

Baird DT. A model for follicular selection and ovulation: lessons from superovulation. *J Steroid Biochem* 1987; **27**: 15–23.

Baird DT, Ledger WL, Glasier AF. Induction of ovulation – cost-effectiveness and future prospects. *Baillière's Clin Obstet Gynaecol* 1990; **4**: 639–50.

Baker TG. Oogenesis and ovulation. In: Austin CR, Short RV, eds. *Reproduction in Mammals* 2nd Edn. Cambridge: Cambridge University Press, 1982; 17–45.

Batista MC, Cartledge TP, Zellmer AW *et al.* Delayed endometrial maturation induced by daily administration of the antiprogestin RU 486: a potential new contraceptive therapy. *Am J Obstet Gynecol* 1992a; **167**: 60–5.

Batista MC, Cartledge TP, Zellmer AW, Nieman LK, Merriam GR, Louriaux DL. Evidence for a critical role of progesterone in the regulation of the midcycle gonadotropin surge and ovulation. *J Clin Endocrinol Metab* 1992b; **74**: 565–70.

Block E. Quantitative morphological investigation of the follicular system in women. *Acta Endocrinol (Copenh)* 1951; **8**: 33–54.

Brzyski RG, Viniegra A, Archer DF. Effects of chronic nocturnal opiate antagonism on the menstrual cycle. *Am J Obstet Gynecol* 1992; **167**: 1780–4.

Buckler HM, Evans CA, Mamtora M, Burger HG, Anderson DA. Gonadotropin, steroid and inhibin levels in women with incipient ovarian failure during anovulatory and ovulating rebound cycles. *J Clin Endocrinol Metab* 1991; **72**: 116–24.

Campbell BK, Mann GE, McNeilly AS, Baird DT. The pattern of ovarian inhibin, estradiol, and androstenedione secretion during the estrous cycle of the ewe. *Endocrinology* 1990; **127**: 227–35.

Collins RL, Hodgen GD. Blockade of the spontaneous midcycle gonadotropin surge in monkeys by RU 486: a progesterone antagonist or agonist? *J Clin Endocrinol Metab* 1986; **63**: 1270–6.

Crowley WF, Jnr., McArthur JW. Stimulation of the normal menstrual cycle in Kallman's syndrome by pulsatile administration of luteinizing hormone-releasing hormone (LH-RH). *J Clin Endocrinol Metab* 1980; **51**: 173–5.

Croxatto HB, Salvatierra AM, Croxatto MD, Fuentealba B. Effects of continuous treatment with low dose mifepristone throughout one menstrual cycle. *Human Reprod* 1993; **8**: 201–7.

Deutinger J, Kirchheimer JC, Reinthaller A, Christ G, Tatra G, Binder BR. Elevated tissue type plasminogen activator in human granulosa cells correlate with fertilising capacity. *Human Reprod* 1988; **3**: 597–9.

di Zerega GS, Hodgen GD. Folliculogenesis in the primate ovarian cycle. *Endocr Rev* 1981; **2**: 27–49.

Djahanbakhch O, McNeilly AS, Hobson BM, Templeton AA. A rapid luteinizing hormone radioimmunoassay for the prediction of ovulation, *Br J Obstet Gynaecol* 1981; **88**: 1016–20.

Fink G. Feedback actions of target hormones on hypothalamus and pituitary with special reference to gonadal steroids. *Ann Rev Physiol* 1979; **41**: 571–85.

Franchimont P, Verstraelen-Proyard J, Hazee-Hagelstein MT, Demoulin RA, Bourguignon JP, Hirstin J. Inhibin: from concept to reality. *Vitamins and Hormones* 1979; **37**: 243–302.

Friedman CI, Barrows H, Moon KH. Hypergonadotropic hypogonadism. *Am J Obstet Gynecol* 1983; **145**: 360–72.

Gauthier G. Olfactogenital dysplasia at puberty. *Acta Neuroveg* 1960; **21**: 345–94.

Gregg DW, Allen MC, Nett TM. Estradiol-induced increase in number of gonadotropin-releasing hormone receptors in cultured ovine pituitary cells. *Biol Reprod* 1990; **43**: 1032–6.

Hammond CB, Wiebe RH, Haney AF, Yancy SG. Ovulation induction with luteinizing hormone-releasing hormone in amenorrhoeic, infertile women. *Am J Obstet Gynecol* 1979; **135**: 924–39.

Hoff JD, Quigley ME, Yen SSC. Hormonal dynamics at midcycle: a re-evaluation. *J Clin Endocrinol Metab* 1983; **57**: 792–6.

Homburg R, Eshel E, Armar NA *et al*. One hundred pregnancies after treatment with pulsatile luteinising hormone releasing hormone to induce ovulation. *Br Med J* 1989; **298**: 809–12.

Illingworth PJ, Reddi K, Smith KB, Baird DT. The souce of inhibin secretion during the human menstrual cycle. *J Clin Endocrinol Metab* 1991; **72**: 667–73.

Kallman FJ, Schoenfeld NA, Barrera SE. The genetic aspects of primary eunuchoidism. *Am J Ment Def* 1944; **48**: 203–36.

Kesner JS, Kaufmann JM, Wilson RC, Kuroda G, Knobil E. The effect of morphine on the electro-physiological activity of the hypothalamic luteinizing hormone releasing hormone pulse generator in the rhesus monkey. *Neuroendocinology* 1986; **43**: 686–8.

Knobil E. The neuroendocrine control of the menstrual cycle. *Rec Prog Horm Res* 1980; **36**: 53–88.

Knobil E, Plant TM, Wildt T, Belchetz PE, Marshall G. Control of the rhesus monkey menstrual cycle: permissive role of hypothalamic gonadotropin-releasing hormone. *Science* 1980; **207**: 1371–3.

Ledger WL, Thomas EJ, Browning D, Lenton EA, Cooke ID. Suppression of gonadotrophin secretion does not reverse premature ovarian failure. *Br J Obstet Gynaecol* 1989; **96**: 196–9.

Ledger WL, Sweeting VM, Hillier H, Baird DT. Inhibition of ovulation by low-dose mifepristone (RU 486). *Hum Reprod* 1992; **7**: 945–50.

Lee SJ, Lenton EA, Sexton L, Cooke ID. The effect of age on the cyclical patterns of plasma LH, FSH, oestradiol and progesterone in women with regular menstrual cycles. *Hum Reprod* 1988; **3**: 851–5.

Levine JE, Ramirez VD. *In vivo* release of luteinizing hormone-releasing hormone estimated with push–pull cannulae from the mediobasal hypothalamus of ovariectomized, steroid-primed rats. *Endocrinology* 1980; **107**: 1782–90.

Levine JE, Ramirez VD. Luteinizing hormone-releasing hormone release during the rat estrous cycle and after ovariectomy, as estimated with push–pull cannulae. *Endocrinology* 1982; **111**: 1439–48.

Leyendecker G, Wildt L, Hansmann M. Pregnancies following chronic intermittent (pulsatile) administration of GnRH by means of a portable pump (Zyklomat) – a new approach to the treatment of infertility in hypothalamic amenorrhoea. *J Clin Endocrinol Metab* 1980; **51**: 1214–17.

Leyendecker G, Waibel-Treber S, Wildt L. The central control of follicular maturation and ovulation in the human. *Oxf Rev Reprod Biol* 1990; **12**: 93–146.

Liu JH, Yen, SSC. Induction of midcycle gonadotropin surge by ovarian steroids in women; an initial evaluation. *J Clin Endocrinol Metab* 1983; **57**: 797–802.

McArdle CA, Schomerus E, Gröner I, Poch A. Estradiol regulates gonadotropin-releasing hormone receptor number, growth and inositol phosphate production in αT_3-1 cells. *Mol Cell Endocrinol* 1992; **87**: 95–103.

McLachlan RI, Healy DL, Robertson DM, Burger HG, de Kretser DM. Circulating immunoactive inhibin in the luteal phase and early gestation of women undergoing ovulation induction. *Fertil Steril* 1987*a*; **48**: 1001–5.

McLachlan RI, Robertson DM, Healy DL, Burger HG, de Kretser DM. Circulating immunoreactive inhibin levels during the normal human menstrual cycle. *J Clin Endocrinol Metab* 1987*b*; **65**: 954–61.

McLachlan RI, Cohen WL, Dahl KD, Bremmer WJ, Soules MR. Serum inhibin levels during the periovulatory interval in normal women: relationships with sex steroid and gonadotropin levels. *Clin Endocrinol* 1990; **32**: 39–48.

MacNaughton J, Banah M, McCloud P, Hee J, Burger J. Age related changes in follicle stimulating hormone, luteinizing hormone, oestradiol and immunoreactive inhibin in women of reproductive age. *Clin Endocrinol* 1992; **36**: 339–45.

Menon M, Preegel M, Katta V. Estradiol potentiation of gonadotropin-releasing hormone responsiveness in the anterior pituitary is mediated by an increase in gonadotropin-releasing hormone receptors. *Am J Obstet Gynecol* 1985; **151**: 534–40.

Monroe SE, Jaffe RB, Midgley AR Jnr. Regulation of human gonadotropins. XII. Increase in serum gonadotropins in response to estradiol. *J Clin Endocrinol Metab* 1972; **34**: 298–305.

Naftolin F, Brown-Grant K, Corker CS. Plasma and pituitary luteinizing hormone and peripheral plasma oestradiol concentrations in the normal oestrous cycle of the rat and after experimental manipulation of the cycle. *J Endocrinol* 1972; **53**: 17–30.

Navot D, Bergh PA, Williams MA *et al.* Poor oocyte quality rather than implantation failure as a cause of age-related decline in female fertility. *Lancet* 1991; **337**: 1375–7.

Nilsson L, Wikland M, Hamberger L. Recruitment of an ovulatory follicle in the human following follicle-ectomy and lute-ectomy. *Fertil Steril* 1982; **37**: 30–4.

Park OK, Ramirez VD. Spontaneous changes in LHRH release during the rat estrous cycle, as measured with repetitive push-pull perfusions of the pituitary gland in the same female rats. *Neuroendocrinology* 1989; **50**: 66–72.

Pauerstein CJ, Eddy CA, Croxatto HD, Hess R, Siler-Khodr TM, Croxatto HB. Temporal relationships of estrogen, progesterone and luteinizing hormone levels to ovulation in women and infrahuman primates. *Am J Obstet Gynecol* 1978; **130**: 876–84.

Pearlstone AC, Fournet N, Gambone JC, Pang SC, Bugalos RP. Ovulation induction in women age 40 and over: the importance of basal follicle-stimulating hormone level and chronological age. *Fertil Steril* 1992; **58**: 674–9.

Permezel JM, Lenton EA, Roberts I, Cooke ID. Acute effects of progesterone and the antiprogestin RU 486 on gonadotropin secretion in the follicular phase of the menstrual cycle. *J Clin Endocrinol Metab* 1989; **68**: 960–5.

Reddi K, Wickings EJ, McNeilly AS, Baird DT, Hillier SG. Circulating bioactive follicle stimulating hormone and immunoreactive inhibin during the normal human menstrual cycle. *Clin Endocrinol* 1990; **33**: 547–57.

Robertson DM, Tsonis CG, McLachlan RI *et al.* Comparison of inhibin immunological and in vitro biological activities in human serum. *J Clin Endocrinol Metab* 1988; **67**: 438–43.

Romeu A, Muasher SJ, Acosta AA, Veech LL, Diaz J, Jones GS *et al.* Results of *in vitro* fertilisation attempts in women 40 years and over: the Norfolk experience. *Fertil Steril* 1986; **47**: 130–6.

Rossmanith WG, Yen SSC. Sleep-associated decrease in luteinizing hormone pulse frequency during the early follicular phase of the menstrual cycle: evidence for an opioidergic mechanism. *J Clin Endocrinol Metab* 1987; **65**: 715–18.

Rossmanith WG, Mortola JF, Yen SSC. Role of endogenous opioid peptides in the initiation of the midcycle luteinizing hormone surge in normally cycling women. *J Clin Endocrinol Metab* 1988; **67**: 695–700.

Rossmanith WG, Wirth U, Sterzik K, Yen SSC. The effects of prolonged opioidergic blockade on LH pulsatile secretion during the menstrual cycle. *J Endocrinol Invest* 1989; **12**: 245–52.

Russell P, Bannatyne P, Shearman RP, Fraser IS, Corbett J. Premature hypergonadotrophic ovarian failure: Clinicopathological study of 19 cases. *Int J Gynaecol Path* 1982; **1**: 185–201.

Sallam HN, Whitehead MI, Collins WP. The incidence of mature follicles in spontaneous and induced ovarian cycles. *Lancet* 1983; **i**: 357.

Sarkar DK, Chiappa SA, Fink G, Sherwood NM. Gonadotropin-releasing hormone surge in pro-oestrous rats. *Nature, London* 1976; **264**: 461–3.

Sauer MV, Paulson RJ, Lobo RA. A preliminary report on oocyte donation extending reproductive potential to women over 40. *N Engl J Med* 1990; **323**: 1157–60.

Strickland S, Beers WH. Studies on the role of plasminogen activator in ovulation. In vitro response of granulosa cells to gonadotropins, cyclic nucleotides and prostaglandins. *J Biol Chem* 1976; **251**: 5694–702.

Tietze C. Reproductive span and rate of reproduction among Hutterite women. *Fertil Steril* 1957; **8**: 89–97.

Van Look PFA, Lothian H, Hunter WM, Michie EA, Baird DT. Hypothalamic-pituitary-ovarian function in perimenopausal women. *Clin Endocrinol* 1977; **7**: 13–31.

Wildt L, Leyendecker G. Induction of ovulation by chronic administration of naltrexone in hypothalamic amenorrhea. *J Clin Endocrinol Metab* 1987; **64**: 1334–6.

Wildt L, Leyendecker G, Sir-Petermann T, Waibel-Trever S. Treatment with naltrexone in hypothalamic ovarian failure; induction of ovulation and pregnancy. *Hum Reprod* 1993; **8**: 350–8.

Ying S-Y. Inhibins, activins and follistatins: gonadal proteins modulating the secretion of follicle-stimulating hormone. *Endocr Revs* 1988; **9**: 267–93.

9

Ovulation 4: Paracrine regulation and ovarian function

M. T. SEPPÄLÄ, M. BRÄNNSTRÖM AND P. O. JANSON

Introduction

Paracrine control involves a mechanism whereby one cell-type influences the activity of another through secretion of bioactive substances (Franchimont, 1986), Autocrine action means that one cell can effect its own bioregulation by secreting messengers to act on the same cell. In order for a substance to be autocrine or paracrine it must be produced locally, its actions on cells should be mediated via receptors, and the action should be detectable *in vivo* (Findlay, 1991). There are many extensive reviews on the subject, and the reader is referred to these for more information (Hsueh *et al.,* 1984; Franchimont, 1986; Adashi, 1990; Findlay, 1991).

As a basis of paracrine interaction, the ovarian follicle contains the oocyte and two somatic cell types, granulosa and theca cells. The ovary also contains transiently migratory cells, such as granulocytes, lymphocytes and macrophages. Androgens and oestrogens produced by the ovary have paracrine regulatory roles in follicular function (Gore-Langton & Armstrong, 1988). In addition to steroid compounds the intraovarian regulatory mechanisms involve growth factors, cytokines, and a great number of other substances (Table 1).

Steroidal autocrine/paracrine regulation

The 'two-cell, two gonadotrophin' model of oestrogen synthesis has been taken as an example of a follicular paracrine system (Armstrong, 1992). Oestradiol-17β, formed in the granulosa cells has direct actions on follicular cells through its activities in various steroidogenic enzymes (see Findlay & Risbridger, 1987). The interaction between granulosa and theca cells in the follicle wall resembles epithelio-mesenchymal interaction (Hillier, 1991). Oestrogens, produced by granulosa cells, may regulate theca cell function (Leung & Armstrong, 1980), by

Table 1. *Putative local regulatory substances in the ovary*

α2 macroglobulin	Interleukin-1
αN-inhibin peptide	Interleukin-6
Activin	Müllerian inhibiting substance
Angiotensin II	Neuropeptide Y
Bradykinin	Oestradiol
Catecholamines	Oxytocin
Epidermal growth factor	Platelet-derived growth factor
Fibroblast growth factor	Progesterone
Follistatin or	Prostaglandins
FSH-suppressing protein	Relaxin
Histamine	Renin
Inhibin	Substance P
Insulin-like growth factor I	β-Endorphin
Insulin-like growth factor	Transforming growth factor β
binding protein	Transforming growth factors α and β
Interferon γ	Tumour necrosis factor α
Interferon α	Vasoactive intestinal peptide

suppressing thecal androgen synthesis in response to the mid-cycle LH surge (Erickson *et al.*, 1985). Oestrogen is an intrafollicular autocrine regulator within the granulosa cell which produces it, as it stimulates proliferation and augments responsiveness of these cells to gonadotrophins. Oestrogen also potentiates FSH-induced steroidogenic enzymes P450aro and P450scc (Richards *et al.*, 1987) and stimulates the expression of inhibin and its subunits (Turner *et al.*, 1989). Steroid-binding sites other than the 'classic' oestrogen receptors may mediate these autocrine actions in the ovary (Hillier, 1991). Granulosa cells contain androgen receptors that mediate the effects of thecal androgens to augment FSH-induced granulosa cell differentiation (Hillier, Knazek & Ross, 1977). The theca interna is regulated by LH and is the principal cellular site of androgen synthesis (Tsang *et al.*, 1979). Androgens can cross the lamina basalis and penetrate the granulosa cell layer to accumulate in follicular fluid (Tsang *et al.*, 1979). Oestrogens promote granulosa cell proliferation, whereas locally produced androgens are engaged in the control of follicular atresia (Louvet *et al.*, 1975).

Although it is well established that steroids subserve paracrine regulatory functions in ovarian follicles, experimental evidence that they participate in the normal ovulatory process is still controversial. However, consensus is emerging from studies on several animal species regarding the importance to ovulation of the preovulatory rise in follicular progesterone synthesis. For example, ovulation is inhibited *in vivo* in rats by systemic administration of an antibody against progesterone (Mori *et al.*, 1977), or by administration of Epostane, an inhibitor of 3-β hydroxysteroid dehydrogenase (Snyder, Beechan & Schane, 1984). Ovulation was also inhibited by a similar inhibitor of 3-β hydroxysteroid dehydrogenase in the *in vitro* perfused ovary and ovulation was restored by administration of progesterone to the perfusion system, indicating that progesterone exerts a local effect on the ovulatory process (Brännström & Janson, 1989). The crucial role of progesterone in ovulation was further highlighted by the findings that the progesterone receptor agonist, RU 486, inhibits ovulation *in vivo* in the mouse (Loutradis *et al.*, 1991) and *in vitro* in the perfused rat ovary when administered concomitantly with the ovulation-inducing dose of hCG but not when administered at 4 hours into the ovulatory process (Brännström, 1993). Follicular progesterone may affect the process of ovulation by locally increasing plasminogen activator activity and kallikreins, substances activating collagenases and bradykinin, respectively (Tanaka *et al.*, 1992). A role of oestrogen in the process of follicular rupture appears to have been ruled out by experiments performed both *in vivo* (Lipner & Wendelken, 1971) and *in vitro* (LeMaire *et al.*, 1982; Morioka *et al.*, 1988).

Insulin-like growth factors (IGFs)

IGF-I and IGF-II are peptides showing structural homology with proinsulin and insulin (Rinderknecht & Humbel, 1978). IGF I is a single-chain polypeptide containing 70 amino acids, with an Mr of 7649. IGF-II consists of 67 amino acids, with an *Mr* of 7471. Receptors for insulin, IGF-I and IGF-II are present on most cells, including ovarian theca and granulosa cells (Poretsky *et al.*, 1985), also in the fetal human ovary (Shifren, Osathanondh & Yeh, 1993). Hyperandrogenism observed in a variety of hyperinsulinemic states has been suggested to be due to an effect of insulin mediated through the insulin receptors, or through type I IGF receptors (Poretsky *et al.*, 1990).

The high affinity for IGF-II of the type I IGF receptor suggests that this receptor may mediate biological responses of both IGF-II and IGF-I (Steele-Perkins *et al.*, 1988). Type I IGF and type IGF-II receptor mRNAs are present in human menopausal ovary and granulosa cells (Hernandex *et al.*, 1992). After binding to the ligand, the human type I IGF receptor undergoes autophosphorylation, and subsequent phosphorylation of endogenous substrates takes place within the cell. This process also mediates IGF-I stimulated glucose uptake, glycogen synthesis and DNA synthesis (Steel-Perkins *et al.*, 1988).

Like many growth factors, IGFs are engaged in the intraovarian regulation system, probably through endocrine, paracrine and autocrine mechanisms (Table

2). The presence of both IGF-I and IGF-II in human follicular fluid has been reported by several investigators (Ramasharma, Cauerera & Li, 1986; Geisthovel *et al.*, 1989). The IGF-I concentration is higher in serum than in follicular fluid (Geisthovel *et al.*, 1989), suggesting synthesis outside the follicle. IGF-I concentrations in follicular fluid are higher in dominant follicles than in cohort follicles, both in spontaneous (Eden *et al.*, 1988) and stimulated cycles (Rabinovici *et al.*, 1990).

The concentrations of IGF-I, IGF-II and insulin in ovarian and peripheral venous blood samples obtained from women undergoing abdominal hysterectomy have revealed a decreased ovarian gradient for IGF-II but not for IGF-I or insulin, suggesting that IGF-II but not IGF-I may be locally regulated by the ovary (Jesionowska *et al.*, 1990). Indeed, human granulosa cells contain IGF-II mRNA but not IGF-I mRNA (Voutilainen & Miller, 1987), and IGF-II is secreted by proliferating granulosa cell cultures from human ovaries (Ramasharma & Li, 1987). Use of 3- and 5-specific antisense RNA probes have revealed the presence of IGF-I mRNAs encoding both E_a and E_b forms of the E-peptide as well as the splicing variants in whole menopausal ovary (Hernandez *et al.*, 1992). Based on immunohistochemical studies the cells in the ovary producing the IGF-I peptide may be the thecal-interstitial cells. El-Roeiy and coworkers (1993) found by studying the expression of the genes encoding the IGFs, their receptors and the localization of their gene products in specific compartments of the human ovary, that IGF-II is synthesized in thecal cells in small antral follicles and in granulosa cells in dominant follicles. Because IGF-II mRNA is detectable in human granulosa cells before ovulation, this peptide probably plays an autocrine-paracrine role in follicle maturation (Geisthovel *et al.*, 1989; Voutilainen & Miller, 1987). While apparently not produced by human granulosa cells, IGF-I stimulates DNA synthesis in human granulosa-luteal cells from both natural and stimulated cycles (Olsson *et al.*, 1990; Angervo *et al.*, 1991). This suggests a role for IGF-I in the regulation of human granulosa cell proliferation. Current data indicate that both endocrine and paracrine actions of IGF-I are likely to modulate granulosa cell function (Adashi *et al.*, 1991; Hernandez *et al.*, 1992).

In some animal species, GH increases intraovarian IGF-I synthesis (Davoren & Hsueh, 1986). In the human, treatment with GH increases serum IGF-I concentration. There are GH receptors on human granulosa calls (Carlsson *et al.*, 1992). In a recent study on cultured human granulosa cells, the addition of GH to the incubation medium resulted in a significant increase in oestradiol accumulation (Mason *et al.*, 1990*a*). Human GH also had a significant additive effect on the dose-related responsiveness to FSH of granulosa cell oestradiol production. It is believed that this action of GH is not mediated by IGF-I, because IGF-I was not detectable in the medium. These studies suggest that GH has a

Table 2. *Ovarian responses to growth factors*

Growth factor	Production	Target cell	Principal effect	Cellular response
EGF	Theca	Granulosa Stroma	± proliferation, depending on the presence or absence of FSH ± differentiation (luteinization)	Enhanced FSH receptor binding and oocyte maturation, variable mitotic activity, attenuated LH receptor induction, inhibition or aromatase
IGF-I	Granulosa (rat) Theca (human) Stroma (human)	Granulosa Theca	+ proliferation + differentiation + differentiation	Enhanced steroidogenesis and proteoglycan production
IGF-II	Granulosa (human)	Granulosa	+ differentiation	Enhanced steroidogenesis
TGFα	Theca	Granulosa	+ proliferation – differentiation	Attenuated steroidogenesis and LH receptor induction
TGFβ	Granulosa Theca	Every compartment of the follicle	± proliferation ± differentiation	Variable effect of DNA-synthesis, attenuated LH receptor induction
bFGF	Theca	Granulosa, mesodermal and neuroectodermal cells	+ proliferation	Increased endothelial cell growth, attenuated steroidogenesis (inhibits aromatase and androgen synthesis)
PDGF		Granulosa	+ proliferation	

direct stimulatory effect on production of oestradiol by the human ovary, independent of the effect of FSH and IGF-I.

IGF-I stimulates oestradiol synthesis in rat and porcine granulosa and granulosa-luteal cells, and it synergizes with FSH to promote granulosa cell steroidogenesis (Adashi *et al.*, 1985; Dor *et al.*, 1992; Mason *et al.*, 1992). Incubation with IGF-I alone increases oestradiol production by human granulosa cells comparable to that caused by FSH, and coincubation with FSH and IGF-I augments oestradiol levels more than either hormone alone (Erickson, Garzo & Magoffin, 1989; Dor *et al.*, 1992; Mason *et al.*, 1992).

The levels of IGF-I are higher in follicles from hyperandrogenaemic women than from controls (Eden *et al.*, 1990). IGF-I may augment androstenedione secretion from ovarian stromal cells (Barbieri *et al.*, 1986). Both insulin and IGF-I stimulate androgen production in incubations of human ovarian stroma and theca. In long-term cultures luteinized human granulosa cells undergo transformation from an initial human FSH and IGF-I responsive state to an hCG responsive state (Christman *et al.*, 1991).

Anovulation in women with polycystic ovary syndrome (PCOS) is thought to result from a disorder in gonadotrophin-mediated follicular maturation which obviously involves paracrine modulation by intra-ovarian factors. Some authors have reported elevated serum IGF-I levels in patients with PCOS (Laatikainen *et al.*, 1990), but this is not the case in all studies (Kazer, Unterman & Glick, 1990). IGF-I stimulates thymidine incorporation in granulosa cells, and GH in combination with FSH stimulates steroidogenesis in granulosa cells obtained from natural, but not stimulated, cycles (Bergh *et al.*, 1991*a,b*). According to a recent hypothesis, PCOS could result from a primary abnormality in the GH–IGF-I axis leading to increased IGF activity at multiple sites (Kazer, 1988). Recent studies suggest that the local activity of IGF-I may be accentuated in PCOS patients, because the circulating level of a local inhibitor, IGFBP-1, is decreased (Suikkari *et al.*, 1989*b*). The median concentration of IGF-I in the follicular fluid from PCOS patients has been found to be higher than that of the controls (Eden *et al.*, 1990) also pointing to augmented local action of IGF-I. In isolated granulosa cells from ovaries of PCOS patients cultured in serum-free medium, FSH and IGF-I stimulate oestradiol production in a dose-dependent manner (Erickson *et al.*, 1990). In the presence of a maximally effective dose of FSH, the cells are more responsive to IGF-I, and in the presence of a maximally effective dose of IGF-I, the stimulatory effect of FSH on oestradiol production is greatly amplified. In synergism with FSH, IGF-I stimulates aromatase activity, enhances proteoglycan biosynthesis, induces luteinizing hormone (LH) receptors, potentiates LH action and increases progesterone secretion (Adashi *et al.*, 1985). In view of all these findings, it is not surprising that patients with PCOS may have explosive responses to superovulation with gonadotrophins.

Treatment with IGF-II has no effect on either basal or FSH-stimulated oestradiol production (Erickson *et al.*, 1990), and treatment with insulin, either alone or in combination with FSH, increases the oestradiol level, but the effect of insulin is seen only at the highest doses tested. *In vitro* experiments with granulosa cells from PCOS patients indicated that 1) physiological concentrations of IGF-I are as effective as FSH in stimulating oestradiol secretion; 2) IGF-I and FSH act synergistically to control the level of oestradiol secretion; and 3) this synergy is not observed with insulin or IGF-II (Erickson *et al.*, 1990).

The effects of IGF-I on regulation of aromatase activity and the synthesis of aromatase cytochrome P-450arom have been studied in granulosa-luteal cells from women undergoing *in vitro* fertilization (IVF) (Steinkampf, Mendelson & Simpson, 1988). IGF-I was found to increase the synthesis of P-450arom. During preovulatory development granulosa cells do not express P450c17 enzyme and are therefore unable to synthesize androgens (Steinkampf, Mendelson & Simpson, 1987). IGF-I and IGF-II stimulate human oocyte maturation (Gomez, Tarin & Pellicer, 1993).

IGF-binding proteins (IGFBPs)

The local actions of IGFs are regulated by IGF-binding proteins (IGFBPs) that bind both IGF-I and IGF-II. At least six different IGFBPs have been identified and their cDNAs have been cloned and sequenced (see Drop *et al.*, 1991). IGFBPs are multifunctional proteins that regulate the transport and presentation of IGFs to cell surface receptors. Before the current nomenclature was established, IGFBP-1 had many names in the literature. N-terminal sequence analyses, and cloning studies indicated that IGFBP-1 is the same as PP12 (placental protein 12) (Koistinen *et al.*, 1986), α_1-PEG (α_1-pregnancy-associated endometrial globulin) (Bell & Keyte, 1988), BP28 (Lee *et al.*, 1988), low molecular weight 34 K IGF-binding protein (Koistinen *et al.*, 1986), and amniotic fluid IGF-binding protein (Povoa *et al.*, 1984).

IGFBP-1 consists of 259 amino acids and has an Mr of 25.3 kDa (Julkunen *et al.*, 1988). The protein binds IGF I with high affinity, similar to that of type I IGF receptor (Koistinen *et al.*, 1987). The IGFBP-1 gene resides in chromosome 7p12-p13 and there is DNA polymorphism in the IGFBP-1 gene (Alitalo *et al.*, 1989).

Human follicular fluid and luteinized granulosa cells contain IGFBP-1/PP12 (Seppälä *et al.*, 1984) and IGFBP-1 mRNA (Koistinen *et al.*, 1990), and human granulosa cells can incorporate radioactive methionine into immunoreactive

IGFBP-1 (Suikkari *et al.,* 1989*a*). Secretion of IGFBP-1 from human granulosa-luteal cells is stimulated by prostaglandin E2 *in vitro* (Julkanen *et al.,* 1989), and there is a positive correlation between follicular fluid oestradiol and IGFBP-1 levels, and between progesterone and IGFBP-1 levels (Seppälä *et al.,* 1984).

Serum IGFBP-1 levels are down-regulated by insulin (Suikkari *et al.,* 1988) which appears to be the main regulator of circulating IGFBP-1 level (Suikkari *et al.,* 1989*b*). Insulin inhibits IGFBP-1 secretion by HepG2 cells, a primary liver cancer cell line (Singh *et al.,* 1990) suggesting that the suppressive action of insulin takes place in the liver. Besides in the liver, recent studies suggest that insulin and IGF-I inhibit IGFBP-1 secretion also at other sites of the body including the ovary (Mason *et al.,* 1993). High levels of circulating IGFBP-1 may reduce IGF-I bio-availability (Holly *et al.,* 1989) and, therefore, a decrease of serum IGFBP-1 concentration by insulin is believed to increase the local IGF-I action (Conover & Lee, 1990).

As an example of local regulation, IGFBP-1 produced by the granulosa cells can inhibit IGF-I stimulated DNA synthesis of the same cells (Angervo *et al.,* 1991), and IGFBP-1 can also inhibit FSH and IGF-I stimulated progesterone secretion from rat and human granulosa cells (Adashi *et al.,* 1992; Mason *et al.,* 1993). These studies indicate that IGFBP-1 has inhibitory autocrine/paracrine actions on the paracrine/endocrine effects of IGF-I on granulosa-luteal cells. IGF-I effectively inhibits IGFBP-1 release from unstimulated human granulosa cells whilst stimulating their oestradiol production (Mason *et al.,* 1993), and this has also been observed for stimulated human granulosa-luteal cells after superovulation for *in vitro* fertilization (IVF) (Dor *et al.,* 1992).

In cultured rat granulosa cells, human IGFBP-1 inhibits FSH-supported progesterone secretion, probably by inhibiting the effect of endogenous rat (IGF-I (Adashi *et al.,* 1992). Previous studies on human granulosa-luteal cells have shown that IGFBP-1/PP12 does not interfere with binding of FSH to its receptor (Seppälä *et al.,* 1984), and IGFBP-1 does not bind FSH (Adashi *et al.,* 1992). Studies on porcine and rat granulosa cells suggest that FSH inhibits IGFBP secretion by the granulosa cells (Adashi *et al.,* 1991; Shimasaki *et al.,* 1990), and according to recent studies the same is true for human granulosa-luteal cells (Dor *et al.,* 1992). Thus, a negative feed-back regulation mechanism seems to exist between IGFBP-1 and FSH into both directions.

Transcripts of IGFBP-2 and IGFBP-3 have also been demonstrated in the human granulosa (Guidice *et al.,* 1991). The most abundant IGFBP in follicular fluid appears to be IGFBP-3 (Holly *et al.,* 1990). Western ligand blotting has revealed five IGF-binding protein bands in follicular fluid migrating parallel with those identified in serum. This suggests that the various IGFBP species previously identified in serum may also be present in follicular fluid. Two bands were found in positions corresponding to the components of the large (150 kDa) binding complex. These were the predominant forms in most follicular fluid samples. At least four different IGFBPs have been demonstrated by ligand analysis in follicular fluid, and each of them has been suggested to be produced independently within the ovary (Holly et al., 1990). However, the use of both Western ligand and Western immunoblot analyses have shown that three of the bands in follicular fluid migrating at 28 kDa, 30 kDa and 60 kDa are accounted for by IGFBP-1 alone (Angervo et al., 1991), emphasizing the importance of using both immunological and ligand-binding criteria for the analysis of IGF-binding protein species in biological fluids. Indeed, simultaneous use of ligand and immunoblot analyses has revealed that IGFBP-3 may be broken down by proteases to several smaller molecular weight fragments which may or may not retain their IGF-binding or immuno-reactive capacity (Koistinen, Seppälä & Koistinen, 1994).

An inhibitor of FSH action on granulosa cells has been purified from porcine follicular fluid. N-terminal sequence analysis of this substance has revealed a high degree of homology with the 53 kDa molecular mass GH-dependent human IGFBP-3. Since both IGF-I and IGF-II are produced locally in the porcine ovary and they exert stimulatory effects on granulosa cells in this species, the local production of this IGFBP is suggested to regulate ovarian follicle growth through its antigonadotrophic effect (Shimasaki et al., 1990; Ui et al., 1989). In human granulosa cells IGFBP-3 has been found to inhibit FSH and IGF-I induced oestradiol and progesterone secretion (Mason et al., 1993).

El-Roeiy and coworkers (1992) studied by immunohistological staining the IGFBPs 1–6 in normal and polycystic ovaries. They concluded that IGFBP-1 is synthesized in granulosa cells of dominant follicles. IGFBP-3 is more widely distributed in theca cells of all follicles, and also in granulosa cells of dominant follicles. They found IGFBPs -2, -4 and -5 in granulosa cells of atretic and PCO follicles, IGFBP-4 and -5 being also localized in thecal and stromal tissues. They found no IGFBP-6 in the human ovary, and there were no distinguishable differences in binding protein expression between atretic follicles of normal and polycystic ovaries.

In studies on normal human ovaries, San Roman and Magoffin (1993) also found that IGFBP-3 is the major binding protein in follicular fluid. Its concentration in leading follicle, decreases as the follicle grows, whereas IGFBPs 2 and 4 are detected in atretic follicles. From these studies it is obvious that the IGF system plays a part in local regulation of follicular maturation and steroidogenesis. Recent studies by Gomez et al. (1993) indicate that the IGFs are able to augment spontaneous maturation in immature human oocytes. The role of IGFBPs in this process is unknown.

Epidermal growth factor (EGF)

EGF is a polypeptide growth factor containing 53 amino acids and having both mitogenic and differentiating effects. The human EGF gene has been localized to chromosome 4q in the same region as another specialized growth factor, T-cell growth factor (Brissenden, Ullrich & Franke, 1984). EGF and TGFα are closely related peptides that bind to the same receptors (Massagué, 1983). Granulosa cells contain hormonally regulated receptors for EGF/TGFα (Feng, Knecht & Catt, 1987), and also the theca cells contain high affinity EGF receptors (Skinner & Coffey, 1988).

Maruo and coworkers (1993) have studied by immunohistochemical staining the localization of EGF and EGF receptors in human ovary. They found no immunostaining for EGF or EGF receptors in primordial follicles. In the preantral follicle, EGF and EGF receptors were found in the oocyte only, the intensity of staining increasing towards the preovulatory stage. In antral follicles, EGF and EGF receptors were observed in the granulosa and theca interna, without appreciable staining in the surrounding stroma. The immunostaining for EGF and EGF receptors in the granulosa and theca interna persisted in corpus luteum and intensified in the midluteal phase. Corpus albicans showed no staining for EGF or EGF receptors. In atretic follicles, the theca interna showed intense staining for EGF and EGF receptors, whereas immunostaining in scattered granulosa cells was negligible (Maruo *et al.*, 1993).

EGF has been found in human preovulatory follicular fluid. There is a significant positive correlation between the levels of EGF in follicular fluid and in serum, whereas no significant relationship exists between intrafollicular levels of EGF and those of progesterone and oestradiol. Serum-free conditioned medium from bovine theca cells, but not from granulosa cells, contains a component that specifically binds to the EGF receptor. This indicates that theca cells produce an EGF-like substance and they respond to EGF by increased cell proliferation (Skinner & Coffey, 1988). Although not itself mitogenic, human alpha fetoprotein can enhance the mitogenic activity of EGF and TGFα and this protein may function to modulate growth factor-mediated proliferation of cultured porcine granulosa cells (Leal, May & Keel, 1990).

EGF/TGFα of thecal origin is probably involved in the paracrine control of granulosa cell responsiveness to FSH in the enhancement of cell proliferation and inhibition of steroidogenesis. EGF alone or in the presence of FSH has no effect on [^{3}H]thymidine incorporation into granulosa cells. However, EGF acts in concert with TGFβ, and with TGFβ plus IGF-I, to promote DNA synthesis. Therefore, EGF has opposite actions on DNA synthesis: it either inhibits or stimulates DNA synthesis depending on the presence or absence of FSH and consequently on the endocrine environment within the follicle (Bendell & Dorrington, 1990).

Testosterone in the absence of FSH results in accumulation of oestradiol in the medium after incubation of granulosa cells from both normal and polycystic ovaries, and this increase can be reversed by the addition of EGF (Mason *et al.*, 1990*b*). Unlike IGF-I, EGF does not increase hybridizable mRNA encoding cytochrome P-450arom when added alone, but it markedly inhibits the action of FSH to stimulate aromatase activity and the synthesis of cytochrome P-450arom (Steinkampf *et al.*, 1988). Thus IGF-I and EGF have opposite actions on aromatase activity. Opposite actions have also been found between the effects of IGF-I and EGF to release IGFBP-1 by human granulosa-luteal cells. While EGF dose-dependently increases IGFBP-1 secretion from human granulosa-luteal cells (Angervo, Koistinen & Seppälä, 1992), IGF-I suppresses it (Mason *et al.*, 1992; Dor *et al.*, 1992).

EGF has been reported to have a luteinizing effect on human granulosa cells. This is suggested by experiments in which exposure of cultured granulosa-luteal cells to EGF has lead to substantial increases in responses to hCG and oestradiol (Richardson, Gadd & Masson, 1989). EGF probably induced luteinization directly, and this may also be mediated indirectly via induction of IGFBP-1 synthesis to counteract the mitogenic effect of IGFs.

Studies by Gomez and his colleagues (1993) have shown that incubation of unstimulated human oocyte–cumulus complexes with EGF significantly increases the percentage of metaphase-II oocytes suggesting that EGF can augment spontaneous maturation of immature oocytes.

Transforming growth factors (TGFs)

Transforming growth factor α (TGFα) is a 50-amino acid polypeptide with 30% sequence homology with EGF. TGFα interacts with the same receptors as EGF (Marquardt *et al.*, 1984). Therefore, TGFα probably affects the same cell types including epithelial cells that respond to EGF (Todaro, Fryling & De Larco, 1980).

Intrafollicular expression of TGFα has been localized to the theca interna (Kudlow *et al.*, 1987). Analysis with a molecular probe has demonstrated TGFα gene expression in theca cells (Skinner & Coffey, 1988). TGFα stimulates the growth of both granulosa and theca cells indicating that TGFα, produced by theca cells, has both paracrine and autocrine actions on cell proliferation within the growing follicle (Skinner *et al.*, 1987). The mode of TGFα action provides an example of a growth factor-mediated mesenchymal–epithelial cell interaction between theca- and granulosa cells.

TGFβs are known as multi-functional regulators of cell growth, differentiation and function which can either stimulate or inhibit cellular proliferation *in vitro* depending on the cell type and presence of other growth factors (Roberts *et al.*, 1988). TGFβs are disulphide-linked homodimeric 25 kDa peptides usually expressed in regions of epithelio-mesenchymal interaction (Derynck *et al.*, 1985). Each monomer consists of 112 amino acids (Flanders *et al.*, 1991). With the identification of mRNAs for three (TGFβ_1, β_2 and β_3) of the five TGFβs in cells of the mammalian ovary (Flanders *et al.*, 1991) the potential roles of TGFβs as intraovarian regulatory substances have become obvious. TGFβs 1, 2, 3 and 5 crossreact with the same receptor sites in many *in vitro* assays. Thus, TGFβ_1 inhibits the growth of endothelial cells more potently than TGFβ_2 (Jennings *et al.*, 1988), whereas TGFβ_3 appears to be active in induction of the mesoderm in certain animal species.

In addition to the five distinct TGFβs, there are peptides in the TGFβ supergene family recognized by their 30% to 40% amino acid homologies to the TGFβs (Flanders *et al.*, 1991). Most cells in culture produce TGFβ and possess TGFβ receptors, and TGFβs inhibit growth of most epithelial cells.

TGFα and TGFβ_1 can modulate the function of cells in every compartment of the ovarian follicle (i.e. oocyte–cumulus, granulosa, and theca–interstitium) Schomberg, 1988). TGFβ is present in the human follicular fluid (Ruegsegger, Veit & Assoian, 1988). Ovarian thecal/interstitial (Skinner *et al.*, 1987) and granulosa cells (Kim & Schomberg, 1989) are sites of TGFβ synthesis. Steroid synthesis in both cell types can be influenced by treatment with TGFβ *in vitro*. Thus TGFβ inhibits androgen synthesis and stimulates progesterone accumulation (Magoffin *et al.*, 1989), and it is a possible mediator of paracrine theca-granulosa cell interaction in the follicle wall. TGFβ may also increase production of FSH in the anterior pituitary (Ying *et al.*, 1986*a*), and potentiate FSH-mediated increase of LH receptor levels, aromatase activity, and progesterone production in cultured mouse (Adashi *et al.*, 1989*a,b*) and rat (Ying *et al.*, 1986*b*) granulosa cells.

In the rat, TGFβ stimulates meiotic maturation by accelerating germinal vesicle breakdown (Feng, Catt & Knecht, 1988). TGFβ has no effect on denuded oocytes, indicating that the effect is mediated by the surrounding cumulus cells. The accelerating effect of TGFβ on oocyte maturation can be inhibited by inhibitors of germinal vesicle breakdown, such as cAMP and hypoxanthine. TGFβ and other growth factors are potent *in vitro* stimulators of oocyte maturation, and they may participate in the selection of dominant follicle and meiotic maturation during follicular development (Feng *et al.*, 1988).

The sensitivity of the theca and interstitial cells to TGFβ action is enhanced by IGF-I (Magoffin, Candedo & Erickson, 1989). Granulosa cells produce factors which enhance thecal production of androgens, and TGFβ1 may play a role in this process (Magoffin *et al.*, 1989). This effect is not a function of cell number, because TGFβ does not have significant effects on granulosa cell number in the presence or absence of FSH (Feng, Catt & Knecht, 1986). TGFβ inhibits EGF-induced mitoses in granulosa cells (Skinner *et al.*, 1987). TGFβ does not alter FSH binding to granulosa cells, while a combination of FSH plus TGFβ gives a two- to four-fold increase in aromatase activity as compared to FSH alone. TGFβ can also increase FSH-stimulated progesterone production (Knecht, Feng & Catt, 1987). TGFβ_1 has turned to be a highly potent inhibitor (greater than 80%) of hCG hormonal action. Cellular radiolabelling studies of TGFβ_1-treated ovarian cells disclosed the accumulation of steroid intermediates proximal to the 17 α-hydroxylation step, suggesting that TGFβ_1 acts at the level of the steroidogenic enzyme 17 α-hydroxylase/17-20-lyase (Hernandez *et al.*, 1990).

TGFβs have an influence on the abundance and architecture of the extracellular matrix (Massagué, 1987). TGFβs may increase deposition of cell-adhesion proteins such as fibronectin, and they may also increase expression of integrin receptors in various mesenchymal and epithelial cell types (Roberts *et al.*, 1988). Granulosa cell differentiation is associated with reduced deposition of fibronectin (Skinner, McKeracher & Dorrington, 1985), and extracellular matrix has an influence on granulosa cell responsiveness to gonadotrophins *in vitro* (Amsterdam *et al.*, 1989). TGFβ inhibits synthesis of various proteases, such as plasminogen activator and collagenase, whereas it increases synthesis and secretion of plasminogen activator inhibitor and tissue inhibitor of metalloproteases (Roberts *et al.*, 1990*a,b*). Both these mechanisms indicate that TGFβ inhibits degradation of matrix proteins.

TGFβ is angiogenic in several *in vivo* assay systems (Roberts *et al.*, 1990*a,b*). Formation of new blood vessels is especially important in functioning of the placenta and in uterine cycling (Flanders *et al.*, 1991). TGFβ is chemotactic for fibroblasts (Postlethwaite *et al.*, 1987) and it increases synthesis of fibronectin and type I collagen (Ignotz & Massaqué, 1986). It is also a potent inhibitor of endothelial cell growth (Jennings *et al.*, 1988). Yet another function of TGFβ is related to its immunosuppressive action. TGFβ inhibits proliferation of both T- and B-lymphocytes and suppresses the secretion of IgG and IgM by B-cells even in the presence of IL-2 (Terranova *et al.*, 1991).

Fibroblast growth factors (FGFs)

FGFs control the proliferation and differentiation of mesodermal and neurecto-dermal cells (Burgess & Maciag, 1989). Basic FGF (bFGF) is abundant in ovaries, whereas acidic FGF (aFGF) is more restricted to brain and other neural tissues (Slack, 1989). Basic fibroblast growth factor is a 146-amino acid polypeptide which acts as a mitogen. Granulosa cell-derived bFGF may be active in an intraovarian autocrine loop concerned with the regulation of growth and maturation of the developing follicle and the corpus luteum. bFGF is thought to play a part as an angiogenic factor in the development of thecal vasculature in the preovulatory follicle and during luteal development (Gospadarowicz & Ferrera, 1989).

In the preovulatory follicle, bFGF effectively inhibits hCG-stimulated androgen synthesis and is also engaged in the local regulation of granulosa cell proliferation and differentiation. The locally derived bFGF may reduce androgen substrate for ovarian oestrogen production. In cultured rat granulosa cells bFGF is not a mitogen, but it inhibits induction of aromatase activity by FSH. It also inhibits FSH-mediated induction of LH receptors and FSH-stimulated progesterone synthesis (Baird & Hsueh, 1986). Therefore bFGF probably exerts autocrine regulatory actions on granulosa cell growth and differentiation. FGF is also an autocrine stimulator of growth of the germinal epithelium, in which TGFβ inhibits the FGF-supported growth (Gospodarowicz, Plouet & Fugii, 1989).

Platelet-derived growth factor (PDGF)

In combination with EGF and IGF-I, PDGF dose-dependently enhances proliferation. This combination also stimulates mitoses in granulosa cells (May, Frost & Bridge, 1990). PDGF causes an acute decrease in the high affinity binding of EGF to cell surface receptors and an increase in phosphorylation state of the EGF receptor at threonine 654. Human receptors for PDGF and EGF have been expressed in Chinese hamster ovary cells that otherwise lack endogenous receptors for these growth factors. In that system neither protein kinase C nor phosphorylation of EGF receptor at threonine 654 are required for the regulation of the apparent affinity of the EGF receptor by PDGF (Countaway, Northwood & Davis, 1989). PDGF and low density lipoprotein (LDL) have facilitative roles in growth factor-stimulated granulosa cell proliferation.

Inhibins and activins

Inhibins are gonadal peptides which suppress pituitary gonadotrophin secretion, preferentially FSH (Mason *et al.*, 1985). A family of structurally related peptides includes inhibin (α/βA), activin-A (βA/βA) and transforming growth factor-β1. There is significant structural homology (30–40%) between these peptides and members of a family of growth factors including TGFβ, mullerian inhibiting substance, decapentaplegic gene complex and vg1 protein, a mesoderm-inducing factor in frog embryos (Roberts *et al.*, 1988). Inhibin is a 32 kD glycoprotein first isolated from porcine ovarian follicular fluid (Ling *et al.*, 1985). It appears as two distinct forms composed of a common α-subunit and one of the two β-subunits βA and βB.

In human follicular fluid inhibin also exists as two major forms: inhibin A and inhibin B (Mason *et al.*, 1985; Mason, Niall & Seeburg, 1986). As in porcine follicular fluid, both are composed of two subunits, similar α-subunits and dissimilar β-subunits. The inhibin subunits are encoded by separate genes (Ling *et al.*, 1986; Mason *et al.*, 1985, 1986) whose expression in granulosa cells is regulated by FSH (Woodruff *et al.*, 1987). Secretion of inhibin by human (Tsonis, Hillier & Baird, 1987) and non-human primate granulosa cells (Hillier, 1991) is regulated by gonadotrophins and sex steroids *in vitro*, FSH stimulating inhibin production by the ovary (Buckler, Healy & Burger, 1989).

Activins are structurally related dimers of the β-subunits representing activin A and activin AB (Ling *et al.*, 1986). While both inhibins suppress the pituitary FSH secretion, the activins stimulate the same.

Besides having systemic endocrine effects, inhibins and activins are believed to subserve local regulatory functions within developing ovarian follicles (De Jongh, 1988; Burger & Findlay, 1989). Binding sites for activin have been demonstrated on granulosa cells (Sugino *et al.*, 1988). Inhibin (α/βA) enhances LH-stimulated androgen secretion in cultured ovarian thecal-interstitial cells and theca explants, whereas activin-A is inhibitory (Hsueh *et al.*, 1987). Inhibin suppresses and activin enhances FSH-stimulated aromatase activity in rat granulosa cells *in vitro* (Ying *et al.*, 1986*a,b*), whereas activin inhibits progesterone secretion and inhibin stimulates the LH-mediated thecal cell androstenedione production (Hsueh *et al.*, 1987; Hillier, 1991). Inhibin also suppresses oocyte maturation (O, Robertson & de Kretser, 1989).

The human preovulatory follicle does not secrete significant amounts of inhibin until the mid-cycle LH surge begins. This is also reflected in circulating inhibin levels which peak in the luteal phase (McLachlan *et al.*, 1987). Significant and sustained increase in peripheral inhibin concentrations occurs mostly during the luteal phase, and regulation of FSH secretion by inhibin occurs primarily in the luteal phase (Reddi *et al.*, 1990). There is no evidence of a primary defect in ovarian inhibin secretion in women with PCOS in terms of either basal or gonadotrophin-stimulated inhibin secretion (Buckler *et al.*, 1988).

In the corpus luteum, inhibin which has been shown to originate from LH/hCG stimulated granulosa-lutein cells (Smith *et al.*, 1992) may contribute to the paracrine modulation of androgen (and hence oestrogen) synthesis in the gland (Hillier *et al.*, 1992). Hillier and Miro (1993) have suggested that activin, acting at early stages of antral follicles, plays a role in follicular recruitment by sensitizing immature granulosa cells to the action of FSH, whereas inhibin is more likely to act in preovulatory follicular selection and maintenance of follicular dominance.

Leukocytes and cytokines

Immunoregulatory and growth factor-related peptides produced by resident leukocytes can modulate the growth and differentiation of diverse non-immunological cell types (Green, 1989). Unlike the testis, the ovary is not considered to be an immunologically privileged site (Adashi, 1990). In the ovary, the presence of large populations of tissue-bound leukocytes and dramatic changes in the specific localization of leukocyte populations within the ovary during different stages of the menstrual cycle have recently been reported (see below). Furthermore, in the rat ovary, the addition of leukocytes to the perfusate significantly increases the number of LH-induced ovulations *in vitro* (Hellberg *et al.*, 1991), suggesting an active role of these cells in the physiology of the ovary. Immunosuppressive mechanisms mediated by non-steroidal factors may also be involved in prevention of activation of the immune system by germ cell antigens and growth factors associated with germ cell proliferation and differentiation (Hedger *et al.*, 1990).

Macrophages are present as resident cells in most organs of the body, and they survive for a long time in tissue. They are important accessory cells in the regulation of lymphocyte proliferation and in the presentation of antigens. Their role in the ovary has been linked to the process of tissue remodelling at ovulation, luteinization and luteolysis, as they are well equipped for these remodelling events with their capacity to secrete cytokines, eicosanoids, vasoactive amines, and tissue remodelling enzymes.

Ovarian macrophage-like cells were first demonstrated in the rat (Bulmer, 1964) and in the guinea-pig (Paavola, 1979). Using specific F4/80 monoclonal antibodies and immunohistochemical staining macrophages were identified in the medullary region of the mouse ovary and in the theca layer of the ovarian follicle (Hume *et al.*, 1984). Monocytes which are undifferentiated precursor cells of the macrophages and tissue specific macrophages were identified in the rat ovary by immunohistochemical methods using antibodies ED1 and ED2, respectively (Brännström, Mayrhofer & Robertson, 1993*a*). These cells were primarily located in the medullary region of the ovary and also in the theca layer of the preovulatory follicle, where their density increased 5-fold at ovulation. A major proportion of the monocytes/macrophages expressed the major histocompatibility (MHC) class II antigen indicating an activated stage. In a subsequent study, Brännström *et al.* (1994*a*) have demonstrated that monocytes/macrophages are the major cell components of the corpus luteum during pregnancy in the rat and that the density of the activated cells increases at the time of luteolysis, indicating an active role of these cells in tissue remodelling during the luteolytic process. Studies on human ovarian tissue have shown the presence of a large number of macrophages in the follicle wall at ovulation (Brännström *et al.*, 1994*b*) and in the corpus luteum (Wang *et al.*, 1992*a*), with an increase towards the stage of luteolysis (Lei, Chegini & Rao, 1991)

An active role of monocytes/macrophages in ovulation is suggested by their ability to migrate towards the interior of the follicle and by their presence in the follicular fluid at oocyte retrieval for IVF (Loukides *et al.*, 1990; Castilla *et al.*, 1990). Moreover, CSF-1 deficient mice, with extremely low numbers of tissue macrophages, have significantly lowered ovulation rates (Robertson, personal communication). In co-incubation studies it has been demonstrated that macrophage-derived products stimulate progesterone production in human granulosa-lutein cells (Halme *et al.*, 1985) and in mouse granulosa cells (Kirsch *et al.*, 1981). This would facilitate ovulation, as progesterone is one of several mediators in this process. In addition, several macrophage-derived products such as plasminogen activator, collagenase, eicosanoids, platelet activating factor and cytokines could possibly directly facilitate the ovulatory process.

A role of macrophages in corpus luteum function is also possible, because macrophages have processes contacting several adjacent luteal cells suggesting cell to cell signalling (Adams & Hertig, 1969). Human peripheral monocytes and macrophages are capable of stimulating progesterone production by autologous luteinized granulosa cells derived from superovulated preovulatory follicles (Halme *et al.*, 1985). These results suggest that peritoneal macrophages may exert luteotrophic effects on granulosa cumulus cells. Macrophages may also be important in tissue degradation and remodelling at the time of luteolysis (Petrovska *et al.*, 1992; Brännström *et al.*, 1994*a*) supporting the initial finding of phagocytosis of luteal cells (Paavola, 1979).

Mast cells and their vasoactive mediator histamine seem to influence the ovulatory process. Mast cells are located around the larger blood vessels in the medulla region in the rat ovary (Jones, Duvall & Guilette, 1980) but are also observed in the thecal layer of the preovulatory follicle in the cow (Nakamura *et al.*, 1987). During ovulation, increased numbers of mast cells are seen in the rat ovary (Gayton *et al.*, 1992). The release of histamine at the time of ovulation is indicated by the decrease in ovarian content of histamine in the hamster ovary at follicular rupture (Krishna & Terranova, 1985) and by the observed degranulation of mast cells in the cow follicle (Nakamura *et al.*, 1987). Mast cells are not present within the corpus luteum tissue of the rat (Jones *et al.*, 1980) and their presence in the corpus luteum of other species has not been reported.

Eosinophilic granulocytes are traditionally considered to be involved mainly in allergic inflammation and in the defence against parasitic infections. The presence of eosinophils in the human ovary has not been studied in any depth. In the pig ovary, eosinophils are the most common leukocyte in the theca layer of the ovulating follicle (Staendert, Zamon & Chew, 1991) and they are also present in high numbers in the theca externa of the sheep follicle (Cavender & Murdoch, 1988). In the sheep ovary, the follicular secretion at ovulation of a specific chemo-attractant against eosinophils (Murdoch & McCormick, 1989) suggests that this leukocyte subtype is important in the ovulatory process or in early luteinization. Possible eosinophil-derived mediators in these events could be the described cationic and major basic proteins (Gleich & Adolphson, 1986), which could promote degradation of connective tissue of the follicle wall. Increased numbers of eosinophils have been observed in corpora lutea of sheep treated with a luteolytic dose of PGF2α (Murdoch, 1987). Cytotoxins released by the eosinophils could cause luteolysis (Murdoch, Steadman & Belden, 1988).

Neutrophilic granulocytes constitute the major proportion of leukocytes recruited into sites of inflammation or injury. These cells are important in the early events of inflammation through their capacity to secrete an array of enzymes and paracrine factors. In particular, collagenase, cytokines, eicosanoids, reactive oxygen metabolites, and platelet activating factor have been linked to tissue remodelling occurring during ovulation and the formation as well as the demise of the corpus luteum. By conventional histological techniques neutrophil-like cells were demonstrated in the ovary of the rabbit (Gerdes *et al.*, 1992) and the sheep (Cavender & Murdoch, 1988). In these studies a distinct preovulatory rise of cells in the theca layer was seen in the ovulating follicle. An immunohistochemical study on the rat ovary showed that the density of neutrophils was increased 3-fold in the medulla and 8-fold in the theca layer at ovulation (Brännström *et al.*, 1993*a*). Moreover, neutrophils were present in high numbers of the human follicle wall at ovulation (Brännström *et al.*, 1994*b*), in keeping with an earlier observation of a preovulatory rise in neutrophil chemotactic activity in human follicular fluid (Herriot, Warnes & Kerin, 1986). Recent studies on the presence of neutrophils in corpus luteum tissue have shown large populations of neutrophils present in the early corpus luteum of the pregnant rat (Brännström *et al.*, 1994*a*) with a decrease towards later stages. This cell type is abundant in the human corpus luteum of the menstrual cycle (Brännström *et al.*, 1994*b*).

Lymphocytes, consisting of two major cell-lineages, B- and T-lymphocytes, are the key cells in production of antibodies, cytotoxicity reactions and in modulating the immune response. Some lymphocytes are subject to steroidal signalling, indicated by detection of oestrogen receptors in certain T lymphocytes (Cohen *et al.*, 1983; Hill, Barbieri & Anderson, 1987). T-lymphocytes have been identified in human preovulatory follicular fluid (Hill *et al.*, 1987) and in the human preovulatory follicle wall (Brännström *et al.*, 1994*b*). Ovarian follicular fluid contains an increased ratio of T-suppressor CD8(+) to T-helper (CD4) cells as compared with peripheral blood (Hill *et al.*, 1987). Adoptive transfer experiments

Table 3. *Human cytokines (adapted from Hill1991)*

Cytokine	Abbreviation	Molecular weight (kd)	Cellular source
Interleukin-1 alpha	Il-1α	15–17	Macrophages, endothelial cells, large granular lymphocytes, **B** lymophocytes, fibroblasts, epithelial cells, astrocytes, keratinocytes, osteoblasts
Interleukin-1 beta	IL-1β	14–16	Macrophages, endothelial cells, large granular lymphocytes, **B** lymphocytes, fibroblasts, epithelial cells, astrocytes, keratinocytes, osteoblasts
Interleukin-2	IL-2	20	T lymphocytes
Interleukin-3	IL-3	20	T lymphocytes
Interleukin-4	IL-4	20	T lymphocytes
Interleukin-5	IL-5	20	T lymphocytes (mouse)
Interleukin-6	IL-6	22–29	Fibroblasts, T lymphocytes
Interleukin-7	IL-7	25	B-lineage cells
Interleukin-8 (or neutrophilactivation protein-1)	IL-8 (NAP-1)	8.4	Macrophages, T lymphocytes, monocytes, endothelial cells, mesangial cells, fibroblasts
Interferon-gamma	IFN-τ	40–50 (dimers of 20 and 24 kD form) (72 or 77 residues, dimer)	T lymphocytes, NK cells
Granulocyte macrophage-colony stimulating-factor	GM-CSF	22	T lymphocytes, endothelial cells, fibroblasts, macrophages
Macrophage-colony stimulating-factor	M-CSF (CSF-1)	47–76	Fibroblasts, monocytes, endothelial cells
Granulocyte-colony-stimulating-factor	G-CSF	19	Macrophages, fibroblasts
Tumour necrosis factor-alpha	TNF-α	17	Macrophages, T lymphocytes, thymocytes, B lymphocytes, NK cells
Tumour necrosis factor-beta (Lymphotoxin)	TNF-β (LT)	25	T lymphocytes

in rodents indicate that CD8(+) cells are required in the gonad for the preventions of autoimmunity (Strelkauskas *et al.*, 1978; Lipscomb *et al.*, 1979). Therefore the high proportion of CD8(+) cells suggests that active immunoregulation occurs in the human ovary to maintain ovarian self-tolerance (Hill, 1991). Cytokine homeostasis must be maintained in the developing follicle and corpus luteum, since overproduction of IFN-γ by activated T-cells can enhance the major histocompatibility complex (MHC) class I and induce MHC class II transplantation antigen expression on granulosa cells (Hill *et al.*, 1990). This may result in ovarian failure and disordered ovulation.

In the rat ovary, T-lymphocytes were present in much lower numbers than neutrophils and macrophages and no changes in their density were seen during the periovulatory period (Brännström *et al.*, 1993a). Some, yet unidentified, lymphocyte-derived products increase progesterone output from cultured granulosa cells of the pig (Hughes *et al.*, 1990), human (Emi *et al.*, 1991) and the rat (Hughes, Pringle & Gorospe, 1991).

Lymphocytes have also been localized in corpus luteum tissue. T-lymphocytes were initially discovered in rabbit corpora lutea of pregnancy, where they were present in numbers of about 10–20% of that of macrophages (Bagavandross *et al.*, 1991), and subsequent studies have shown low and constant numbers of these cells in the human corpus luteum of the menstrual cycle (Wang *et al.*, 1992a; Brännström *et al.*, 1994b) and in the rat corpus luteum of pregnancy (Brännström *et al.*, 1994a). We have not been able to detect any B-lymphocytes in human corpus luteum tissue, and there are extremely low numbers of natural killer lymphocytes (Brännström *et al.*, 1994b). Lymphocytes are rich sources of several cytokines, which have the capacity to influence the function of corpus luteum cells. There are indications that factors secreted by lymphocytes may work in a luteotrophic fashion, as demonstrated by the ability of these cells to stimulate steroidogenesis in luteinized human granulosa cells during coculture conditions (Emi *et al.*, 1991).

Interleukin-1 (IL-1) is a pleiotropic, pro-inflammatory cytokine produced by immune cells, endothelial cells, epithelial cells and fibroblasts (Table 3). IL-1 exists in two forms, IL-1α and IL-β, individually regulated products of different genes, but recognising the same cell surface receptors and thereby having identical biological activities. Among the immune cells, tissue macrophages secrete large amounts of IL-1 upon activation but this cytokine is also secreted by neutrophils, B-lymphocytes and natural killer cells (Dinarello, 1991). IL-1 interferes with the *in vitro* secretion of anterior pituitary hormones LH, FSH, thyrotrophin, GH and prolactin (Bernton *et al.*, 1987). The effects of IL-1 at the level of the ovary may depend on the differentiation status of the cells. An immunohistochemical study in the mouse ovary showed that the expression of IL-1 and IL-1 receptors during follicular development are confined to the theca-interstitial tissue, with the exception of very intense staining for the type 1 receptor in the cytoplasm and plasma membrane of the growing oocyte (Simon *et al.*, 1994*a*). The effects of IL-1 on undifferentiated granulosa and theca cells seem to be mainly inhibitory. IL-1β inhibits FSH-induced development of LH receptors, and suppresses oestradiol and progesterone secretion from undifferentiated rat granulosa cells (Gottschall *et al.*, 1988, 1989; Kasson & Gorospoe, 1989). In the pig, it was shown that IL-1 inhibits hCG-stimulated and basal progesterone production from granulosa cells of small follicles (Fukuoka *et al.*, 1987), while having a proliferative effect on the cells (Fukuoka *et al.*, 1989*a*). Thus, the ability of IL-1 to inhibit granulosa cell differentiation is inversely correlated to its ability to promote granulosa cell growth (Fukuoka *et al.*, 1989*a*). The antigonadotropic activity of IL-1 involves sites of action both proximal and distal to cAMP generation (Fukuoka *et al.*, 1989*b*). The effect of IL-1 on theca-interstitial cells of immature rats is also inhibitory, since it suppresses hCG-induced androgen production of these cells (Hurwitz *et al.*, 1991*a*). Intraovarian IL-1 may play a dual role in the developing ovarian follicle, by acting on both the granulosa and theca-interstitial cells, to inhibit differentiation and promote cell growth.

Significant amounts of IL-1 bioactivity (Khan *et al.*, 1988) and immunoreactivity (Watanabe *et al.*, 1994) have been detected in human follicular fluid of IVF patients. The circulating IL-1 levels are also elevated during the luteal phase of normally cycling women (Cannon & Dinarello, 1985). Furthermore, a complete IL-1 system, with its ligands, receptor and antagonist, has been identified in the human ovary (Hurwitz *et al.*, 1992). Several studies have indicated a crucial role of intraovarian IL-1 in the ovulatory process. The ovulating rat ovary produces IL-1 bioactivity (Brännström *et al.*, 1994*c*) and the mRNA for IL-1β increases 4-5 fold in the rat ovary at ovulation (Hurwitz *et al.*, 1991*b*). At this ovulatory stage, the expression of IL-1 is initially confined to the theca layer, but just before follicle rupture the expression of the receptor is also seen in the granulosa (Simon *et al.*, 1994*a*). Several *in vitro* studies on preovulatory ovarian cells and tissues have shown that IL-1 induces production of ovulatory mediators such as progesterone (Sjögren, Holmes & Hillensjö,1991; Brännström *et al.*, 1993*b*), prostaglandins (Brännström *et al.*, 1993*b*), and proteoglycanase (Hurwitz *et al.*, 1993). The strongest evidence for IL-1 as an ovulatory mediator is its capability to induce ovulation in the *in vitro* perfused rat (Brännström *et al.*, 1993*c*) and rabbit ovary (Takehara *et al.*, 1994), as well as the capacity of the IL-1 receptor antagonist to inhibit ovulation in the rat ovary *in vitro* (Simon *et al.*, 1994*b*). With immunohistochemical methods, IL-1 and its type 1 receptor have been localized in the granulosa luteal cells during the luteinization process (Simon *et al.*, 1994*a*). However, IL-1 seems to have no effect on luteal steroidogenesis (Wang *et al.*, 1991; Nothnick & Pate, 1990) while stimulating prostaglandin production (Nothnick & Pate, 1990). IL-1 activity in human pelvic macrophages is subject to hormonal regulation by gonadal steroids (Pacifii *et al.*, 1989). Low concentrations of progesterone upregulate macrophage IL-1 gene expression, whereas higher concentrations significantly inhibit IL-1 activity (Polan, Carding & Loukides, 1988).

Interleukin-6 is a 26 kD multifunctional cytokine important in the regulation of proliferation and function of lymphocytes and is an inducer of acute phase protein synthesis. IL-6 is produced by a variety of lymphohaematopoietic cells, such as T-lymphocytes, B-lymphocytes, and macrophages, as well as in other cells such as endothelial cells and fibroblasts. IL-6 mRNA was identified in the mouse ovary by *in situ* hybridization techniques and was localized close to the vasculature of the growing follicles (Motro *et al.*, 1990), supporting its role in angiogenesis. We found large quantities of IL-6 bioactivity being secreted from the perfused rat ovary with no detectable variations dependent on the stage of the ovary (Brännström *et al.*, 1994c). IL-6 may have a paracrine role in the regulation of steroidogenesis, as it was recently demonstrated that this cytokine is secreted by rat granulosa cells and that IL-6 inhibits FSH-induced progesterone production (Gorospe, Hughes & Spangelo, 1992). An inhibitory effect by IL-6 on bovine granulosa cell proliferation and FSH-induced oestradiol production was also recently reported (Alzipar & Spicer, 1993).

Tumor necrosis factor α (TNFα) was originally named after its oncolytic activity. *TNFα* is a 157-amino acid polypeptide with a molecular mass of 17 kDa under reducing conditions (Pennica *et al.*, 1984) and 45 kDa under non-reducing conditions (Aggarwal *et al.*, 1985). TNFα is a product of several different cell lineages, and it has a range of functions as a pleiotrophic regulator of growth, differentiation and function of immune- and non-immune cells in physiological as well as pathophysiological processes.

In the human ovary, TNFα immunoreactivity is localized to follicular and luteal compartments (Roby *et al.*, 1990). Immunoreactive TNFα appears in the healthy follicle at the time of antrum formation. In the corpus luteum, TNF α is found in the large lutein-like cells and paraluteal cells, and also in the cytoplasm of the small paraluteal cells (Terranova *et al.*, 1991). Messenger RNA of TNFα has been detected in rat ovaries (Sancho-Tello *et al.*, 1992) and its presence has been demonstrated in human follicular fluid (Wang *et al.*, 1992b), follicular fluid of cows (Zolti *et al.*, 1990), and in the perfusate of ovulating rat ovaries (Brännström *et al.*, 1994c).

In immature rats, TNFα attenuates differentiation of cultured granulosa cells through neutralization of FSH action at sites proximal to cAMP generation (Emoto & Baird, 1988). TNFα appears to act as an FSH antagonist as it inhibits

FSH-induced aromatization and accumulation of several progestagen species including progesterone, 20α-dehydroprogesterone, 5α-pregnanediol, and pregnanolone (Adashi *et al.*, 1989*a*; Adashi, 1990). TNFα inhibits FSH-stimulated cholesterol side chain cleavage and 3β-hydroxysteroid dehydrogenase/isomerase (Adashi, 1990; Adashi *et al.*, 1990). Both theca and granulosa cells are targets of TNFα. In the human granulosa-luteal cells, TNFα enhances hCG-stimulated progesterone production, probably through increased hCG binding (Terranova *et al.*, 1991), and it stimulates prostaglandin production (Wang *et al.*, 1992*b*).

TNFα may also regulate the androgen-producing theca interstitial cells. Treatment with increasing concentrations of TNFα inhibits hCG-induced accumulation of androsterone by modulating the activity of steroidogenic enzyme 17α-hydoxylase/17:201yase (Andreani *et al.*, 1991).

Recent studies suggest that TNFα is involved in the ovulatory process. TNFα is expressed in the preovulatory follicle (Chen *et al.*, 1993) and the ovulating *in vitro* perfused rat ovary secretes TNFα like bioactivity (Brännström *et al.*, 1994*c*). TNFα immunoreactivity is present in human follicular fluid (Wang *et al.*, 1992*b*) and there is a preovulatory rise of bioactive TNFα in bovine follicular fluid (Zolti *et al.*, 1990). This cytokine also has the capacity to induce follicular production of the ovulatory mediators progesterone and prostaglandins (Brännström *et al.*, 1993*b*; Roby & Terranova, 1989). TNFα enhances hCG-stimulated progesterone production by granulosa cells, probably by increasing hCG binding (Terranova *et al.*, 1991). A direct ovulation-promoting effect at the ovarian level was demonstrated by the ability of TNFα to enhance the LH-induced ovulation rate in the *in vitro* perfused rat ovary (Brännström, Wang & Norman, 1992).

TNFα has been suggested to be one of several luteolytic factors. Immunoreactive TNFα is present in the corpus luteum of several species (Roby & Terranova, 1989) and the secretion of bioactive TNFα has been demonstrated from lipopolysacharide-stimulated regressing rabbit corpus luteum (Bagavandoss *et al.*, 1991). Moreover, TNFα inhibits progesterone synthesis of bovine corpora lutea cells, while stimulating prostaglandin secretion (Fairchild, Benyo & Pate, 1992). *In vivo* experiments in the pig have shown that locally administered TNFα induces functional luteolysis (Wuttke, 1993).

Interferons (IFNs) are a heterogeneous group of peptides with antiviral, antiproliferative and immunoregulatory actions (Pestka, 1983). IFN-γ inhibits the FSH-induced steroidogenesis and LH-receptor formation of rat granulosa cells *in vitro,* with IFNα having no effect (Gorospe, Tuchel & Kasson, 1988). This finding was later extended to show that recombinant IFNγ inhibits FSH-induced inhibin secretion from undifferentiated granulosa cells of the rat (Xiao & Findlay, 1992). IFN-γ has an inhibitory effect on progesterone production by human luteal cells stimulated by hCG (Wang *et al.*, 1992*c*) and in luteinized human granulosa cells after controlled superovulation for IVF (Fukuoka *et al.*, 1992). The cellular origin of IFNs in the ovary and their mechanisms of action are presently unknown.

Prostaglandins and leukotrienes

Ovulation

There is abundant evidence suggesting that prostaglandins are critically involved in the process of ovulation. In several species both the granulosa and theca cells produce prostaglandins in response to LH, and inhibitors of prostaglandin synthesis can inhibit follicular rupture through a local mechanism in the ovarian follicle. There are conflicting reports in the literature as to which of the prostaglandins is the most important for ovulation, and there are species differences in this respect. The mechanisms by which prostaglandins exert their ovulatory effects are not clear. There may be several prostaglandin-induced alterations operating simultaneously, such as the effects on follicular microcirculation, chemotactic effects on leukocytes, effects on follicular steroidogenesis, plasminogen activator, collagen breakdown, and on neuromuscular mechanisms. In addition, prostaglandins may cause a release of oxygen-free radicals and be related to other compounds of an inflammation-like reaction, such a bradykinin and histamine. The role of prostaglandins in ovulation has recently been reviewed by Brännström and Janson (1991) and by Wallach and Dharmarajan (1992).

Leukotrienes are formed from arachidonic acid by the action of lipoxygenase enzymes, the activities of which have been detected in the rat ovary and in human granulosa cells. The involvement of lipoxygenase products in ovulation in rats was deduced from the findings that hCG significantly increased follicular lipoxygenase activity, and a non-specific lipoxygenase inhibitor reduced ovulation upon intrabursal injection (Reich *et al.*, 1983). Other experiments in rats have failed to show any effect of a lipoxygenase inhibitor on ovulation (Tanaka *et al.*, 1991), and a recent report described an increased rate of ovulations in rabbits, possibly by diverting arachidonic acid from the lipoxygenase pathway (Hellberg *et al.*, 1990). Although the role of leukotrienes for ovulation is still unclear, these compounds deserve further attention. For example, in the rat, lipoxygenase inhibitors have been shown to inhibit collagenolysis induced by hCG and to suppress ovarian content of neutrophil leukocytes. Furthermore, leukotrienes C4 and D4 have been shown to stimulate human endothelial cells to synthesize platelet activating factor, which has been shown to be of importance for ovulation in the rat. Leukotriene B4 can induce chemotaxis of leukocytes in inflamed tissues (Espey, Tanaka & Okamura, 1989*a*) and other lipoxygenase products have been shown to promote endothelial proliferation and angiogenesis (Tanaka *et al.,* 1989). Recent reviews on lipoxygenase products and ovulation have been published by Brännström and Janson (1991) and by Espey (1992).

Corpus luteum function

It is well established that the steroid-producing function of the corpus luteum is highly dependent on LH/hCG stimulation, but spontaneous regression of the gland cannot be explained simply by inadequate gonadotrophin stimulation. Prostaglandin F2α is involved in this altered luteal cell responsiveness to LH. In several domestic animal species it appears that luteolysis is induced by prostaglandin F2α released by the oestrogen-primed, non-pregnant uterus in response to luteal oxytocin (Auletta & Flint, 1988). Prostaglandin F2α acts as a luteolysin by blocking the luteotrophic actions of LH, possibly either by inducing loss of LH receptors or by inhibiting the gonadotrophin delivery to luteal cells (Behrman *et al.,* 1978), or perhaps by interfering with post-receptor signalling (Thomas, Dorflinger & Behrman, 1978). In women and non-human primates the luteolytic process is independent of the uterus, and a theory has been put forward that functional luteolysis in the human is preprogrammed at the cellular level and luteal regression occurs by default in the absence of luteal rescue by hCG in early pregnancy (Fisch *et al.,* 1988).

Other lines of evidence suggest, however, a paracrine and/or autocrine mechanism for the initiation of luteal regression also in the human; prostaglandin F2α is produced locally in the ovary (Patwardhan & Lanthier, 1985), the luteal cells contain receptors for this prostaglandin (Powell, Hammarström & Samuelsson, 1979), and prostaglandin F2α has been shown to inhibit basal and hCG stimulated progesterone synthesis in the corpus luteum both *in vitro* (Dennefors, Sjögren & Hamberger, 1982) and *in vivo* (Bennegård *et al.,* 1992). The human corpus luteum has also been reported to secrete oxytocin and to have oxytocin receptors (Fuchs *et al.,* 1990). A recent study by Bennegård *et al.* (1992) strongly indicates an autocrine and/or paracrine mechanism involving both oxytocin and prostaglandin F2α in regression of the human corpus luteum. When injected locally into the corpus luteum of women with normal menstrual cycles, oxytocin caused a rise in prostaglandin F2α metabolites coinciding with a fall in serum progesterone level. This response was completely abolished by an inhibitor of prostaglandin synthesis, indicating that the luteolytic effect of oxytocin is prostaglandin-mediated. Other paracrine/autocrine factors are also likely to be involved in luteolysis. For example, reactive oxygen species are generated by luteal cells responding to stimulation by LH. Such locally produced oxygen radicals may act directly to abolish luteal progesterone synthesis and luteal responsiveness to LH (Behrman, Alen & Pepperell, 1991).

Histamine

As a part of the inflammation-like reaction of preovulatory follicles in response to gonadotrophin stimulation there is release of histamine originating from mast cells around the ovarian vessels (Krishna & Terranova, 1985; Schmidt, Owman & Sjöberg, 1988). Histamine has been reported to induce ovulation in *in vitro* perfused rabbit and rat ovaries (Schmidt, Owman & Sjöberg, 1986), and antihistamines (both H1 and H2 receptor antagonists) can block ovulation in rat ovaries (Schmidt *et al.*, 1986). These findings, indicating that histamine is a paracrine mediator of the process of ovulation, are contradicted by the observations in rabbits (Kitai *et al.*, 1985; Yoshimura & Wallach, 1987) and sheep (Halterman & Murdoch, 1986), in which antihistamines failed to inhibit ovulation. Furthermore, other studies using indomethacin have suggested that the action of prostaglandins and histamine are not interdependent in the ovulatory process (Kitai *et al.*, 1985; Schmidt *et al.*, 1986). Thus, the role of histamine in ovulation needs further clarification.

Bradykinin

Several studies have shown that there is an increase in kinin-forming enzymes in the ovary during ovulation (Smith & Perks, 1983; Espey *et al.*, 1989*b*). Like histamine, vasoactive bradykinin induces ovulation in perfused rabbit ovaries (Yoshimura *et al.*, 1988) and potentiates the effect of LH on ovulation in perfused rat ovaries (Brännström & Hellberg, 1989). The mechanism by which bradykinin affects ovulation may involve mediation by prostaglandins, since it has been shown that kinin activates phospholipase A_2 (Espey *et al.*, 1989*b*) and stimulates formation of ovarian prostaglandins F2α and I_2 (Yoshimura *et al.*, 1988; Hellberg *et al.*, 1991).

Miscellaneous substances

Alpha 2-macroglobulin

Alpha 2-macro-globulin (α-2M) is a broad spectrum protease inhibitor which functions as a carrier of specific growth factors, activin and cytokines including TGFβ, bFGF, IL-1, IL-6. Before ovulation, α-2M mRNA is not detectable in granulosa cells and it appears in luteinizing follicles 12 hours after injection of an ovulatory dose of hCG and is maintained in the corpus luteum. The changes in α-2M mRNA in follicles or developing corpus luteum do not reflect the amount of α-2M protein present in the follicles, as the protein (188K monomer) is present in small antral and preovulatory follicles even though mRNA is not detectable (Gaddy-Kurten *et al.*, 1989).

Prorenin

Prorenin is present at high concentrations in preovulatory follicular fluid. Its biosynthesis and secretion from the ovary are regulated by gonadotrophins (Itskovitz *et al.*, 1991). Renin is probably derived from the granulosa cell.

Relaxin

This polypeptide is composed of α- and β chains derived by posttranslational cleavage from preprorelaxin. There are two relaxin genes, H1 and H2, in the human genome encoding different amino acid sequences. In addition to the ovary, relaxin is produced in decidualized endometrium and the trophoblast. Human corpus luteum transcribes the H2 relaxin gene, whereas the H1 gene is expressed in decidua (Hansell, Bryant-Greenwood & Greenwood, 1991). An intra-ovarian role of relaxin before ovulation is suggested by several findings. The preovulatory pig follicle secretes relaxin (Bryant-Greenwood *et al.*, 1989), and LH stimulates relaxin secretion from cultured pig granulosa cells (Loeken *et al.*, 1983). In addition, a recent study has shown that theca cells release relaxin and this release is increased prior to ovulation (Evans *et al.*, 1983). Relaxin may be important in tissue remodelling in the follicular wall at ovulation, as it increases granulosa cell production of collagen-degrading enzymes, plasminogen activator and collagenase *in vitro* (Too, Bryant-Greenwood & Greenwood, 1984) and stimulates thecal collagenolytic activity in the human follicle wall (Norström & Tjugum, 1986). This is also indicated by a study demonstrating that recombinant human relaxin induces ovulations in the *in vitro* perfused rat ovary (Brännström & MacLennan, 1993).

Acknowledgements

Original studies were supported by grants from the Academy of Finland, the University of Helsinki and the Nordisk Forsknings komitté.

References

Adams EC, Hertig AT. Studies on the human corpus luteum. I. Observations of the ultra structure of development and regression of the luteal cells during the menstrual cycle. *J Cell Biol* 1969; **41**: 696-715.

Adashi EY. the potential relevance of cytokines to ovarian physiology: the emerging role of resident ovarian cells of the white blood series. *Endocrine Rev* 1990; **11**: 434–64.

Adashi EY, Resnick CE, D'Ercole AJ, Svoboda M, Van Wyk JJ. Insulin-like growth factors as intraovarian regulators of granulosa cell growth and function. *Endocr Rev* 1985; **6**: 400–20.

Adashi EY, Resnick CE, Croft C, Payne D. Tumor necrosis factor α inhibits gonadotropin hormonal action in nontransformed ovarian granulosa cells. *J Biol Chem* 1989*a*; **264**: 11591–7.

Adashi EY, Resnick CE, Hernandez ER, May JV, Purchio AF, Twardzik DR. Ovarian transforming growth factor-β (TGF-β): Cellular site(s) and mechanism(s) of action. *Mol Cell Endocrinol* 1989*b*; **61**: 247–56.

Adashi EY, Resnick CE, Packman JN, Hurwitz A, Payne DE. Cytokine-mediated regulation of ovarian function: tumor necrosis factor alpha inhibits gonadotropin-supported progesterone accumulation by differentiating and luteinized murine granulosa cells. *Am J Obstet Gynecol* 1990; **164**: 889–99.

Adashi EY, Resnick CE, Hurwitz A, Ricciarelli E, Hernandez ER, Rosenfield RG. Ovarian granulosa cell-derived insulin-like growth factor binding proteins: modulatory role of follicle-stimulating hormone. *Endocrinology* 1991; **128**: 754–60.

Adashi EY, Resnick CE, Ricciarelli E, Hurwitz A, Kokia E, Botero L, Tedeschi C, Hernandez ER, Koistinen R, Rutanen EM, Seppälä M. Local tissue modification of follicle stimulating hormone action. In: Genazzani AR, Petraglia F, eds. *Hormones in Gynecological Endocrinology*. Carnfors, UK: Parthenon Publishing, 1992: 255–60.

Aggarwal BB, Kohr, WJ, Hass PE, Moffat B, Spencer SA, Henzel WJ, Bringham TS, Nedwin GE, Goeddel DV, Harkins RN. Human tumor necrosis factor production, purification and characterization. *J Biol Chem* 1985; **260**: 2345–54.

Alitalo T, Kontula K, Koistinen R, Aalto-Setälä K, Julkunen M, Jänne OA, Seppälä M, de la Chapelle A. The gene encoding human low-molecular weight insulin-like factor binding protein (IGF-BP25): regional localization to 7p12-p13 and description of a DNA polymorphism. *Hum Genet* 1989; **83**: 335–8.

Alpizar E, Spicer LJ. Effects of interleukin-6 on proliferation and FSH-induced estradiol production by bovine granulosa cells *in vitro*: dependence on size of follicle. *Biol Reprod* 1993; **49**: 38–43.

Amsterdam A, Rotmensch S, Furman A, Venter EA, Vlodavsky I. Synergistic effect of human chorionic gonadotropin and extracellular matrix on *in vitro* differentiation of human granulosa cells: progesterone production and gap junction formation. *Endocrinology* 1989; **124**: 1956–64.

Andreani CL, Payne DW, Packman JN, Resnick CE, Hurwitz A, Adashi EY. Cytokine-mediated regulation of ovarian function. *J Biol Chem* 1991; **266**: 6761–6.

Angervo M, Koistinen R, Suikkari A-M, Seppälä M. Insulin-like growth factor binding protein-1 inhibits the DNA amplification induced by insulin-like growth factor I in human granulosa-luteal cells. *Hum Reprod* 1991; **6**: 770–3.

Angervo M, Koistinen R, Seppälä M. Epidermal growth factor stimulates production of insulin-like growth factor binding protein-1 in human granulosa-luteal cells. *J Endocrinol* 1992; **134**: 127–31.

Armstrong DT. Local regulation of corpus luteum development and function. In: Coelingh Bennink HJT *et al.*, eds. *Local regulation of ovarian function.* An Eric K Fernström Symposium. Parthenon Publishing 1992; 211–32.

Auletta FJ, Flint APF. Mechanisms controlling corpus luteum function in sheep, cows, non-human primates and in women especially in relation to the time of luteolysis. *Endocrine Rev* 1988; **9**: 88–105.

Bagavandross P, Wiggins RC, Kunkel SL, Remick DG, Keyes PL. Tumor necrosis factor production and accumulation of inflammatory cells in the corpus luteum of pseudopregnancy and pregnancy in rabbits. *Biol Reprod* 1991; **42**: 367–76.

Baird A, Hsueh AJW. Fibroblast growth factor as an intraovarian hormone: differential regulation of steroidogenesis by an angiogenic factor. *Regul Pept* 1986; **16**: 243–50.

Barbieri RL, Makris A, Randall RW, Daniels G, Kistner RW, Ryan KJ. Insulin stimulates androgen accumulation in incubation of ovarian stroma obtained from women with hyperandrogenism. *J Clin Endocrinol Metab* 1986; **62**: 904–10.

Behrman HR, Grinwich DL, Hicheno M, McDonald GJ. Effect of hypophysectomy, prolactin and $PGF_{2\alpha}$ on LH and prolactin-binding *in vivo* and *in vitro* in the corpus luteum. *Endocrinology* 1978; **103**: 349–447.

Behrman HR, Alen RF, Pepperell JR. Cell-to-cell interactions in luteinization and luteolysis. In: Hillier SG, ed. *Ovarian Endocrinology.* Blackwell Scientific Publications. 1991; 190–225.

Bell SC, Keyte JW. N-terminal amino acid sequence of human pregnancy-associated endometrial alpha-1 globulin, an endometrial insulin-like growth factor (IGF) binding protein – evidence for two small molecular weight IGF binding proteins. *Endocrinology* 1988; **123**: 1202–4.

Bendell JJ, Dorrington JH. Epidermal growth factor influences growth and differentiation of rat granulosa cells. *Endocrinology* 1990; **127**: 533–40.

Bennegård B, Hahlin M, Hamberger L. Oxytocin and prostaglandin $F_{2\alpha}$ in human luteolysis. In: Coelingh Bennink HJT *et al.*, *Local regulation of ovarian function.* An Eric K Fernström Symposium. Parthenon Publishing 1992, 323–26.

Bergh C, Carlsson B, Olsson JH, Billig H, Hillensjo T. Effects of insulin-like growth factor I and growth hormone in cultured human granulosa cells. *Ann NY Acad Sci* 1991*a*; 626: 169–76.

Bergh C, Olsson JH, Hillensjo T. Effect of insulin-like growth factor I on steroidogenesis in cultured human granulosa cells. *Acta Endocrinol* 1991*b*; 125: 177–85.

Bernton EW, Beach JE, Holaday JW, Smallridge R, Fein HG. Release of multiple hormones by a direct action of interleukin-1 on pituitary cells. *Science* 1987; **238**: 519–21.

Brännström M. Inhibitory effect of mifepristone (RU 486) on ovulation in the isolated perfused rat ovary. *Contraception* 1993; **48**: 393–402.

Brännström M, Hellberg P. Bradykinin potentiates LH-induced follicular rupture in the rat ovary perfused *in vitro*. *Hum Reprod* 1989; **4**: 475–81.

Brännström M, Janson PO. Progesterone is a mediator in the ovulatory process in the *in vitro* perfused rat ovary. *Biol Reprod* 1989; **40**: 1170–7.

Brännström M, Janson PO. The biochemistry of ovulation. In: Hillier SG, ed. *Ovarian Endocrinology*. Blackwell Scientific Publications, 1991; 133–66.

Brännström M, MacLennan AH. Relaxin induces ovulation in the *in vitro* perfused rat ovary. *Hum Reprod* 1993; **8**: 1011–14.

Brännström M, Wang L, Norman RJ. Stimulatory effects of cytokines on the ovulatory process in the rat ovary perfused *in vitro*. *Proc 35th Annual Meeting of the Endocrine Society of Australia* 1992 p. 121 (abstract).

Brännström M, Mayrhofer G, Robertson S. Localization of leukocyte subsets in the rat ovary during the periovulatory period. *Biol Reprod* 1993*a*; **48**: 277–86.

Brännström M, Wang L, Norman RJ. Effects of cytokines on prostaglandin production and steroidogenesis of rat preovulatory follicles *in vitro*. *Biol Reprod* 1993*b*; **48**: 165–71.

Brännström M, Wang L, Norman RJ. Ovulatory effect of interleukin-1β on the rat ovary perfused *in vitro*. *Endocrinology* 1993*c*; **132**: 399–404.

Brännström M, Giesecke L, van den Heuvel CJ, Moore IC, Robertson SA. Leukocyte subpopulations in the rat corpus luteum during pregnancy and pseudopregnancy. *Biol Reprod* 1994*a*; **50**: 1161–7.

Brännström M, Pascoe V, Norman RJ, McClure N. Localization of leukocytye subsets in the human follicle wall and in the corpus luteum throughout the menstrual cycle. *Fertil Steril* 1994*b*; **61**: 488–495.

Brännström M, Norman RJ, Seamark RF, Robertson SA. Rat ovary produces cytokines during ovulation. *Biol Reprod* 1994*c*; **50**: 88–94.

Brissenden JE, Ullrich A, Francke U. Human chromosomal mapping of genes for insulin-like growth factors I and II and epidermal growth factors. *Nature, London* 1984; **310**: 781–4.

Bryant-Greenwood GD, Jeffrey R, Ralph MM, Seamark RF. Relaxin production by the porcine ovarian Graafian follicle *in vitro*. *Biol Reprod* 1989; **23**: 792–800.

Buckler HM, McLachlan RI, MacLachlan VB, Healy DL, Burger HG. Serum inhibin levels on polycystic ovary syndrome: basal levels and response to luteinizing hormone-releasing hormone agonist and exogenous gonadotrophin administration. *J Clin Endocrinol Metab* 1988; **66**: 798–803.

Buckler HM, Healy DL, Burger HG. Purified FSH stimulates production of inhibin by the human ovary. *J Endocrinol* 1989; **122**: 279–85.

Bulmer D. The histochemistry of ovarian macrophages in the rat. *J Anat* 1964; **98**: 313–19.

Burger HG, Findlay JK. Potential relevance of inhibin to ovarian physiology. *Semin Reprod Endocrinol* 1989; **7**: 69–78.

Burgess WH, Maciag T. The heparin-binding (fibroblast) growth factor family of proteins. *Annu Rev Biochem* 1989; **58**: 575–606.

Cannon JG, Dinarello CA. Increased plasma interleukin-1 activity in women after ovulation. *Science* 1985; **227**: 1247–9.

Carlsson B, Bergh C, Bentham J, Olsson JH, Norman MR, Billig H, Roos P, Hillensjo T. Expression of functional growth hormone receptors in human granulosa cells. *Hum Reprod* 1992; **7**: 1205–9.

Castilla JA, Sampalo A, Molina R, Samaniego F, Mozas J, Vergara F, Garrido F, Herruzo AJ. Mononuclear cell subpopulations in human follicular fluid from stimulated cycles. *Am J Immunol Reprod* 1990; **22**: 127–9.

Cavender JL, Murdoch WJ. Morphological studies of the microcirculatory system of periovulatory ovine follicles. *Biol Reprod* 1988; **39**: 989–97.

Chen H, Marcinkiewicz JL, Sancho-tello M, Hunt JS, Terranova PF. Tumor necrosis factor α gene expression in mouse oocytes and follicular cells. *Biol Reprod* 1993; **48**: 707–14.

Chrisman GM, Randolph JF, Peegel H, Menon KM. Differential responsiveness of luteinized human granulosa cells to gonadotropins and insulin-like growth factor I for induction of aromatase activity. *Fertil Steril* 1991; **55**: 1099–105.

Cohen JHM, Danel L, Cordier G, Saez S, Revillard JP. Sex steroid receptors in peripheral T cells: absence of androgen receptors and restriction of estrogen receptors to OKT8-positive cells. *J Immunol* 1983; **131**: 2767–71.

Conover CA, Lee PDK. Insulin regulation of insulin-like growth factor-binding protein production in cultured Hep G2 cells. *J Clin Endocrinol Metab* 1990; **70**: 1062–7.

Countaway JL, Northwood IC, Davis RJ. Mechanism of phosphorylation of the epidermal growth factor receptor at threonine 669. *J Biol Chem* 1989; **264**: 10828–35.

Davoren JB, Hsueh A-JW. Growth hormone increases ovarian levels of immunoreactive somatomedin-C/insulin-like growth factor 1 *in vivo*. *Endocrinology* 1986; **118**: 888–90.

De Jong FH. Inhibin. *Physiol Rev* 1988; **68**: 555–607.

Dennefors B, Sjögren A, Hamberger L. Progesterone and adenosine 3-5' monosphoshate formation by isolated human corpora lutea of different ages; influence of human chorionic gonadotropin and prostaglandins. *J Clin Endocrinol Metab* 1982; **55**: 102–10.

Derynck R, Jarrett JA, Chen EY, Eaton DH, Bell JR, Assoian RK, Roberts AB, Sporn MB, Goeddel DV. Human transforming growth factor-beta cDNA sequence and expression in tumor cell lines. *Nature London,* 1985; **316**: 4377–9.

Dinarello CA. Interleukin-1 and interleukin-1 antagonism. *Blood* 1991; **77**: 1627–35.

Dor J, Costritschi N, Pariente C, Rabinovici J, Maschiach S, Lunenfeld B, Kaneti H, Seppälä M, Koistinen R, Karasik A. Insulin-like growth factor-I and follicle-stimulating hormone suppress insulin-like growth factor binding protein-1 secretion by human granulosa-luteal cells. *J Clin Endocrinol Metab* 1992; **74**: 539–42.

Drop SLS, Brinkman A, Kortleve DJ, Groffen CAH, Schuller A, Zwarthoff EC. The evolution of the insulin-like growth factor binding protein family. In: Spencer EM, ed. *Modern Concepts of Insulin-Like Growth Factors.* New York: Elsevier, 1991: 311.

Eden JA, Jones J, Carter GD, Alaghband-Zadeh J. A comparison of follicular fluid levels of insulin-like growth factor I in normal dominant and cohort follicles, polycystic and multicystic ovaries. *Clin Endocrinol* 1988; **29**: 327–35.

Eden JA, Jones J, Carter GD, Alaghband-Zadeh J. Follicular fluid concentrations of insulin-like growth factor I, epidermal growth factor, transforming growth factor-alpha and sex-steroids in volume matched normal and polycystic human follicles. *Clin Endocrinol* 1990; **32**: 395–405.

El-Roeiy A, Chen X, Roberts VJ, LeRoith D, Roberts CT, Yen SSC. Expression of insulin-like growth factor-I (IGF-I) and IGF-II and the IGF-I, IGF-II, and insulin receptor genes and localization of the gene products in the human ovary. *J Clin Endocrinol Metab* 1993; **77**: 1411–18.

El-Roiey A, Roberts VJ, Shimasaki S, Ling N, Yen SSC. Localization and expression of insulin-like growth factor binding proteins (IGFBPs) 1-6 in normal and polycystic (PCO) human ovaries. *Proc 48th Annual Meeting of the American Fertility Society,* November 2-5, 1992. Abstract No. 0-020.

Emi N, Kanzaki H, Yoshida M, Takakura K, Kariya M, Okamoto N, Imai K, Mori T. Lymphocytes stimulate progesterone production by cultured human granulosa luteal cells. *Am J Obstet Gynecol* 1991; **165**: 1469–74.

Emoto N, Baird A. The effect of tumor necrosis factor/cachectin on follicle-stimulating hormone-induced aromatase-activity in cultured rat granulosa cells. *Biochem Biophys Res Commun* 1988; **153**: 792–8.

Erickson GF, Magoffin DA, Dyer CA, Hofeditz C. The ovarian androgen producing cells: a review of structure/function relationships. *Endocr Rev* 1985; **6**: 371–99.

Erickson GF, Garzo VG, Magoffin DA. Insulin-like growth factor-I regulates aromatase activity in human granulosa and granulosa luteal cells. *J Clin Endocrinol Metab* 1989; **69**: 716–24.

Erickson GF, Magoffin DA, Cragun JR, Chang RJ. The effects of insulin and insulin-like growth factors-I and II on estradiol production by granulosa cells of polycystic ovaries. *J Clin Endocrinol Metab* 1990; **70**: 894–902.

Espey LL. Ovulation as an inflammatory process. In: Coelingh Bennink HJT *et al.*, eds. *Regulation of Ovarian Function*. An Eric K Fernström Symposium. Parthenon Publishing 1992, 183–200.

Espey LL, Tanaka N, Okamura H. Increase in ovarian leukotrienes during hormonally induced ovulation in the rat. *Am J Physiol* 1989*a*; **256**: E753–9.

Espey LL, Tanaka N, Wihu V, Okamura H. Increase in ovarian kallikrein activity during ovulation in the gonadotrophin-primed immature rat. *J Reprod Fertil* 1989*b*; **87**: 503–8.

Evans G, Wathes DC, King GJ, Armstrong DT, Porter DG. Changes in relaxin production by the theca during the preovulatory period of the pig. *J Reprod Fertil* 1983; **69**: 677–83.

Fairchild, Benyo D, Pate JL. Tumor necrosis factor α alters bovine luteal cell capacity and viability. *Endocrinology* 1992; **130**: 854–60.

Feng P, Catt KJ, Knecht M. Transforming growth factor β regulates the inhibitory actions of epidermal growth factor during granulosa cell differentiation. *J Biol Chem* 1986; **261**: 14167–70.

Feng P, Knecht M, Catt K. Hormonal control of epidermal growth factor receptors by gonadotrophins during granulosa cell differentiation. *Endocrinology* 1987; **120**: 1121–6.

Feng P, Catt K, Knecht M. Transforming growth factor-beta stimulates meiotic maturation of the rat oocyte. *Endocrinology* 1988; **122**: 181–6.

Findlay JK. The ovary. *Baill Clin Endocrinol Metab* 1991; **5**: 755–69.

Findlay KK, Risbridger GP. Intragonadal control mechanisms. *Baill Clin Endocrinol Metab* 1987; **1**: 223–43.

Fisch B, Margara RA, Winston RML, Hillier SG. Cellular basis of luteal steroidogenesis in the human ovary. *J Endocrinol* 1988; **122**: 303–11.

Flanders KC, Marascalco BA, Roberts AB, Sporn MB. Transforming growth factor β: a multifunctional regulatory peptide with actions in the reproductive system. In: Schomberg DW, ed. *Growth Factors in Reproduction*. New York: Springer-Verlag, 1991: 23–37.

Franchimont P. Paracrine control. *Baill Clin Endocrinol Metab* 1986; **15**: ix–xiii.

Fuchs A-R, Behrens O, Helmer H, Vangstad A, Ivanisevic M, Grifo J, Barros C, Fields M. Oxytocin and vasopressin binding sites in human and bovine ovaries. *Am J Obstet Gynecol* 1990; **163**: 1961–5.

Fukuoka M, Mori T, Taii S, Yasuda K. Interleukin-1 inhibits luteinization of porcine granulosa cells in culture. *Endocrinology* 1987; **122**: 367–9.

Fukuoka M, Yasuda K, Taii S, Takakura K, Miro T. Interleukin stimulates growth and inhibits progesterone secretion in cultures of porcine granulosa cells. *Endocrinology*, 1989*a*; **124**: 884–90.

Fukuoka M, Taii S, Yasuda K, Takakura K, Mori T. Inhibitory effects of interleukin-1 of LH-stimulated adenosine 3,5-monophosphate accumulation by cultured porcine granulosa cells. *Endocrinology* 1989*b*; **125**: 136–43.

Fukuoka M. Yashuda K, Emi N, Fujiwara H, Iwai M, Takakura K, Kanzaki H, Mori T. Cytokine modulation of progesterone and estradiol secretion in cultures of luteinized human granulosa cells. *J Clin Endocrinol Metab* 1992; **75**: 254–8.

Gaddy-Kurten D, Hickey GJ, Fey GH, Gauldie J, Richards JS. Hormonal regulation and tissue-specific localization of alpha 2-macroglobulin in rat ovarian follicles and corpora lutea. *Endocrinology* 1989; **125**: 2985–95.

Gayton F, Aceitero J, Bellido C, Sanchez-Criado JE. Estrus cycle-related changes in mast cells numbers in several ovarian compartments in the rat. *Biol Reprod* 1992; **45**: 27–33.

Geisthovel F, Moretti-Rojas I, Asch RH, Rojas FJ. Expression of insulin-like growth factor-II (IGF-II) messenger ribonucleic acid (mRNA), but not IGF-I mRNA, in human preovulatory granulosa cells. *Hum Reprod* 1989; **4**: 899–902.

Gerdes U, Gåfvels M. Bergh A, Cajander S. Localized increases in ovarian vascular permeability and leukocyte accumulation after induced ovulation in rabbits. *J Reprod Fertil* 1992; **95**: 539–50.

Gleich GJ, Adolphson CR. The eosinophilic leukocyte: structure and function. *Adv Immunol* 1986; **39**: 177–253.

Gomez E, Tarin JJ, Pellicer A. Oocyte maturation in humans: the role of gonadotropins and growth factors. *Fertil Steril* 1993; **60**: 40–6.

Gore-Langton RE, Armstrong DT (1988). Follicular steroidogenesis and its control. In: Knobil E, Neill JD, eds. *The Physiology of Reproduction*. New York: Raven Press, 1988: 331–85 (vol. 1).

Gorospe WC, Tuchel T, Kasson BG. γ-Interferon inhibits rat granulosa cell differentiation in culture. *Biochem Biophys Res Commun* 1988; **157**: 891–7.

Gorospe WC, Hughes FM, Spangelo BL. Interleukin-6: effects on and production by rat granulosa cells *in vitro*. *Endocrinology* 1992; **130**: 1750–2.

Gospodarowicz RE, Ferrara N. Fibroblast growth factor and the control of pituitary and gonad development and function. *J Steroid Biochem* 1989; **32**: 183–91.

Gospodarowicz D, Plouet J, Fugii DK. Ovarian germinal epithelial cells respond to basic fibroblast growth factor and express its gene: implications for early folliculogenesis. *Endocrinology* 1989; **125**: 1266–76.

Gottschall PE, Katsuura G, Arimura A. Interleukin-1 suppresses FSH-induced estradiol secretion from cultured ovarian granulosa cells. *J Reprod Immunol* 1989; **15**: 281–90.

Gottschall PE, Katsuura G, Hoffman ST, Arimura A. Interleukin 1: an inhibitor of LH receptor formation in cultured rat granulosa cells. *FASEB J* 1988; **2**: 2492–6.

Green AR. Peptide regulatory factors: multi-functional mediators of cellular growth and differentiation. *Lancet* 1989; **i**: 705–7.

Guidice LC, Milki AA, Milkowski DA, El Danasouri I. Human granulosa contain messenger ribonucleic acids encoding insulin-like growth factor-binding proteins (IGFBPs) and secrete IGFBPs in culture. *Fertil Steril* 1991; **56**: 475–80.

Halme J, Hammond MG, Syrop CH, Talbert LM. Peritoneal macrophages modulate human granulosa-luteal cell progesterone production. *J Clin Endocrinol Metab* 1985; **61**: 912–16.

Halterman SD, Murdoch WJ. Ovarian function in ewes treated with antihistamines. *Endocrinology* 1986; **119**: 2417–21.

Hansell DJ, Bryant-Greenwood GD, Greenwood FC. Expression of human relaxin H1 gene in the decidua, trophoblast, and prostate. *J Clin Endocrinol Metab* 1991; **72**: 899–904.

Hedger MP, Qin JX, Robertson DM, de Kretser DM. Intragonadal regulation of immune system functions. *Reprod Fertil Dev* 1990; **2**: 263–80.

Hellberg P, Holmes PV, Brännström M, Olofsson J, Janson PO. Inhibitors of lipoxygenase increase the ovulation rate in the *in vitro* perfused luteinizing hormone-stimulated rabbit ovary. *Acta Physiol Scand* 1990; **138**: 557–64.

Hellberg P, Larson L, Olofson I, Hedin L, Brännström M. Stimulatory effects of bradykinin on the ovulatory process in the *in vitro*-perfused rat ovary. *Biol Reprod* 1991; **44**: 2669–74.

Hernandez ER, Hurwitz A, Payne DW, Dharmarajan AM, Purchio AF, Adashi EY. Transforming growth factor-beta 1 inhibits ovarian androgen production: gene expression, cellular localization, mechanism(s), and site(s) of action. *Endocrinology* 1990; **127**: 2804–11.

Hernandez ER, Hurwitz A, Vera A, Pellicer A, Adashi EY, LeRoith D, Roberts CT. Expression of the genes encoding the insulin-like growth factors and their receptors in the human ovary. *J Clin Endocrinol Metab* 1992; **74**: 419–25.

Herriot DM, Warnes GM, Kerin JF. Pregnancy-related chemotactic activity of human follicular fluid. *Fertil Steril* 1986; **45**: 196–201.

Hill JA. Cellular immune mechanisms of early reproductive failure. *Semin Perinatol* 1991; **15**: 225–9.

Hill JA, Barbieri RL, Anderson DJ. Detection of T8 (suppressor/cytotoxic) lymphocytes in human ovarian follicular fluid. *Fertil Steril* 1987; **47**: 460–5.

Hill JA, Welch WR, Faris HMP *et al*. Induction of class II major histocompatibility complex (MHC) antigen expression in human granulosa cells by gamma-interferon: a potential mechanism of autoimmune ovarian failure. *Am J Obstet Gynecol* 1990; **162**: 534–40.

Hillier SG. Cellular basis of follicular endocrine function. In: Hillier SG, ed. *Ovarian Endocrinology*. Oxford: Blackwell Scientific Publications, 1991: 73–106.

Hillier SG, Miro F. Inhibin, activin, and follistatin. Potential roles in ovarian physiology. *Ann N Acad Sci* 1993; **687**: 29–38.

Hillier SG, Knazek RA, Ross GT. Androgenic stimulation of progesterone production by granulosa cells from preantral ovarian follicles: further *in vitro* studies using replicate cell cultures. *Endocrinology* 1977; **100**: 1539–49.

Hillier SG, Yong EL, Baird DT, Fisch B. Steroid synthesis in the corpus luteum. In: Coelingh Bennink HJT *et al.*, eds. *Local regulation of ovarian function*. an Eric K Fernström Symposium, Parthenon Publishing 1992, 287–96.

Holly JMP, Smith CP, Dunger DB *et al*. Levels of the small insulin-like growth factor-binding protein are strongly related to those of insulin in prepubertal and pubertal children but only weakly so after puberty. *J Endocrinol* 1989; **121**: 383–7.

Holly JM, Eden JA, Alaghband-Zadeh J *et al*. Insulin-like growth factor binding proteins in follicular fluid from normal dominant and cohort follicles polycystic and multicystic ovaries. *Clin Endocrinol* 1990; **33**: 53–64.

Hsueh AJ, Adashi EY, Jones BPC, Wlesh T Jr. Hormonal regulation of the differentiation of cultured ovarian granulosa cells. *Endocrin Rev* 1984; **5**: 76–127.

Hsueh AJW, Dahl KD, Vaughan J *et al*. Heterodimers and homodimers of inhibin subunits have different paracrine action in the modulation of luteinizing hormone-stimulated androgen biosynthesis. *Proc Natl Acad Sci* 1987; **84**: 5082–6.

Hughes FM, Lane T, Chen TT, Gorospe WC. Effects of cytokines on porcine granulosa cell steroidogenesis *in vitro*. *Biol Reprod* 1990; **43**: 812–17.

Hughes FM, Pringle CM, Gorospe WC. Production of progestin-stimulatory factor(s) by enriched populations of rat T- and B-lymphocytes. *Biol Reprod* 1991; **44**: 922–6.

Hume DA, Halpin D, Charlton H, Gardo S. The mononuclear phagocyte system of the mouse defined by immunohistochemical localization of antigen F4/80: macrophages of endocrine organs. *Proc Natl Acad Sci USA* 1984; **81**: 4174–7.

Hurwitz A, Payne DW, Packman JN *et al*. Cytokine-mediated regulation of ovarian function: interleukin-1 inhibits gonadotropin-induced androgen biosynthesis. *Endocrinology* 1991*a*; **129**: 1250–59.

Hurwitz A. Ricciarelli E, Botero L, Rohen RM, Hernandez ER, Adashi EY. Endocrine and autocrine mediated regulation of rat ovarian (theca-interstitial) interleukin-1β gene expression: gonadotropin dependent preovulatory acquisition. *Endocrinology* 1991*b*; **129**: 3427–9.

Hurwitz A, Louikides J, Ricciarelli E, Botero L, Katz E, McAllister JM, Garcia JE, Rohan R, Adashi EY. Human intraovarian interleukin-1 (IL-1) system: highly compartmentalized and hormonally dependent regulation of the genes encoding IL-1, its receptor, and its receptor antagonist. *J Clin Invest* 1992; **88**: 1746–54.

Hurwitz A, Dushnik M, Solomon H, Ben-chetri A, Finci-Yeshkel Z, Mildiwsky A, Mayer M, Adashi EY, Yagel S. Cytokine-mediated regulation of rat ovarian function: interleukin-1 stimulates the accumulation of a 92-kilodalton gelatinase. *Endocrinology* 1993; **132**: 2709–14.

Ignotz RA, Massagué J. Transforming growth factor-beta stimulates the expression of fibronectin and collagen and their incorporation into extracellular matrix. *J Biol Chem* 1986; **261**: 4337–45.

Itskovitz J, Tubattu S, Rosenwaks Z, Liu HC, Sealey JE. Relationship of follicular-fluid prorenin to oocyte maturation, steroid levels, and outcome of *in vitro* fertilization. *J Clin Endocrinol Metab* 1991; **72**: 165–71.

Jalkanen J, Suikkari A-M, Koistinen R, Bützow R, Ritvos O, Seppälä M, Ranta T. Regulation of insulin-like growth factor-binding protein-1 production in human granulosa-luteal cells. *J Clin Endocrinol Metab* 1989; **69**: 1174–9.

Jennings JC, Mohan S, Linkhart TA, Widstrom R, Baylink DJ. Comparison of the biological activities of TGF-β1 and TGF-β2: Differential activity in endothelial cells. *J Cell Physiol* 1988; **137**: 167–72.

Jesionowska H, Hemmings R, Guyda HJ, Posner BI. Determination of insulin and insulin-like growth factors in the ovarian circulation. *Fertil Steril* 1990; **53**: 88–91.

Jones RE, Duvall D, Guilette LJ. Rat ovarian mast cells: distribution and cyclic changes. *Anat Rec* 1980; **197**: 489–90.

Julkunen M, Koistinen R, Aalto-Setälä K, Seppälä M, Jänne OA, Kontula K. Primary structure of human insulin-like growth factor-binding protein/placental protein 12 and tissue-specific expression of its mRNA. *FEBS Lett* 1988; **236**: 295–302.

Kasson BG, Gorospe WC. Effects of interleukins 1, 2 and 3 on follicle-stimulating hormone-induced differentiation of rat granulosa cells. *Mol Cell Endocrinol* 1989; **62**: 103–11.

Kazer R. The etiology of polycystic ovary syndrome (PCO). *Med Hypotheses* 1988; **30**: 151–5.

Kazer RR, Unterman TG, Glick RP. An abnormality of the growth hormone/insulin-like growth factor-I axis in women with polycystic ovary syndrome. *J Clin Endocrinol Metab* 1990; **71**: 958–62.

Khan SA, Schmidt K, Hallin P, DiPauli R, De Geyter CH, Nieschlag E. Human testis cytosol and ovarian follicular fluid contain high amounts of interleukin-1-like factor(s). *Mol Cell Endocrinol* 1988; **58**: 221–30.

Kim I-C, Schomberg DW. The production of transforming growth factor-β by rat granulosa cell cultures. *Endocrinology* 1989; **124**: 1345–51.

Kirsch TM, Friedman RL, Vigel RL, Flickinger GL. Macrophages in corpora lutea of mice: characterization and effects on steroid secretion. *Biol Reprod* 1981; **25**: 629–38.

Kitai H, Kobayashi Y, Santulli R. Wright KH, Wallach EE. The relationship between prostaglandins and histamine in the ovulatory process as determined with the *in vitro* perfused rabbit ovary. *Fertil Steril* 1985; **43**: 646–51.

Knecht M, Feng P, Catt K. Bifunctional role for transforming growth factor-β during granulosa cell development. *Endocrinology* 1987; **120**: 1243–9.

Koistinen H, Seppälä M, Koistinen R. Different forms of insulin-like growth factor-binding protein-3 detected in serum and seminal plasma by immunofluorometric assay with monoclonal antibodies. *Clin Chem* 1994; **40**: 531–7.

Koistinen R, Kalkkinen N, Huhtala M-L, Seppälä M, Bohn H, Rutanen E-M. Placental protein 12 is a decidual protein that binds somatomedin and has an identical N-terminal amino acid sequence with somatomedin-binding protein from human amniotic fluid. *Endocrinology* 1986; **118**: 1375–8.

Koistinen R, Huhtala M-L, Stenman U-H, Seppälä M. Purification of placental protein PP12 from human amniotic fluid and its comparison with PP12 from placenta by immunological, physicochemical and somatomedin-binding properties. *Clin Chim Acta* 1987; **164**: 293–303.

Koistinen R, Suikkari A-M, Tiitinen A, Kontula K, Seppälä M. Human granulosa cells contain insulin-like growth factor binding protein (IGFBP-1) mRNA. *Clin Endocrinol* 1990; **32**: 635–40.

Krishna A, Terranova PF. Alteration in mast cell degranulation and ovarian histamine in the proestrous hamster. *Biol Reprod* 1985; **32**: 1211–17.

Kudlow JE, Kobrin MS, Purchio AF *et al.* Ovarian transforming growth factor-α gene expression: immunohistochemical localization to the theca-interstitial cells. *Endocrinology* 1987; **121**: 1577–9.

Laatikainen T, Anttila L, Suikkari A-M, Ruutiainen K, Erkkola R, Seppälä M. Effect of naloxone on plasma insulin, insulin-like growth factor I, and its binding protein 1 in patients with polycystic ovarian disease. *Fertil Steril* 1990; **54**: 434–7.

Leal JA, May JV, Keel BA. Human alpha fetoprotein enhances epidermal growth factor proliferative activity upon porcine granulosa cells in monolayer culture. *Endocrinology* 1990; **126**: 669–71.

Lee Y-L, Hintz RL, James PM *et al.* Insulin-like growth factor (IGF) binding protein complementary deoxyribonucleic acid from human HP G2 hepatoma cells: predicted protein sequence suggests an IGF binding domain different from those of the IGF and IGF II receptors. *Mol Endocrinol* 1988; **2**: 404–11.

Lei RM, Chegini N, Rao CHV, Quantitative cell composition of human and ovine corpora lutea from various reproductive states. *Biol Reprod* 1991; **44**: 1148–56.

LeMaire WJ, Janson PO, Källfelt BJ, Holmes PV, Cajander S, Bjersing L, Ahrén K. The prevalidity decline in the follicular estradiol is not required for ovulation in rabbit. *Acta Endocrinol* 1982; **101**: 452–7.

Leung PCK, Armstrong DT. Interactions of steroids and gonadotrophins in the control of steroidogenesis of the ovarian follicle. *Annu Rec Physiol* 1980; **42**: 71–82.

Ling N, Ying S-Y, Ueno N, Esch F, Denoroy L, Guillemin R. Isolation and partial characterizarion of a *Mr* 32 000 protein with inhibin activity from porcine follicular fluid. *Proc Natl Acad Sci USA* 1985; **82**: 7217–21.

Ling N, Ying SY, Ueno N *et al*. Pituitary FSH is released by the heterodimer of the beta subunits from two forms of inhibin. *Nature* 1986; **321**: 779–82.

Lipner H, Wendelken L. Inhibition of ovulation by inhibition of steroidogenesis in immature rats. *Proc Soc Exp Biol Med* 1971; **136**: 1141–5.

Lipscomb HL, Gardner PJ, Sharp G. The effect of neonatal thymectomy on the induction of autoimmune orchitis in rats. *J Reprod Immunol* 1979; **1**: 209–17.

Loeken MR, Channing CP, D'Eletto R, Weiss G. Stimulatory effect of LH upon relaxin secretion by cultured porcine granulosa cells. *Endocrinology* 1983; **112**: 769–71.

Loukides JA, Loy RA, Edwards R, Honig J, Visintin I, Polan ML. Human follicular fluids contain tissue macrophages. *J Clin Endocrinol Metab* 1990; **71**: 1363–7.

Loutradis D, Bletsa R, Aravantinos L, Kallianidis K, Michalas S, Psychoyos A. Preovulatory effects of the progesterone anatagonist mifepristone (RU 486) in mice. *Hum Reprod* 1991; **6**: 1238–40.

Louvet JP, Hasman SM, Schreiber JR, Ross GT. Evidence for a role of androgens in follicular maturation. *Endocrinology* 1975; **97**: 366–72.

Magoffin DA, Candedo B, Erickson GF. Transforming growth factor-β promotes differentiation of ovarian thecal-interstitial cells but inhibits androgen production. *Endocrinology* 1989; **125**: 1951–8.

Marquardt H, Rose TM, Webb NR *et al*. Rat transforming growth factor type I: structure and relation to epidermal growth factor. *Science* 1984; **223**: 1079–82.

Maruo T, Ladines-Llave CA, Samoto T, Matsuo H, Manalo AS, Ito H, Mochizuki M. Expression of epidermal growth factor and its receptor in the human ovary during follicular growth and regression. *Endocrinology* 1993; **132**: 924–31.

Mason AJ, Hayflick JS, Ling N *et al*. Complementary DNA sequences of ovarian follicular fluid inhibin show precursor structure and homology with transforming growth factor-β. *Nature London*, 1985; **318**: 659–63.

Mason AJ, Niall HD, Seeburg PH. Structure of two human ovarian inhibins. *Biochem Biophys Res Commun* 1986; **135**: 957–64.

Mason HD, Martikainen H, Beard RW, Anyaoku V, Franks S. Director gonadotropic effects of growth hormone on oestradiol production by human granulosa cells *in vitro*. *J Endocrinol* 1990a; **126**: R1-4.

Mason HD, Margara R, Winston RML, Seppälä M, Koistinen R, Franks S. Insulin-like growth factor-I inhibits production of IGF binding protein-1 while stimulating estradiol secretion in granulosa cells from normal and polycystic ovaries. *J Clin Endocrinol Metab* 1993; **76**: 1275–9.

Mason HD, Willis D, Holly JMT, Cwyfan-Hughes SC, Seppälä M, Franks S. Inhibitory effects of insulin-like growth factor-binding proteins on steroidogenesis by human granulosa cells in culture. *Mol Cell Endocrinol* 1992; **89**: R1-R4.

Massagué J. Epidermal growth factor-like transforming growth factor. II. Interaction with epidermal growth factor receptors in human placenta membranes and A431 cells. *J Biol Chem* 1983; **258**: 12614–3620.

Massagué J. The TGF-β family of growth and differentiation factors. *Cell* 1987; **49**: 437–8.

May JV, Frost JP,Bridge AJ. Regulation of granulosa cell proliferation: facilitative roles of platelet-derived growth factor and low density lipoprotein. *Endocrinology* 1990; **126**: 2896–905.

McLachlan RI, Robertson DM, Healy DL, Burger HG, De Kretser DM. Circulating immunoreactive inhibin levels during the normal human menstrual cycle. *J Clin Endocrinol Metab* 1987; **65**: 954–61.

Mori T, Suzuki A, Nishimura T, Kambegawa A. Inhibition of ovulation in immature rats by antiprogesterone antiserum. *J Endocr* 1977; **73**: 185–6.

Morioka N, Brännström M, Koos RD, LeMaire WJ. Ovulation in the perfused ovary *in vitro*: further evidence that estrogen is not required. *Steroids* 1988; **45**: 173–83.

Motro B, Itin A, Sachs L, Keshet E. Pattern of interleukin-6 gene expression *in vivo* suggests a role for this cytokine in angiogenesis. *Proc Natl Acad Sci USA* 1990; **87**: 3092–6.

Murdoch WJ. Treatment of sheep with prostaglandin F_{2a} enhances production of a luteal chemoattractant for eosinophils. *Am J Reprod Immunol Microbiol* 1987; **15**: 52–6.

Murdoch WJ, McCormick RJ. Production of low molecular weight chemoattractants for leukocytes by periovulatory ovine follicles. *Biol Reprod* 1989; **40**: 86–90.

Murdoch WJ, Steadman LE, Belden EL. Immunoregulation of luteolysis. *Med Hypotheses* 1988; **27**: 197–9.

Nakamura Y, Smith M, Krishna A, Terranova PF. Increased number of mast cells in the dominant follicle of the cow: relationships among luteal, stromal, and hilar regions. *Biol Reprod* 1987; **37**: 546–9.

Norström A, Tjugum J. Hormonal effects on collagenolytic activity in the isolated human ovarian follicular wall. *Gynecol Obstet Invest* 1986; **22**: 12–16.

Nothnick WB, Pate JL. Interleukin-1β is a potent stimulator of prostaglandin synthesis in bovine luteal cells. *Biol Reprod* 1990; **43**: 898–903.

O W-S, Robertson DM, de Kretser DM. Inhibin as an oocyte meiotic inhibitor. *Mol Cell Endocrinol* 1989; **62**: 307–11.

Olsson JH, Carlsson B, Hillensjö T. Effect of insulin-like growth factor-I on deoxyribonucleic acid synthesis in cultured granulosa cells. *Fertil Steril* 1990; **54**: 1052–7.

Paavola LG. The corpus luteum of the guinea pig. Fine structure of macrophages during pregnancy and postpartum luteolysis and the phagocytosis of luteal cells. *Am J Anat* 1979; **154**: 337–64.

Pacifici R, Rifas L, McCracken R, Vered I, McMurtry C, Avioli LV, Peck WA. Ovarian steroid treatment blocks a postmenopausal increase in blood monocyte interleukin 1 release. *Proc Natl Acad Sci* 1989; **86**: 2398–402.

Patwardhan VV, Lanthier A. Luteal phase variations in endogenous concentrations of prostaglandins PGE and PGF and in the capacity for their *in vitro* formulation in the human corpus luteum. *Prostaglandins* 1985; **30**: 91–6.

Pennica D, Nedwin GE, Hayflick JS, Seeburg PH, Derynck R, Palladino MA, Kohr WJ, Aggarwal BB, Goeddel DV. Human tumor necrosis factor: precursor structure, expression and homology to lymphotoxin. *Nature London*, 1984; **312**: 724–9.

Pestka S. The human interferons - from protein purification and sequence to cloning and expression in bacteria: before, between and beyond. *Arch Biochem Biophys* 1983; **221**: 1–37.

Petrovska M, Sedlak R, Nouza K, Presl J, Kinsky R. Development and distribution of the white blood cells within various structures of the human menstrual corpus luteum; examined using an image analysis system. *Am J Reprod Immunol* 1992; **28**: 77–80.

Polan ML, Carding S, Loukides J. Progesterone modulates interleukin-1β (IL-1β) mRNA production by human pelvic macrophages. *Fertil Steril* 1988; **50**: S4.

Poretsky L, Bhargava G, Levitan E. Type I insulin-like growth factor receptors in human ovarian stroma. *Horm Res* 1990; **33**: 22–6.

Poretsky L, Grigorescu F, Seibel M, Moses AC, Flier JS. Distribution and characterization of insulin and insulin-like growth factor I receptors in normal human ovary. *J Clin Endocrinol Metab* 1985; **61**: 728–34.

Postlethwaite AE, Keskioja J, Moses HL, Kang AH. Stimulation of the chemotactic migration of human fibroblasts by transforming growth factor beta. *J Exp Med* 1987; **165**: 251–6.

Povoa G, Enberg G, Jörnvall H, Hall K. Isolation and characterization of a somatomedin-binding protein from mid-term human amniotic fluid. *Eur J Biochem* 1984; **144**: 199–204.

Powell WS, Hammarström S, Samuelsson B. Prostaglandin $F_{2\alpha}$ receptor in human corpora lutea. *Lancet* 1979; **6**: 1120–2.

Rabinovici J, Dandekar P, Angle MJ, Rosenthal S, Martin MC. Insulin-like growth factor I (IGF-I) levels in follicular fluid from human preovulatory follicles: correlation with serum IGF-I levels. *Fertil Steril* 1990; **54**: 428–33.

Ramasharma K, Caverera CM, Li CH. Identification of insulin-like growth factor II in human seminal and follicular fluids. *Biochem Biophys Res Commun* 1986; **140**: 536–42.

Ramasharma K, Li GH. Human pituitary and placental hormones control human insulin-like growth factor secretion in human granulosa cells. *Proc Natl Acad Sci USA* 1987; **84**: 2643–7.

Reddi K, Wickings EJ, McNeilly AS, Baird DT, Hillier SG. Circulating bioactive follicle stimulating hormone and immunoreactive inhibin levels during the normal human menstrual cycle. *Clin Endocrinol* 1990; **33**: 547–57.

Reich R, Kohen F, Naor Z, Tsafriri A. Possible involvement of lipoxygenase products of arachidonic acid pathway in ovulation. *Prostaglandins* 1983; **26**: 1011–21.

Richards JS, Jahnsen T, Hedin L, Lifka J, Taroosh S, Durica JM, Goldring N. Ovarian follicular development: from physiology to molecular biology. *Recent Prog Horm Res* 1987; **43**: 231–70.

Richardson MC, Gadd SC, Masson GM. Augmentation by epidermal growth factor of basal and stimulated progesterone production by human luteinized granulosa cells. *J Endocrinol* 1989; **121**: 397–402.

Rinderknecht E, Humbel RE. The amino acid sequence of human insulin-like growth factor I and its structural homology with proinsulin. *J Biol Chem* 1978; **253**: 2769–76.

Roberts AB, Flanders KC, Kondaiah P, Thompson NL, Va Obberghen-Schilling E, Wakefield L, Rossi P, de Crombrugghe B, Heine U, Sporn MB. Transforming growth factor β: biochemistry and roles in embryogenesis, tissue repair and remodeling, and carcinogenesis. *Recent Prog Horm Res* 1988; **44**: 157–93.

Roberts AB, Kondaiah P, Rosa R. Watanabe S, Good P, Danielpour D, Roche NS, Rebbert ML, Dawid IB, Sporn MB. Mesoderm induction in Zenopus laevis distinguishes between the various TGF-β isoforms. *Growth Factors* 1990a; **3**: 277–86.

Roberts AB, Rosa F, Roche NS, Coligan JE, Garfield M, Rebbert ML, Kondaiah P,

Danielpour D, Kehrl JH, Wahl SM. Isolation and characterization of TGF-β2 and TGF-β5 from medium conditioned by Zenopus XTC cells. *Growth Factors* 1990*b*; **2**: 135–47.

Roby KF, Terranova PF. Localization of tumor necrosis factor (TNF) in rat and bovine ovary using immunocytochemistry and cell blot: evidence for granulosal production. In: Hirshfield AN, ed. *Growth Factors and the Ovary*, Plenum Press, New York 1989; 273–8.

Roby KF, Weed J, Lyles R, Terranova PF. Immunologic evidence for a human ovarian tumor necrosis factor alpha. *J Clin Endocrinol Metab* 1990; **71**: 1096–102.

Ruegsegger Veit C, Assoian RK. Identification of transforming growth factor-β in human ovarian follicular fluid [Abstract]. *Endocrinology* 1988; **122**(suppl): 1227.

San Roman GA, Magoffin DA. Insulin-like growth factor-binding proteins in healthy and atretic follicles during natural menstrual cycles. *J Clin Endocrinol Metab* 1993; **76**: 625–32.

Sancho-Tello M, Perez-Roger I, Imakawa K, Tilzerm L, Terranova PF. Expression of tumor necrosis factor α in the rat ovary. *Endocrinology* 1992; **130**: 1359–64.

Schmidt G, Owman C, Sjöberg NO. Histamine induces ovulation in the isolated perfused rat ovary. *J Reprod Fertil* 1986; **78**: 159–66.

Schmidt G. Owman C, Sjöberg NO. Cellular localization of ovarian histamine, its cyclic variations, and histaminergic effects on ovulation in the rat ovary perfused *in vitro*. *J Reprod Fertil* 1988; **82**: 409–17.

Schomberg DW. Growth factors and reproduction. In: Hodgen GD, Rosenwaks Z, Spieler JM, eds. *Nonsteroidal Gonadal Factors*. Norfolk, CT: Jones Institute press, 1988; 330-8.

Seppälä M, Wahlström T, Koskimies AI, Tenhunen A, Rutanen EM, Koistinen R, Huhtaniemi I, Bohn H, Stenman UH. Human preovulatory follicular fluid, luteinized cells of hyperstimulated preovulatory follicles and corpus luteum contain placental protein 12 (PP12). *J Clin Endocrinol Metab* 1984; **58**: 505–10.

Shifren JL, Osathanondh R, Yeh J. Human fetal ovaries and uteri: developmental expression of genes encoding the insulin, insulin-like growth factor I, and insulin-like growth factor II receptors. *Fertil Steril* 1993; **59**: 1036–40.

Shimasaki S, Shimonaka M, Ui M, Inouye S, Shibata F, Ling N. Structural characterization of a follicle-stimulating hormone action inhibitor in porcine ovarian follicular fluid. *J Biol Chem* 1990; **265**: 2198–202.

Simon C, Frances A, Piquette G, Polan ML. Immunohistochemical localization of the interleukin-1 system in the mouse ovary during follicular development, ovulation and luteinization. *Biol Reprod* 1994*a*; **50**: 449–57.

Simon C, Tsafriri A, Chun S-Y, Piquette N, Dang W, Polan ML. Interleukin-1 receptor antagonist suppresses hCG-induced ovulation in the rat. *Biol Reprod* 1994*b*; in press.

Singh A, Hamilton-Fairley D, Koistinen R, Seppälä M, Franks S, Reed MJ. Effect of insulin-like growth factor-type I (IGF-I) and insulin on the secretion of sex hormone binding globulin and IGF-I binding protein (IBP-I) by human hepatoma cells. *J Endocrinol* 1990; **124**: R1-R3.

Sjögren A, Holmes PV, Hillensjö T. Interleukin-1α modulates LH stimulated cAMP and progesterone release from human granulosa cells *in vitro*. *Hum Reprod* 1991; **6**: 910–13.

Skinner MK, McKeracher HL, Dorrington JH. Fibronectin as a marker of granulosa cell cytodifferentiation. *Endocrinology* 1985; **117**: 886–92.

Skinner MK, Coffey RJ Jr. Regulation of ovarian cell growth through the local production of transforming growth factor-alpha by theca cells. *Endocrinology* 1988; **123**: 2632–8.

Skinner MK, Keski-Oja J, Osteen KG, Moses HL. Ovarian thecal cells produce transforming growth factor-β which can regulate granulosa cell growth. *Endocrinology* 1987; **121**: 786–92.

Slack JMW. Peptide regulatory factors in embryonic development. *Lancet* 1989; **i**: 1312–15.

Smith C, Perks AM. Changes in plasma kininogen levels in rats before ovulation, and after treatment with luteinizing hormone and oestradiol-17β. *Acta Endocrinol* 1983; **104**: 123–8.

Smith KB, Millar MR, McNeilly AS, Illingworth PJ, Hillier SG, Baird DT. Localization and production of immunoreactive inhibition by the human corpus luteum. In: Coelingh Bennink HJT *et al.*, eds. *Local Regulation of Ovarian Function*. an Eric K Fernström Symposium, Parthenon Publishing 1992; 313–16.

Snyder BW, Beechan GD, Schane HP. Inhibition of ovulation in rats with epostane, an inhibitor of 3β-hydroxysteroid dehydrogenase. *Proc Soc Exp Biol Med* 1984; **176**: 238–42.

Staendert FS, Zamon CS, Chew BP. Quantitative and qualitative changes in blood leukocytes in the porcine ovary. *Am J Reprod Immunol* 1991; **215**: 163–8.

Steele-Perkins G, Turner J, Edman JC, Hari J, Pierce SB, Stover C, Rutter WJ, Roth RA. Expression and characterization of a functional human insulin-like growth factor I receptor. *J Biol Chem* 1988; **263**: 11486–92.

Steinkampf MP, Mendelson CR, Simpson ER. Regulation by follicle-stimulating hormone of the synthesis of aromatase cytochrome P-450 in human granulosa cells. *Mol Endocrinol* 1987; **1**: 465–71.

Steinkampf MP, Mendelson Cr, Simpson ER. Effects of epidermal growth factor and insulin-like growth factor I on the levels of mRNA encoding aromatase cytochrome P-450 of human ovarian granulosa cells. *Mol Cell Endocrinol* 1988; **59**: 93–9.

Strelkauskas AJ, Callery RT, McDowell J, McDowell J, Borel Y, Schlossman SF. Direct evidence for loss of human suppressor cell during active autoimmune disease. *Proc Natl Acad Sci USA* 1978; **75**: 5150–4.

Sugino H, Nakamura T, Hasegawa Y, Miyamoto K, Igarashi M, Eto Y, Shibai H, Titani K. Identification of a specific receptor for erythroid differentiation factor on follicular granulosa cell. *J Biol Chem* 1988; **263**: 15249–52.

Suikkari A-M, Koivisto VA, Rutanen E-M, Yki-Järvinen H, Karonen S-L, Seppälä M. Insulin regulates the serum levels of low molecular weight insulin-like growth factor-binding protein. *J Clin Endocrinol Metab* 1988; **66**: 266–72.

Suikkari A-M, Jalkanen J, Koistinen R, Bützow R, Ritvos O, Ranta T, Seppälä M. Human granulosa cells synthesize low molecular weight insulin-like growth factor-binding protein. *Endocrinology* 1989*a*; **124**: 1088–90.

Suikkari A-M, Koivisto VA, Koistinen R, Seppälä M, Yki-Järvinen J. Dose–response characteristics for suppression of low molecular weight plasma insulin-like growth factor-binding protein by insulin. *J Clin Endocrinol Metab* 1989*b*; **68**: 135–40.

Takehara Y, Dharmarajan AM, Kaufman G, Wallach EE. Effect of interleukin-1β on ovulation in the *in vitro* perfused rabbit ovary. *Endocrinology* 1994; **134**: 1788–93.

Tanaka N, Espey LL, Okamura H. Increase in ovarian 15-hydroxyeicosatetraenoic acid during ovulation in the gonadotropin-primed immature rat. *Endocrinology* 1989; **125**: 1373–7.

Tanaka N, Espey LL, Kawano T, Okamura H. Comparison of inhibitory actions of indomethacin and epostane on ovulation in rats. *Am J Physiol* 1991; **260**: E170–4.

Tanaka N, Espey LL, Stacy S, Okamura H. Epostane and indomethacin, actions on ovarian kallikrein and plasminogen activator activities during ovulation in the gonadotropin-primed immature rat. *Biol Reprod* 1992; **46**: 665–70.

Terranova PF, Roby KF, Sancho-Tello M, Weed J, Lyles R. (1991). Tumor necroris factor α: Localization and actions within the preovulatory follicle. In: Schomberg DW, ed. *Growth Factors in Reproduction*. New York: Springer-Verlag 1991; 63–78.

Thomas JP, Dorflinger LV, Behrman HV. Mechanisms of the rapid antigonadotrophic action of prostaglandins in cultured luteal cells. *Proc Natl Acad Sci USA* 1978; **75**: 1344–8.

Todaro GJ, Fryling C, DeLarco JE. Transforming growth factors produced by certain human tumor cells: polypeptides that interact with epidermal growth factor receptors. *Proc Natl Acad Sci USA* 1980; **77**: 5158–62.

Too CK, Bryant-Greenwood GD, Greenwood FC. Relaxin increases the release of plasminogen activator, collagenase, and proteoglycanase from rat granulosa cells *in vitro*. *Endocrinology* 1984; **115**: 1043–50.

Tsang BK, Moon YS, Simpson, CW, Armstrong DT. Androgen biosynthesis in human ovarian follicles: cellular source, gonadotropic control, and adenosine 3'5'-monophosphate mediation. *J Clin Endocrinol Metab* 1979; **48**: 153–8.

Tsonis CG, Hillier SG, Baird DT. Production of inhibin bioactivity by human granulosa-lutein cells: stimulation by LH and testosterone *in vitro*. *J Endocrinol* 1987; **112**: R11–14.

Turner IM, Saunders PTK, Shimasaki S, Hillier SG (1989). Regulation of inhibin subunit gene expression by FSH and estradiol in cultured rat granulosa cells. *Endocrinology* 1989; **125**: 2790–2.

Ui M, Shimonaka M, Shimasaki S, Ling N. An insulin-like growth factor-binding protein in ovarian follicular fluid blocks follicle-stimulating hormone-stimulated steroid production by ovarian granulosa cells. *Endocrinology* 1989; **125**: 912–16.

Voutilainen R, Miller WL. Coordinate tropic hormone regulation of mRNAs for insulin-like growth factor II and the cholesterol side-chain-cleavage enzyme P450 Scc, in human steroidogenic tissues. *Proc Natl Acad Sci USA* 1987; **84**: 1590–

Wallach EE, Dharmarajan AM. Prostaglandins and ovulation. In: Coelingh Bennink *et al.*, eds. *Local Regulation of Ovarian Function*. An Eric K Fernström Symposium. Parthenon Publishing, 1992; 183–200.

Wang L, Robertson S, Seamark RF, Norman RJ. Lymphokines, inducing interleukin-2, alter gonadotropin-stimulated progesterone production and proliferation of human granulosa cells *in vitro*. *J Clin Endocrinol Metab* 1991; **72**: 824–31.

Wang LJ, Pascoe V, Petrucco OM, Norman RJ. Distribution of leukocyte subpopulations in the human corpus leteum. *Hum Reprod* 1992*a*; **7**: 197–206.

Wang LJ, Brännström M, Robertson SA, Norman RJ. Tumor necrosis factor α in the human ovary: presence in follicular fluid and effects on cell proliferation and prostaglandin production. *Fertil Steril* 1992*b*; **58**: 934–40.

Wang HZ, Lu SH, Han ZJ, Zhan W, Sheng WX, Sun ZD, Gong YT. Inhibitory effect of interferon and tumor necrosis factor in human luteal function *in vitro*, *Fertil Steril* 1992*c*; **58**: 934–40.

Watanabe H, Nagai K, Yamaguchi M, Ikenoue T, Mori N. Concentration of interleukin-1β correlates with prostaglandin E2 and F2α in human pre-ovulatory follicular fluid. *Hum Reprod* 1994; **9**: 9–12.

Woodruff TK, Meunier H, Jones PB, Hsueh AJW, Mayo KE. Rat inhibin: molecular cloning of α- and β-subunit complementary deoxyribonucleic acids and expression in the ovary. *Mol Endocrinol* 1987; **1**: 561–9.

Wuttke W, Jarry H, Pitzel L, Knake I, Spiess S. Luteotrophic and luteolytic actions of ovarian peptides. *Hum Reprod* 1993; **8**(suppl 2): 141–6.

Xiao S, Findlay JK. Modulation of differentiation of rat granulosa cells *in vitro* by interferon-γ. *J Endocrinol* 1992; **133**: 131–9.

Ying S-Y, Becker A, Baird A, Ling N, Ueno N, Esch F, Guillemin R. Type beta transforming growth factor (TGF-β) is a potent stimulator of the basal secretion of follicle stimulating hormone (FSH) in a pituitary monolayer system. *Biochem Biophys Res Commun* 1986*a*; **135**: 950–6.

Ying S-Y, Becker A, Ling N, Ueno N, Guillemin R. Inhibin and beta type transforming growth factor (TGF-β) have opposite modulating effects on the follicle stimulating hormone (FSH)-induced aromatase activity of cultured rat granulosa cells. *Biochem Biophys Res Commun* 1986*b*; **136**: 969–75.

Yoshimura Y, Wallach EE. Studies on the mechanism(s) of mammalian ovulation. *Fertil Steril* 1987; **47**: 22–34.

Yoshimura Y, Espey LL, Hsoi L, Adachi T, Atlas SJ, Ghodaonkar RB, Dubin NH, Wallach EE. The effect of bradykinin on ovulation and prostaglandin production by the perfused rabbit ovary. *Endocrinology* 1988; **122**: 2540–6.

Zolti M, Meirom R, Shemesh M, Woollach D, Maschiach S, Shore L, Rafael ZB. Granulosa cells as a source and target organ for tumor necrosis factor-α. *FEBS Lett* 1990; **261**: 253–5.

10

Oocyte transport

H. B. CROXATTO AND M. VILLALÓN

Since oocytes, the only cells endowed with the potential to form new individuals, are stored in ovarian follicles, and the progeny must separate from the maternal body, a pathway and appropriate mechanisms exist to achieve this end. Oocyte transport is a fundamental part of this process.

In mammals, the oocyte needs to be fertilized to form a new individual, a process that usually starts in the genital tract and continues in it until birth. Fertilization turns the oocyte into a zygote, whose successful cleavage and differentiation make up preimplantation development of an embryo. Transport of this changing structure within the genital tract lasts until the blastocyst is fixed to the site of implantation. Oocytes which remain unfertilized can experience spontaneous activation which, to some extent, mimics development but does not lead to viable embryos. These, as well as fertilized oocytes whose development is arrested prior to implantation, undergo cytolysis and in some species, before their disintegration or expulsion, they are transported to the site of implantation very much like normally developing embryos.

Irrespective of the fate of ovulated oocytes, they gain or lose diverse egg coatings as they traverse different segments of the genital tract. Thus, their size and external surface as well as their biological properties change, and this may influence the behaviour of the genital tract and consequently affect the way they are transported.

The journey of oocytes from their site of storage to their final destination, be it implantation or oviposition, is a continuum but, for the purpose of its analysis in mammals, it can be divided into four main steps: a) oocyte release from the follicle, b) oocyte pick-up by the fimbria, c) tubal or oviductal transport, and d) uterine transport.

Each one of these steps will be reviewed after a brief description of the common anatomical features of the oviduct. The term egg will be used indistinctively to refer to the oocyte or any biological entity derived from it which is transported within the female genital tract.

Reviews and recent publications on each topic will be cited rather than all the original findings.

Anatomy of the oviduct

In accordance with different anatomical, physiological and biochemical requirements, the genital tract is composed of distinct communicating compartments arranged in line. Their features comply with various necessities: to convey an adequate number of sperm with fertilizing capacity to encounter the oocyte; to recognize, nurture and transport the developing egg; to dispose of excess or faulty gametes and embryos; to relay embryonic signals to distant organs; to sustain the implanted embryo and later deliver the fetus; to limit the access of microorganisms from the external opening into the innermost segments. Different parts at different times contribute to this aggregate of functions in response to endocrine, paracrine, autocrine and neural signals.

The oviduct is the tubular organ that connects the ovary to the uterus. Depending on the species, the distal end may open to the abdominal cavity or into a bursa that surrounds the ovary. The proximal end opens to the uterine cavity. The length and shape of the oviduct varies considerably among species. In the human, the length of the extrauterine portion of the oviduct measures from 6 to 15 cm and is fairly straight, while in small rodents it measures a few millimetres and is highly coiled.

It is customary to distinguish four segments along the oviduct. From the distal (ovarian) to the proximal (uterine) end, these segments are: the fimbria and infundibulum, the ampulla, the isthmus, and the intramural segment. A short segment connecting the ampulla and the isthmus is known as the ampullary–isthmic junction (AIJ) and the very end connecting with the uterus is the utero-tubal junction (UTJ). There are no sharp limits between the segments.

Each oviduct is wrapped by the abdominal serosa which, after encircling the tube, forms the mesosalpinx, that loosely connects the oviduct to the posterior peritoneum. The two serosal sheets of the mesosalpinx enclose a thin smooth muscle layer, as well as supporting ligaments, nerves, lymphatics and blood vessels.

The major part of the oviductal wall is composed of an intricate layer of smooth muscle fibres, the myosalpinx and an innermost highly folded mucosa, the endosalpinx. The oviductal segments differ considerably in the amount of circular smooth muscle, the degree of folding and cellular composition of the mucosa as well as in their autonomic innervation. For reviews on the comparative aspects of the gross and fine structure of the oviducts; the reader is referred to Nilsson & Reinius (1969), Beck & Boots (1974) and Hunter (1988).

The mucosa is lined by a cylindrical monostratified epithelium containing

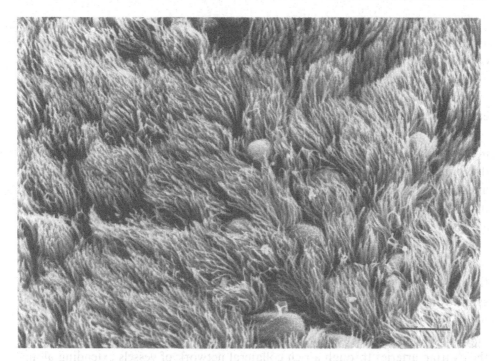

Fig. 1. Scanning electron micrograph of the mucosal surface of the rabbit fimbria. The vast majority of the cells are ciliated. A few dome-shaped cells that correspond to secretory cells are visible. The average length of each cilium is 6–8 μm. Notice that no mucus is present on the surface of the epithelium probably due to the few secretory cells normally found in this segment of the oviduct but also to some artefact related to the fixation procedure. The bar in the lower right corner is 7 μm.

ciliated, secretory, 'peg' and basal cells. Ciliated cells tend to be more numerous in the ampulla than in the isthmus, where secretory activity is more prominent (Jansen, 1984). Morphological and functional changes of the tubal epithelium have been described in association with the hormonal fluctuations of the ovarian cycle (Fredericks, 1986).

The distal segment of the oviduct, the fimbria and infundibulum, is an expansion of the mucous membrane which adopts diverse forms across the species (funnel-shaped, flower-shaped or simple eversion) having in common the highest density of ciliated cells (Fig. 1), and the thinnest layer of muscle fibres. The active stroke of the cilia beat in centripetal direction converging towards the entrance to the ampulla.

The ampulla is the longest segment in the human and the shortest in rodents. It is characterized by the great abundance and complexity of mucosal folds which fill the lumen leaving only a virtual space, and is surrounded by a thin layer of smooth muscle.

The characteristic increase in the thickness of the smooth muscle of the isthmus as compared to that of the ampulla, marks the AIJ with a distinct change in consistency in the middle third of the oviduct. Also, beginning at this point and extending throughout the remainder of the isthmus, the mucosa is reduced to a few primary folds, and the cross-sectional diameter occupied by the mucosal epithelium is drastically decreased.

In the isthmus, the smooth muscle forms a sheath several times thicker than in the ampulla, and is organized in layers. For instance, in humans there is a thin inner longitudinal layer that runs at the foot of the mucosal folds; an intermediate circular layer that occupies the largest proportion of the wall thickness; and a thick outer helicoidally orientated longitudinal layer which forms a continuum with the interserosal muscle of the mesosalpinx.

At their caudal end, the oviducts penetrate the uterine wall to form the intramural segment. The most consistent morphological features of this segment, the narrow lumen and the drastic increase in the thickness of the surrounding smooth muscle, are probably responsible for the high resistance to the passage of fluids found at the UTJ in some species.

In the mammalia, the oviduct receives its blood supply from the uterine and the ovarian arteries through a rich collateral network of vessels extending along the mesosalpingeal side of the tube. Interconnecting capillary networks in the muscle layers and in the mucosa of the tube resolve into venous vessels that follow the course of the arterial supply (Verco, 1991). The close relationship between arteries and veins in the ovarian pedicle provides the anatomical basis for a local counter-current transfer system of hormonal signals between the ovary and the tube (Hunter, 1988).

The tube is innervated by sympathetic and parasympathetic nerves and afferent visceral nerves (Hodgson & Eddy, 1975). The application of histochemical fluorescence methods for detecting catecholamines has revealed that the sympathetic innervation of the ampulla is sparse and reduced to vascular terminals whereas that of the isthmus is abundant and supplies the circular muscle layer (Owman *et al.*, 1976). There is also evidence for the presence of peptidergic terminals (Sjöberg & Helm, 1991). The functional relationship between the innervation, the myosalpinx and oocyte transport are discussed under smooth muscle cells and regulation of oviductal transport.

Oocyte release from the follicle and uptake by the fimbria

The transit of the oocyte from the follicle into the tubal lumen takes from a few minutes to a few hours at most. The ovary, the oviduct and their connecting ligaments play an active role in this process which requires follicular rupture with extrusion of the cumulus, the encounter of the latter with the fimbria, and the action of a mucociliary current that drives it into the infundibulum.

Follicular rupture results from the concerted action of enzymes that degrade the intercellular matrix in the apex, and of tonic contraction of smooth muscle cells that sustain the pressure as the debilitated follicle wall yields (see chapters on ovulation in this volume). Oocyte release from the follicle may fail under a variety of circumstances, even when follicular rupture does occur (Croxatto & Ortiz, 1989).

In small rodents, the follicular content is emptied into the periovarian bursa, into which the fimbria protrudes and this ensures the cumulus–fimbria encounter. In the human, in which the follicular content is voided into a large space, the peritoneal cavity, ovum pick-up from the surface of the ruptured follicle is not ensured. During ovulation, the distal end of the tube and the ovary move actively using the tubo-ovarian ligaments as a bascule. These movements allow the fimbria to sweep the surface of the ovary enhancing the probability of capturing the cumulus oophorus whose mucus matrix and elasticity allow the cilia to pull very effectively, detach and carry the oocyte in cumulus into the infundibulum. However, normal or near normal fertility has been observed in animals following microsurgical disruption of the tubo-ovarian anatomic relationships, including fimbriectomy, thus challenging the functional importance of this arrangement (for review see Croxatto & Ortiz, 1989).

There is clinical and experimental evidence which suggests two modalities of ovum pickup. In the first, the fimbria encounters the cumulus still adhering to the ovarian surface and effects its transfer directly from that site to the infundibulum. In the other, the fimbria takes up an oocyte which has detached from the ovarian surface, and is freely floating in the intervisceral spaces of the pelvis. The ability of the fimbria to pick up particles from the intervisceral space has been demonstrated in rabbits and in women (Diaz *et al.*, 1976, Gómez & Croxatto, 1977; Uher, Rypácvek & Presl, 1990). The second modality is more prone to result in delayed pick-up and also in transmigration of the oocyte from the ovulating ovary to the contralateral oviduct. This is believed to be a back-up mechanism and to occur infrequently in women (Croxatto & Ortiz, 1989).

Oviductal transport

Methods of study

Investigators have used several techniques to determine the gross and detailed time course of oviductal transport. These techniques seek specific information on how many eggs remain or where the eggs are in the oviduct at known intervals from ovulation or after being transferred to the oviduct.

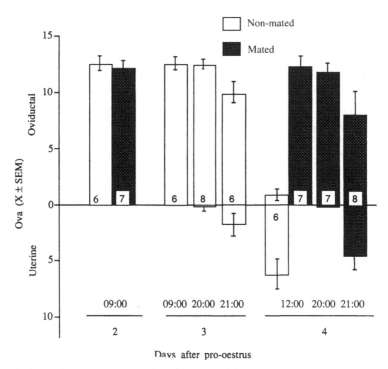

Fig. 2. Distribution of ova at various times after ovulation (Day 1) in mated and non mated rats. Mated rats were caged overnight with fertile males in the evening of pro-oestrus (Day 0) and the non mated were kept isolated. Mating was confirmed by the finding of sperm in the vagina the following morning and the finding of embryos at autopsy. At the indicated times the oviducts and uterus were removed and flushed separately to count the ova. Notice unfertilized oocytes in non mated females begin to enter the uterus at 21:00 on day 3 while embryos enter the uterus 24 hours later in mated rats. Figures at the foot of the bars indicate number of animals autopsied at each time.

The approximate location of eggs is usually established by systematic flushing of segments of the genital tract in situ or after its removal. The flushings collected into separate dishes are examined under a stereoscopic microscope to count and classify the eggs. Division of the tract in two segments, oviduct and uterus, affords a gross estimation of transport by assessing the proportion of eggs that have crossed the UTJ. The accuracy increases as the interval between time points is shortened (Fig. 2) or as the tract is divided into smaller segments (Fig. 3). The precise location of each egg within the oviduct can be established in some cases without dislodging them from the lumen. For instance, in the mouse, the eggs can be located, counted and classified when the oviducts, slightly compressed between glass slides, are examined with the microscope while being transilluminated.

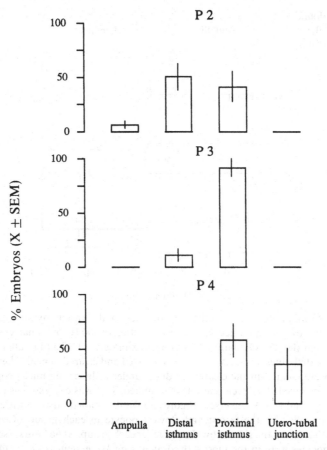

Fig. 3. Segmental distribution of embryos in the rat oviduct from the second (P2) through the fourth (P4) day of pregnancy. After mating as described in legend of Fig. 2 the oviducts were removed at the indicated times and were divided into four segments using a dual operator surgical microscope. Each segment was flushed to count the embryos. The total number recovered from each oviduct was taken at 100%. Passage from the ampulla to distal isthmus takes place right after midnight of P1 (not shown). Notice the high proportion of embryos in the proximal isthmus on P3.

The thicker walls of the rabbit oviduct do not allow the eggs inside to be seen unless they are stained or the oviducts are cleared in benzyl-benzoate (Longley & Black, 1968). Once the exact distance travelled from the fimbria by each egg, and the length of the oviduct have been measured, transport can be expressed quantitatively as mean per cent of total length travelled by eggs at a given time point (Fig. 4).

Stained cumulus masses (Blandau, 1969; Villalón *et al.*, 1991) or egg surrogates that can be seen through the wall of the oviduct have been

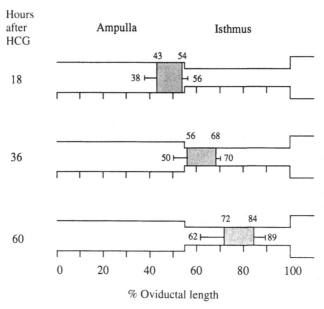

Fig. 4. Percentage distance travelled by oocytes in the rabbit oviduct at three intervals after ovulation induction by an i.v. injection of 100 IU of human chorionic gonadotropin (HCG). Ovulation occurs approximately 10–12 hours after HCG. At the indicated times oviducts were removed, fixed and cleared in benzyl benzoate. Oocytes were located in the cleared oviducts under a dissecting microscope and the distance travelled by each one was determined. This was expressed as per cent of total oviductal length traversed. Figures above the shaded area are the average per cent travelled by the fastest and slowest oocyte in each group of oviducts ($n = 4$–6). Figures on the sides show the range for each group. At 66 hours essentially all oocytes were in the uterus. (Redrawn from Pauerstein et al., 1974.)

introduced in living anaesthetized animals (Moore & Croxatto, 1988b) or in vitro (Hodgson, Talo & Pauerstein, 1977) to observe their motions within the lumen.

Asynchronous transfer of embryos or transfer of alien eggs or microspheres of diverse materials and diameters (Diaz et al., 1976; Moore & Croxatto, 1988a, b) to the oviduct followed by assessment of their location at various time points have been used to explore mechanical and biological aspects of oviductal transport. Assessment of myosalpingeal activity with concomitant measurement of the motions of the luminal contents has greatly improved our understanding of the mechanics of oocyte transport (Talo, 1980, 1991).

Well thought-out microsurgical interventions which alter the gross structure or anatomical relationships of the oviductal segments have yielded valuable information on the relative importance of different oviductal components for egg transport (for review see Land, 1987).

Table 1. *Approximate duration (hours) of oviductal egg transport*

Opposum	24	Rhesus monkey[a]	72
Pig	48	Baboon[f]	71
Guinea pig[a]	48–72	Human[g]	80
Rabbit[b]	55	Rat	88
Hamster[c]	60	Goat	98
Ewe[d]	66	Horse[h]	144
Mouse	72	Cat	144–168
Cow	72	Dog	192–240
		Bat[i]	188

Data from a. Maia *et al.*, 1977; b. Pauerstein *et al.*, 1974; c. Bastianns, 1973; d. Holst, 1974; e. Eddy *et al.*, 1975; f. Eddy *et al.*, 1976; g. Croxatto *et al.*, 1978; h. Betteridge *et al.*, 1982; i. Rasweiler, 1979. All others from review in Croxatto & Ortiz, 1975.

Duration and time course

The total duration of oviductal transport is the time taken by the egg to reach the uterine lumen since it was released from the follicle. This differs between species and ranges from 1 to 12 days (Table 1). For a given species, this is fairly constant among individuals observed under the same physiological condition. Obviously, this indicates it is a highly programmed and controlled process. On the other hand, the duration of transport can differ among conspecific individuals under different conditions, i.e. mated versus non-mated (see Fig. 2). This suggests that the programme is not fixed but only, in part or wholly, amenable to physiological regulation.

It is well established that eggs do not traverse the entire length of the oviduct at a uniform speed. In all mammals in which this has been examined, transport through the ampullary segments takes minutes and eggs stay close to the AIJ from many hours to several days. After crossing the AIJ, progress through the isthmus may be fast or slow but fairly regular and in some species eggs stays close to the UTJ for a while before entering the uterus. During transport through the ampulla or isthmus or while staying close to the junctions, eggs move back and forth for variable short distances at a speed that far exceeds the average speed of their net transport towards the uterus.

The proportion of time spent by the ova in each segment varies considerably among the species (Fig. 5) and bears no constant relationship with the relative

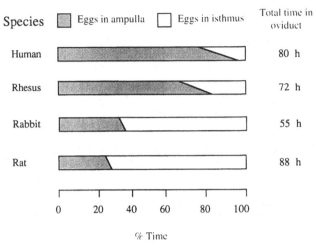

Fig. 5. Relative time spent by oocytes or embryos in the ampulla and isthmus of the oviduct in two primates and two species widely used in studies on oviductal transport. The ampulla represents approximately two-thirds of the length of the oviduct in the primates, about one half in the rabbit and one third in the rat. (Data from: Croxatto & Oritz, 1989 (human), Eddy *et al.,* 1975 (rhesus) Pauerstein *et al.,* 1974 (rabbit); Croxatto *et al.,* 1991 (rat).)

length of the segments or to that of the entire oviduct. In the human, the egg spends 90% of the time in the ampulla, while, in rodents, the eggs spend only 25% of the time in that segment.

The time course of oviductal transport has been described in detail in the rabbit, the mouse, the rat and the hamster. In these four polyovular species, progress towards the uterus is transitorily arrested when eggs in cumulus reach the AIJ. Most stages of fertilization and the loss of cumulus cells occur at this point. Once eggs pass the AIJ they tend to travel close together. Rabbit eggs acquire a thick mucin coat as they traverse the isthmus.

In rats, mice and hamsters, whose oviducts are highly coiled most of the time, eggs occupy one or two adjacent isthmic loops. Observations in the living oviduct *in situ* or *in vitro* show that eggs are moving all the time. Their back and forth movements reshuffles them intermittently. Eggs from two adjacent segments may join in a single group and segregate again in two groups with a different mix. Eggs are seen to occupy a bolus of fluid trapped between luminal constrictions. The lumen appears distended where the bolus lays. Sometimes the bolus is displaced as such, carrying the eggs within. At other times, the fluid is forced through a constricted lumen in one or in opposite directions, and this causes segregation of the eggs that previously moved together.

Gate-like behaviour of the ampullary isthmic junction

When eggs in cumulus or ovum surrogates are transferred to the infundibulum shortly after ovulation, they are transported up to the AIJ where they mix with native eggs. Subsequently, they travel together. If transfer to the infundibulum is increasingly delayed with respect to ovulation, the time they have to wait near the AIJ to enter the isthmus becomes shorter and shorter. If transfer of alien eggs or surrogates is postponed until the native eggs have crossed the AIJ, they experience no delay at the AIJ, and they reach them in the isthmus in a short time. With further postponement of transfer, a time comes when surrogates or alien eggs reach the AIJ and do not pass beyond even for several days. This has been observed in rabbits (Weinberg & Pauerstein, 1980) and rats (Moore & Croxatto, 1988*b*) and has led to the concept that the AIJ behaves as a gate which is closed at the time of ovulation, opens several hours or days later pending on the species, remains open for a while after the eggs enter the isthmus and closes again to remain shut probably until the next ovulatory episode. Closing the gate soon after the eggs enter the isthmus probably helps the mechanics of transport in that segment and also isolates an environment for oviductal embryo development in those species in which most of it occurs beyond the AIJ.

Mechanical effector cells of the oviduct

Smooth muscle cells

Smooth muscle, ciliated and secretory cells are recognized as the oviductal mechanical effector cells that generate the forces that move or prevent the eggs from moving or progressing within the lumen. Cause–effect relationships between the contractile activity of the myosalpinx and progression or non-progression of oocytes within the oviduct have been sought by a variety of *in vivo* and *in vitro* techniques, yet very little is known to explain how muscle contractions of the tubal wall integrate their action in time and space to account for the pattern of egg transport.

The smooth muscle of the oviduct demonstrates both phasic and tonic activity. Detailed measurements of transport of supravitally stained eggs in cumulus inside the oviduct by cinematographic recording and computer image analysis have revealed that phasic muscle contractions of the tube are responsible for the typical random pendular motions of the egg which have been observed in the oviducts of a variety of species, including primates (Verdugo *et al.*, 1976; Hodgson, Talo & Pauerstein, 1977; Villalón *et al.*, 1991). These pendular motions are produced by contractions of the circular smooth muscle (Hodgson *et al.*, 1977).

Recordings of myoelectric activity show that along the wall of excised human oviducts there are multiple pacemaker sites. During observation, these pacemakers change location and periods of short-ranged directed (biased) propagation of the myoelectrical activity alternate with periods of complete randomness of propagation (Talo, 1991). Directional propagation of myoelectric activity and the corresponding movement of material within the lumen take place through very short tubal lengths at speeds that can reach up to one or two mm/s. Contractions last for only a few seconds before reversing direction, resulting in a characteristic to and fro pattern of intraluminal motion and very slow rates of net oviductal transport (Hodgson *et al.*, 1977; Talo, 1991). However, indirect quantitative evidence indicates that oviductal motility can be partially derandomized resulting in biased contraction-driven egg motions in the rabbit oviduct (Verdugo, 1982).

The sole measurement of oviductal motility at a single point by intra- or extra-luminal sensors has no predictive value for the speed of oviductal transport, although peristaltic activity of the oviduct has been cited in the past as the basic mechanism of oocyte transport.

In summary, the movement of material within the lumen is determined by the frequency and distance that phasic contractions of the circular muscle propagate along the oviduct. On the other hand, junctional pauses of net tubal transport are probably due to the tonic activity of the myosalpinx in the next segment and to the uneven increases of smooth muscle mass along the tubal wall. More data on the time–space characteristics of tonic and phasic contractions related to various patterns of oocyte transport are needed for better understanding of the mechanics of oocyte transport through the oviduct.

The phasic and/or tonic behaviour of the myosalpinx can be independently affected by hormones or neurotransmitters, and longitudinal and circular muscle fibres can respond differently to the same substance.

Oestradiol (E_2) and progesterone (P) receptors and uptake of these steroids have been found to occur in the oviduct of all species examined. Quantitative studies of both steroid receptors at different times of the ovarian cycle and in different segments of the oviduct and immunocyto-chemical localization studies reveal that E_2 and P receptors are localized in secretory, stromal and smooth muscle cells and that their levels are subject to differential regulation (Brenner, West & McClelland, 1990).

Within physiological conditions, steroids do not cause immediate contraction or relaxation of smooth muscle, but they change the cell membrane potential

(Nozaki & Ito, 1987) and the responsiveness of the muscle cell to inotropic substances. Sex steroids also concentrate in sympathetic ganglia innervating the genital tract (Thompson *et al.*, 1985) and part of their action on oviductal contractility may be mediated through the extrinsic innervation.

In general, oestrogen potentiates and progesterone inhibits contractility of oviductal smooth muscle. These steroid actions are probably exerted by regulating the synthesis and/or release of sympathetic agonists and prostaglandins and the turnover of their corresponding receptors (for review see Harper, 1994).

The oviducts receive long and short postganglionic sympathetic fibres. The circular muscle is innervated mainly by short fibres, and receive most of the sympathetic nerve endings which contain catecholamines and neuropeptides. The content and turnover of these neurotransmitters and their receptors (Owman *et al.*, 1976) and the responsiveness of the myosalpinx to adrenergic agents are modulated by sex steroids (Nozaki & Ito, 1987). This affords a complex control system in which the same agent has different effects. For instance, norepinephrine, a dual α- and β-receptor agonist with preferential α-receptor stimulation, causes contraction or relaxation of the myosalpinx depending on the tubal segment, the muscle layer, and the type of steroidal domination. Such variations may help to explain many controversial results observed in the past on the control of muscle activity by catecholamines.

Several neuropeptides have been shown to occur in the oviduct of the human and other species. They include: neuropeptide Y, vasoactive intestinal peptide and substance P (Sjöberg & Helm, 1991). Gamma-aminobutyric acid has been found in high concentrations in the rat oviduct but it is localized in the epithelium rather than the nerve terminals (Celotti *et al.*, 1991). These substances affect the contractile activity of oviductal muscle.

Prostaglandins (PGs) are among the most widely distributed paracrine messengers, and they have a powerful effect on the smooth muscle cells of the mammalian oviduct (for review see Harper, 1994).

The content, distribution and effect of PGs varies, depending upon the species, the segment of the tube, type of prostaglandin and the pre-existing steroid levels. In the rabbit, for example, the number of binding sites of $PGF_{2\alpha}$ and PGE_2 in the myosalpinx changes in the various segments of the tube and at different times after ovulation. Also it has been shown that oestrogen potentiates the synthesis of $PGF_{2\alpha}$ and the stimulation of tubal contractions produced by $PGF_{2\alpha}$. Conversely, progesterone inhibits the local synthesis and the response of tubal smooth muscle to $PGF_{2\alpha}$ and it potentiates the inotropic effect of PGE_1 on the proximal isthmus. The observed pharmacological effects are consistent with contractile patterns and tubal transport during periods of oestrogen and/or progesterone dominance in the rabbit.

In the monkey, the effect of PGs depends upon the time in the cycle. During the preovulatory phase, PGE_1 and PGE_2 have no effect on spontaneous tubal contractions, but during the luteal phase they clearly suppress spontaneous tubal contractions. On the other hand, $PGF_{2\alpha}$ has no effect on contractility during the follicular phase, but it stimulates contractions immediately before and during ovulation.

Human oviducts not only contain prostaglandins, but they are responsive to them. Studies conducted both *in vivo* and *in vitro* show that, with some exceptions, $PGF_{2\alpha}$ stimulates the PGE_2 inhibits contractions in the different tubal segments at various times during the menstrual cycle. The evidence, obtained so far, clearly indicates that prostaglandins are involved in the control of tubal contractility and that their synthesis and effects are modulated by ovarian steroids.

Ciliated cells

Various densities of ciliated cells have been found in the mucosa lining the internal surface of the oviduct in vertebrates (Nilsson & Reinius, 1969). It is now well established that, with a few species variations, oestrogen influences the development, persistence and density of cilia in the mucosa of the oviduct.

In primates, the density of oviductal cilia or the height of the ciliated epithelium undergoes cyclic variations in relation to the menstrual cycle. The oviductal epithelium is low (10 μm) in periods of progesterone domination; its height doubles in periods of oestrogen domination; and it shows signs of atrophy in late menopausal state (macaque: Brenner, 1969; human: Verhage & Jaffe, 1986).

The involvement of oviductal cilia in oocyte transport was postulated very early but only recently it was shown that, in the absence of muscle contractions, ciliary activity is sufficient to drive the ovum throughout the ampulla of the rabbit and the rat (Halbert, Tam & Blandau, 1976; Halbert, Becker & Szal, 1989). Although ciliary action is sufficient to power tubal transport, it may not be essential. Some women suffering from immotile cilia syndrome, who are assumed to have no ciliary activity in their tubes, have intrauterine pregnancies (Afzelius, Camner & Mossberg, 1978; McComb *et al.*, 1986). These findings have been subject to controversial interpretations, owing to the idea that the role of muscle and cilia in the oviduct are mutually exclusive. This apparent paradox can be explained on the basis of redundancy in oviductal function i.e. both muscle contractions and ciliary movement might not be necessary, yet each could be sufficient to ensure the transport of gametes (Villalón & Verdugo, 1991).

Cilia beat in a pro-uterine direction along the different segments of the tube. The regulation of ciliary movements in the oviduct has only recently begun to be explored. The frequencies of ciliary beat in various sections of the human and rabbit oviduct change throughout the ovarian cycle. Direct hormonal actions on ciliated cells cannot be unequivocally established by measuring ciliary movements in the intact oviduct because hormones can affect secretory activity and change the rheological properties of the secreted mucus. Such variations of the fluid load may, in turn, indirectly change the movement of cilia.

The recent introduction of a validated method for measuring ciliary movement, based on laser Doppler spectroscopy, and the development of a mucus-free tissue culture preparation of oviductal ciliated cells have made possible study of the control of ciliary motion. Using these techniques, it was unequivocally demonstrated that ciliated cells of the rabbit oviduct are responsive to hormones. For instance, PGs, $F_{2\alpha}$, E_1 and E_2 and ATP in concentrations equivalent to those found *in vivo* have been shown to stimulate oviductal ciliary activity. Beta-adrenergic agonists also stimulate oviductal ciliary motion and, although ovarian steroids do not cause immediate changes in ciliary activity, preliminary data suggest that either oestrogen or progesterone alone strongly potentiate and both combined inhibit β-adrenergic stimulation (Villalón & Verdugo, 1991).

Secretory cells

Fluid present in the lumen of the oviduct is formed by transudation from the blood and active secretion from the oviductal mucosa and varies in composition, rheological properties and volume depending on the stage of the sex cycle. The volume of the fluid is greatest near ovulation and minimal during the luteal phase. As described in an earlier section, fluid displacements caused by contractions serve to move the eggs in the isthmus. In humans and rabbits, tenacious mucus that fills the isthmus around the time of ovulation and that disappears several days later might be important for timing the entrance of oocytes into this segment (Jansen, 1984).

Regulation

As stated in a previous section, oocyte transport is a regulated process. Premature arrival or transfer of the embryos to the uterus is followed by decreased rate of implantation at least in rodents and rabbits. On the other hand, embryos retained in the oviduct by mechanical or hormonal manipulations stop developing and lose viability. The idea that there is an optimal time for embryos to move from the oviductal to the uterine milieu is widely held as a teleological argument in favour of the existence of regulatory mechanisms that determine the time of their passage into the uterus.

Three possible regulatory pathways have been investigated: a) endocrine regulation exerted by the ovarian sex steroids, b) nervous regulation through the autonomic innervation of the oviduct and c) paracrine regulation exerted by the embryo. Studies reported in the literature do not allow us to examine the relative participation of all three regulatory mechanisms in any single species.

While the role of sex steroids has been examined with great detail in the rat, mouse and rabbit, the role of the sympathetic innervation has been examined extensively only in the rabbit and the role of the embryo has been studied in equines (Hunter, 1988), bats (Rasweiler, 1979) and more recently in rats, mice and hamsters (Ortiz *et al.*, 1991*a, b*).

The concept that ovarian steroids control oviductal transport arose from experiments designed to assess the effects of ovariectomy or exogenous hormones on this process. It became clear that diverse species reacted differently to these manipulations and that, within a species, the same hormone could exert qualitatively different effects on oviductal transport pending on the dose and time of administration (Greenwald, 1967). Most of the work involving exogenous steroids did not differentiate physiological from pharmacological effects. More recently selective hormone deficits have been produced or simulated either by inhibiting hormone synthesis and secretion or neutralizing the hormone in the circulation by means of antibodies or by intercepting the hormone at the receptor level by means of antihormones (Croxatto *et al.*, 1991). In these experiments it is assumed that the effects observed are the mirror image of what the hormone does to oviductal transport when acting at physiological concentration. As an example, if the experimental deficit results in accelerated transport, this is interpreted to mean that at physiological levels the hormone is acting to slow down oviductal transport. From this type of experiment, it is now fairly well established that oestrogens and progestins have opposite effects on oocyte transport, and act disparately in different species. Endogenous oestradiol speeds up oviductal transport in the rat and has the opposite effect in rabbits (Bigsby, Duby & Black, 1986). Endogenous progesterone delays oviductal transport in the rat and has the opposite effect in mice (Vinijsanun *et al.*, 1990). That sex steroids control the rate of oocyte transport in rodents by virtue of a direct action upon the oviduct has been demonstrated by comparing the local versus the systemic effective dose (Zenteno *et al.*, 1989 and Fig. 6).

The precise role of endogenous steroids in the regulation of egg transport in other species including the human is unknown although it is suspected

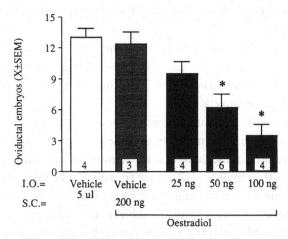

Fig. 6. Accelerated oviductal transport of embryos caused by intraoviductal (I.O.) injection of oestradiol. Rats on day one of pregnancy subjected to laparotomy under anaesthesia received, in the infundibulum of each oviduct, an injection of 5 μl of vehicle (ethanol:glycerol:saline; 20:30:50) with or without oestradiol. One group treated I.O. with vehicle alone received 200 ng oestradiol subcutaneously (s.c.). Notice a significant decrease in the number of embryos remaining in the oviducts on day 2 of pregnancy in animals which received 50 or 100 ng oestradiol I.O. The vehicle alone or 200 ng oestradiol s.c. had no effect (Data from Forcelledo M.L., observations unpublished.)

in those in which the effect of pharmacological doses has been observed. In the human, acute administration of fairly large doses of oestradiol or progesterone in the immediate postovulatory period failed to alter the recovery of oocytes from the tubes up to the time at which they would normally pass into the uterus (Croxatto *et al.,* 1979). This indicates that neither one of these hormones accelerates tubal transport in the human. It remains to be seen whether or not they delay passage of the oocyte beyond the AIJ or UTJ. Until now there is no direct evidence that sex steroids control tubal transport in the human. Indirect evidence stems from studies focused on smooth muscle, (Maia & Coutinho, 1976), ciliary (Critoph & Dennis, 1977) and secretory activity (Jansen, 1984) under different endocrine conditions. The association of tubal ectopic pregnancy with progestin-only contraceptive use (World Health Organization, 1985) suggests a relationship between sex steroid hormonal balance and tubal transport. Similarly, the alleged association of subnormal progesterone production by the corpus luteum during the early stages of ectopic pregnancy has been interpreted in the same manner (Pulkkinen & Jaakola, 1989). For the time being, both clinical observations constitute only a weak indication that tubal transport is under sex steroid hormone control in the human.

The chain of biochemical events that link the intracellular increase in oestradiol or progesterone to the final mechanical effect of moving the eggs at a faster or slower rate, or to lock them within one of the oviductal segments remains to be unveiled.

In spite of the profuse autonomic innervation of the oviduct, the responsiveness of the myosalpinx to nerve stimulation and the assortment of neurotransmitters found in the nerve terminals, there is little or no evidence that any of these play a significant role in the regulation of oocyte transport. The majority of the relevant studies on this topic were performed in the rabbit and the conclusions may not apply to other species. Various forms to achieve denervation of the oviduct failed to affect the pattern of egg transport in the rabbit. Systemic administration of adrenergic agonist or antagonists caused minimal alteration of normal or abnormal patterns of transport (Hodgson & Eddy, 1975). In most of those experiments, the endogenous sex steroid levels were not controlled, and therefore one cannot discriminate a direct interference with the neurotransmitter function in the myosalpinx from an indirect effect mediated through pituitary-gonadal dysfunction. If, on the other hand, the nervous control is exerted through the balance between neurotransmitters that have opposite effects, complete removal of nerve terminals may have no overt effects on oocyte transport. It is tempting to speculate that the innervation may serve to control oviductal functions relevant to reproduction only under special field conditions, i.e. those that threaten survival or afford enhancement of genetic diversity, that so far have not been simulated in the laboratory. The effects of various forms of stress on embryo transport in intact rats and mice have been very mild and of little if any consequence for fertility (Cárdenas, 1988) and denervation of the oviduct had no deleterious effect on fertility in these rodents (Roche, Parkington & Gibson, 1985).

That eggs regulate their transport through the oviduct is not a widespread concept. For a while the reports describing that unfertilized oocytes stayed in the oviduct instead of being transported to the uterus in the horse and one species of bat remained as a curiosity. More recently, less drastic but still clear differences in the transport of fertilized and unfertilized eggs have been described in rodents. Studies in the rat showed a pronounced difference in the timing of egg passage into the uterus between mated and non mated females (Fig. 2). This raised the question of whether the different rate of transport was due to the differences in the endocrine milieu or in the type of egg being transported. When the two types of eggs were produced in separate groups of pseudopregnant females by insemination with fertile or infertile sperm, the difference in oviductal transport between oocytes and embryos almost disappeared. On the other hand, similar experiments performed in hamsters showed that, even when the same animal was transporting fertilized ova in one side and unfertilized ova in the other, the former entered the uterus approximately 24 h earlier. Since the endocrine milieu was the same for both oviducts, it follows that the different transport resulted from local asymmetrically distributed factor(s) associated either with the condition of the eggs being transported or with the condition of the sperm inseminated (Ortiz *et al.*, 1991*b*).

Further exploration of these possibilities was conducted by transferring hamster oocytes or hamster zygotes to the oviducts of separate groups of rats on their first day of pregnancy. At autopsy on day four of pregnancy, the distribution of native and transferred eggs in the genital tract differed between the two groups. Where unfertilized hamster eggs had been transferred, almost all eggs, native and transferred, were recovered from the oviduct, as in control pregnant rats. In the group transporting rat and hamster embryos, more than half of the native and transferred eggs were recovered from the uterus. The fact that rat embryos entered the uterus earlier in the presence of hamster embryos, in conjunction with the previous results suggests that, in response to a signal produced by hamster embryos, the hamster and the rat oviduct transport the eggs to the uterus faster than they would if they were transporting only unfertilized eggs or rat embryos, respectively. When one-cell or four-cell rat embryos were transferred to the oviducts of recipient rats on day one of pregnancy, embryo passage into the uterus started earlier in the group transporting more advanced embryos. Thus, advanced rat embryos also influence the timing of their entrance to the uterus. The oviductal transport of oocytes and embryos in mice mated with vasectomized and fertile males, respectively, was also different but there is no evidence yet that this is a local phenomenon (Ortiz *et al.*, 1991*b*).

The nature of the putative signal produced by the embryo to time its entrance to the uterus was recently investigated in mares. Equine embryos were found to produce PGE_2 in increasing amounts since day 5 after ovulation, that is shortly before entering the uterus (Weber *et al.*, 1991*a*). Subsequently, it was demonstrated that a continuous intraoviductal infusion of PGE_2 started on day 3 after ovulation, but not a control infusion, stimulated the passage of embryos and unfertilized oocytes to the uterus by day 4 (Weber *et al.*, 1991*b*). These results suggest a role for embryonic PGE_2 in the differential transport of oocytes and embryos by the oviduct of the mare.

Another indication that the oviduct reacts to the presence of eggs is provided by the different behaviour of rat oviductal contractility and prostaglandin production *in vitro* when eggs are present or have been removed from the lumen (Viggiano *et al.*, 1990). In addition, the early pregnancy factor (EPF) component originated in the mouse and rabbit oviduct is apparently produced in response to platelet activating factor (PAF) or other unidentified ovum factor secreted by fertilized oocytes (Sueoka *et al.*, 1989).

The possibility that the oviduct can recognize embryonic signals is beginning to be explored in relationship to the regulation of egg transport as well as to the systemic embryo-maternal dialogue. In the former process the oviduct may act as a target and in the second as a relay station that amplifies or transduces the embryonic signals that must reach distant targets.

Uterine transport

Once the eggs enter the uterus they can be retained or expelled. At least in rats (Ortiz *et al.*, 1991*a*) and rabbits (Adams, 1980) premature arrival of eggs in the uterus is followed by their rapid expulsion to the vagina. At the normal time eggs are due to enter, the uterus shifts from an expulsive to a retentive state. Retention of embryos in the uterus is more important the longer the eggs remain free in the lumen prior to attachment to the endometrium. During retention embryos are not still. In mono- and polytocous animals, which have uterine horns, embryos are transported throughout the full length of the uterus and when there is luminal continuity between the two horns, they migrate from one to the other. This has been particularly well illustrated in the horse (Ginther, 1986). The single embryo enters one uterine horn on day 6 after ovulation and becomes visible by ultrasound on day 9. Until day 15 in which fixation occurs, the embryo moves continuously along the horn, in and out of the uterine body and the other horn. In the words of Ginther: 'The mobile embryonic vesicle blocks luteolysis in all parts of the uterus and at the same time distributes estrogens or some other substance that gradually increases uterine tone.' The ultimate destination is not a random location, but the flexure of the caudal portion of either horn where fixation and orientation of the embryonic vesicle occur.

In the pig, after the embryos enter the uterus they remain near the tip of the uterine horn for 4 days. Then, for the following 6 days, they migrate continuously along the horns, entering the horn opposite the one of origin until they are fixed regularly spaced. It appears that the whole length of the uterus needs the proximity of embryos or their signals to deactivate the luteolytic mechanism. If embryos are prevented from entering a significant section of the uterus in the period of mobility, pregnancy will not continue (Dziuk, 1985).

In polyovular species, embryos are transported within the uterus in a way that results in their dispersion throughout the length of the uterine horn. This is just the opposite to what happens in the oviduct where they tend to travel together. At the time of fixation, the blastocysts are spaced in many species more regularly than expected by chance.

Acknowledgements

We are grateful to Mrs Emma Muñoz for the skilful typing of this chapter. The support of the Rockefeller Foundation and the Human Reproduction Program of the World Health Organization made possible much of authors' work reported here.

References

Adams CE. Retention and development of eggs transferred to the uterus at various times after ovulation in the rabbit. *J Reprod fertil* 1980; **60**: 309–15.

Afzelius BA, Camner P, Mossberg B. On the function of cilia in the female reproductive tract. *Fertil Steril* 1978; **29**: 72–4.

Bastiaans LA. Effecten van enkele oestrogene en progestatieve stoffen op ovumtransport en zwangerschap bij de goudhamster, mesocricetus auratus (waterhouse) (Thesis). Nijmegen: Katholieke Universiteit te Nijmegen, 1973, 83 pp.

Beck LR, Boots LR. The comparative anatomy, histology and morphology of the mammalian oviduct. In: Johnson AD, Foley CW, eds. *The Oviduct and its Functions.* New York: Academic Press, Inc, 1974: 1–51.

Betteridge KJ, Eaglesome MD, Mitchell D, Flood PF, Beriault R. Development of horse embryos up to twenty two days after ovulation: observations on fresh specimens. *J Anat* 1982; **135**: 191–209.

Bigsby M, Duby RT, Black DL. Effects of passive immunization against estradiol on rabbit ovum transport. *Int J Fertil* 1986; **31**: 240–5.

Blandau RJ. Gamete transport-comparative aspects. In: Hafez ESE, Blandau RJ, eds. *The Mammalian Oviduct.* Chicago: The University of Chicago Press, 1969: 129–62.

Brenner RM, West NB, McClellan MC. Estrogen and progestin receptors in the reproductive tract of male and female primates. *Biol Reprod* 1990; **42**: 11–9.

Cárdenas H. El transporte ovular en condiciones de estrés (Thesis) Santiago: P. Universidad Católica de Chile, 1988, 83 pp.

Celotti F, Apud J, Negri-Cesi P *et al.* Gabaergic and cholinergic systems of the oviduct. *Arch Biol Med Exp* 1991; **24**: 257–268.

Critoph F, Dennis KJ. Ciliary activity in the human oviduct. *Br J Obstet Gynaecol* 1977; **84**: 216–18.

Croxatto HB, Ortiz ME. Egg transport in the Fallopian tube. *Gynecol Invest* 1975; **6**: 215–25.

Croxatto HB, Ortiz ME, Díaz S, Hess R, Balmaceda J, Croxatto H-D. Studies on the duration of egg transport by the human oviduct. II, ovum location at various intervals following luteinizing hormone peak. *Am J Obstet Gynecol* 1978; **132**: 629–34.

Croxatto HB, Ortiz ME, Díaz S, Hess R. Attempts to modify ovum transport in women. *J Reprod Fertil* 1979; **55**: 231–7.

Croxatto HB, Ortiz ME. Oocyte pickup and oviductal transport. In: Capitanio GL, Asch RH, De Cecco L, Croce S, eds. *Gift: from Basics to Clinics*. New York: Raven Press, 1989: 137–47.

Croxatto HB, Ortiz ME, Forcelledo ML, Fuentealba B, Noé G, Moore G, Morán F, Cárdenas H. Hormonal control of ovum transport through the rat oviduct. *Arch Biol Med Exp* 1991; **24**: 403–410.

Díaz J, Vásquez, J, Díaz S, Díaz F, Croxatto HB. Transport of ovum surrogates by the human oviduct. In: Harper MJK, Pauerstein CJ, Adams CE, Coutinho EM, Croxatto HB, Paton DM, eds. *Ovum Transport and Fertility Regulation*. Copenhagen: Scriptor, 1976: 404–15.

Dziuk P. Effect of migration, distribution and spacing of pig embryos on pregnancy and fetal survival. *J Reprod Fertil* 1985; **33**: 57–63.

Eddy CA, García RG, Kraemer DC, Pauerstein CJ. Detailed time course of ovum transport in the rhesus monkey (*Macaca mulatta*). *Biol Reprod* 1975; **13**: 363–9.

Eddy CA, Turner TT, Kraemer DC, Pauerstein CJ. Pattern and duration of ovum transport in the baboon (*Papio anubis*). *Obstet Gynecol* 1976; **47**: 658–64.

Fredericks CM. Morphological and functional aspects of the oviductal epithelium. In: Siegler AM, ed. *The Fallopian Tube*. New York: Futura Publishing Company, Inc. 1986: 67–80.

Ginther OJ. *Ultrasonic Imaging and Reproductive Events in the Mare*. 3rd edn. Wisconsin: Equiservices, 1986.

Gómez CV, Croxatto HB. A study of the time course of egg retention activity in the rabbit oviduct. *J Reprod Fertil* 1977; **50**: 69–73.

Greenwald GS. Species differences in egg transport in response to exogenous estrogen. *Anat Rec* 1967; **157**: 163–72.

Halbert SA, Tam PY, Blandau RJ. Egg transport in the rabbit oviduct: the roles of cilia and muscle. *Science* 1976; **191**: 1052–3.

Halbert SA, Becker DR, Szal SE. Ovum transport in the rat oviductal ampulla in the absence of muscle contractility. *Biol Reprod* 1989; **40**: 1131–6.

Harper MJK. Gamete and zygote transport. In: Knobil E, Neill J *et al.*, eds. *The Physiology of Reproduction*. New York: Raven Press, 1994: 123–87.

Hodgson BJ, Eddy CA. The autonomic nervous system and its relationship to tubal ovum transport – a reappraisal. *Gynecol Invest* 1975; **6**: 162–85.

Hodgson BJ, Talo A, Pauerstein CJ. Oviductal ovum surrogate movement: interrelation with muscular activity. *Biol Reprod* 1977; **16**: 394–6.

Holst PJ. The time of entry of ova into the uterus of the ewe. *J Reprod Fertil* 1974; **36**: 427–8.

Hunter RHF. *The Fallopian Tubes*. New York: Springer-Verlag, 1988.

Jansen RPS. Endocrine response in the Fallopian tube. *Endocr Rev* 1984; **5**: 525–51.

Land JA. Tubal microsurgery. II. Experimental use. *Gynecol Obstet Invest* 1987; **23**: 145–50.

Longley WJ, Black DL. Comparisons of methods for locating ova in the oviduct of the rabbit. *J Reprod Fertil* 1968; **16**: 69–72.

Maia H, Coutinho M. Motility of the human oviduct *in vivo*. In: Harper MJK, Pauerstein CJ, Adams CE, Coutinho EM, Croxatto HB, Paton DM, eds. *Ovum Transport and Fertility Regulation*. Copenhagen: Scriptor, 1976: 221–7

Maia H, Salinas LA, Fernández E, Pauerstein CJ. Time course of ovum transport in guinea pigs. *Fertil Steril* 1977; **28**: 863–5.

McComb P, Langley L, Villalón M, Verdugo P. The oviductal cilia and Kartagener's syndrome. *Fertil Steril* 1986; **46**: 412.

Moore GD, Croxatto HB. Synthetic microspheres transferred to the rat oviduct on day 1 of pregnancy mimic the transport of native ova. *J Reprod Fertil* 1988a; 82: 735–42.

Moore GD, Croxatto HB. Effects of delayed transfer and treatment with oestrogen on the transport of microspheres by the rat oviduct. *J Reprod Fertil* 1988b; 83: 795–802.

Nilsson O, Reinius S. Light and electron microscopic structure of the oviduct. In: Hafez ESE, Blandau RJ, eds. *The Mammalian Oviduct*. Chicago: The University Chicago Press, 1969: 57–83.

Nozaki M, Ito Y. Changes in physiological properties of rabbit oviduct by ovarian steroids. *Am J Physiol* 1987; **21**: R1059–65.

Ortiz ME, Bastías G, Darrigrande O, Croxatto HB. Importance of uterine expulsion of embryos in the interceptive mechanism of postcoital oestradiol in rats. *Reprod Fertil Dev* 1991a; **3**: 333–7.

Ortiz ME, Gajardo G, Mosso L *et al.* Differential transport of fertilized and unfertilized eggs. *Arch Biol Med Exp* 1991b; **24**: 393–401.

Owman CH, Falck B, Johansson EDB *et al.* Autonomic nerves and related amine receptors mediating motor activity in the oviduct of monkey and man. A histochemical, chemical and pharmacological study. In: Harper MJK, Pauerstein CJ, Adams CE, Coutinho EM, Croxatto HB, Paton DM, eds. *Ovum Transport and Fertility Regulation*. Copenhagen: Scriptor, 1976: 256–75.

Pauerstein CJ, Anderson V, Chatkoff ML, Hodgson BJ. Effect of estrogen and progesterone on the time-course of tubal ovum transport in rabbits. *Am J Obstet Gynecol* 1974; **120**: 299–308.

Pulkkinen MO, Jaakola U-M. Low serum progesterone levels and tubal dysfunction – a possible cause of ectopic pregnancy. *Am J Obstet Gynecol* 1989; **161**: 934–6.

Rasweiler JJ, IV. Differential transport of embryos and degenerating ova by the oviducts of the long-tongued bat. *Glossophaga soricina*. *J Reprod Fertil* 1979; **55**: 329–34.

Roche PJ, Parkington HC, Gibson WR. Pregnancy and parturition in rats after sympathetic denervation of the ovary, oviduct and utero-tubal junction. *J Reprod Fertil* 1985; **75**: 653–61.

Sjöberg N-O, Helm G. Adrenergic and peptidergic neuromuscular systems in the Fallopian tube. *Arch Biol Med Exp* 1991; **24**: 241–7.

Sueoka K, Dharmarajan AM, Miyazaki T, Atlas SJ, Wallach EE. *In vivo* and *in vitro* determination of components of rabbit early pregnancy factors. *J Reprod Fertil* 1989; **87**: 47–53.

Talo A. Myoelectrical activity and transport of unfertilized ova in the oviduct of the mouse *in vitro*. *J Reprod Fertil* 1980; **60**: 53–8.

Talo A. How the myosalpinx works in gamete and embryo transport. *Arch Biol Med Exp* 1991; **24**: 361–75.

Thompson SA, Radde L, Farley DB, Rosazza JP, Van Orden DE. Immunocytochemical localization of tissue-bound oestradiol in rat paracervical ganglion. *Histochem J* 1985; **17**: 493–506.

Uher J, Rypácek F, Presl J. Transport of novel ovum surrogates in the human Fallopian tube: a clinical study. *Fertil Steril* 1990; **54**: 278–82.

Verco CJ. Mammalian oviduct vasculature and blood flow. *Arch Biol Med Exp* 1991; **24**: 229–239.

Verdugo P, Blandau RJ, Tam PY, Halbert SA. Stochastic elements in the development of deterministic models of egg transport. In: harper MJK, Pauerstein CJ, Adams CE, Coutinho EM, Croxatto HB, Paton DM, eds. *Ovum Transport and Fertility Regulation*. Copenhagen: Scriptor, 1976: 126–37.

Verdugo P. Stochastic analysis of ovum transport: the effects of prostaglandin E_2. In: Brokaw CJ, Verdugo P, eds. *Mechanism and Control of Ciliary Movement*. New York: Alan R. Liss, Inc., 1982: 85.

Verhage HG, Jaffe RC. Hormonal control of the mammalian oviduct: morphological features and the steroid receptor system. In: Siegler Am, ed. *The Fallopian Tube*. New York: Futura Publishing Company, Inc., 1986: 107–17.

Viggiano M, Zicari JL, Gimeno AL, Gimeno MAF. Influence of ova within rat oviducts on spontaneous motility and on prostaglandin production. *Prost Leukot Essent Fatty Acids* 1990; **41**: 13–17.

Villalón M, Verdugo P. Control of ciliary movement in mammalian oviductal ciliated cells. *Arch Biol Med Exp* 1991; **24**: 377–84.

Villalón M, Verdugo P, Boling JL, Blandau RJ. The transport of cumulus egg masses through the ampullae of the oviducts in the pigtailed, *Macaca Nemestrina*. *Arch Biol Med Exp* 1991; **24**: 385–91.

Vinijsanun A, Martin L, Wang DY, Fantl VE. Effects of monoclonal antibody against progesterone, on embryo transport, development and implantation in laboratory mice. *Reprod Fertil Dev* 1990; **2**: 395–405.

Weber JA, Freeman DA, Vanderwall DK, Woods GL. Prostaglandins E_2 secretion by oviductal transport-stage equine embryos *Biol Reprod* 1991*a*; **45**: 540–3.

Weber JA, Freeman DA, Vanderwall DK, Woods GL. Prostaglandin E_2 hastens oviductal transport of equine embryos. *Biol Reprod* 1991*b*; **45**: 544–6.

Weinberg L, Pauerstein CJ. Transport of ova transferred to rabbit oviducts at varying intervals after human chorionic gonadotropin injection. *Fertil Steril* 1980; **33**: 77–81.

World Health Organization. A multicenter case-control study of ectopic pregnancy. *Clin Reprod Fertil* 1985; **3**: 131–43.

Zenteno J, Silva C, Cárdenas H, Croxatto HB. Effect of oestradiol delivered from a perioviducal device on ovum transport in mice. *J Reprod Fertil* 1989; **86**: 545–8.

11

Factors affecting oocyte quality

R. HOMBURG AND M. SHELEF

The assessment of oocyte quality is, of necessity, indirect. The good-quality oocyte may prove its true worth by being fertilized and producing a normal pregnancy capable of surviving through to viability. This positive result leaves us in no doubt, but a negative outcome may involve many other factors that do not necessarily incriminate a faulty oocyte.

The capacity of the oocyte to be fertilized may be assessed directly by its exposure to proven fertile sperm in ideal *in vitro* conditions. An oocyte problem, rather than a sperm problem, may be identified by the failure of fertilization of the oocyte in question when other oocytes from the same collection, or from another woman in a 'cross' test, are successfully fertilized by the same sperm sample.

The process of human *in vitro* fertilization (IVF) and the increasingly more sophisticated laboratory techniques involved, have given us the tools to attempt an assessment of oocyte quality and the possibility of examining factors that affect this quality which, in effect, is 'fertilizability' and the capacity to produce a normal embryo.

The morphology of the oocyte can now be well defined and classified and it is not surprising that a great deal of effort has been made to correlate the morphological evaluation of the oocyte with the chances of fertilization and a successfully implanting embryo. As oocytes may be collected for IVF at various stages of meiotic maturity, the assessment of their nuclear maturity has become a valid factor influencing fertilization and implantation rates. Thus the direct visualization of the oocyte for the assessment of oocyte quality and the effect of the various superovulation induction protocols on the appearance of the oocyte will be discussed.

There is now little doubt that increasing age has a deleterious effect on the chances to conceive and retention of the pregnancy and even less doubt that it is advantageous to be young and healthy. It is possible that age influences the quality of the oocytes directly, although it is also reasonable to assume that advancing years will also affect the potential of the endometrium or other conditions of the uterus to accept the pregnancy. There may also be a tenuous connection between age and the prevalence of so-called zona hardening which may be regarded as a morphologically seen physical barrier affecting the chances of fertilization.

The gonadotrophic control of the ovary and the fluctuations of luteinizing hormone (LH) and the follicle-stimulating hormone (FSH) that are involved in generating unifollicular maturation and development and then ovulation, have been well documented. In this chapter we discuss the endocrine control of the oocyte rather than of the ovary. Increasing amounts of data from studies in animals and, more recently, in man, suggest that control of oocyte maturation is one of the physiological processes that may readily become disrupted, with serious consequences, both for fertility and for the successful outcome of pregnancy.

This notion may be extended to thoughts on the importance of the environment in which conception occurs. These influences may be regarded as general endocrine or local intra-follicular. The penetration of drugs (e.g. gonadotrophin-releasing hormone agonists [GnRH-a] or anti-oestrogens) also have a potential influence on the immediate environment of the oocyte. In summary, this latter approach moves away from the purely quantitative (i.e. induction of ovulation or superovulation) to an appreciation of the quality of fertility therapy.

Determination of oocyte nuclear maturity

Since the innovation of IVF techniques we have the opportunity, at first hand, to examine the nuclear maturity of the oocyte and to investigate the influence of the stages of maturity on oocyte quality.

With any stimulation strategy, a cohort of oocytes at various stages of maturation is collected for IVF or related procedures and an assessment of nuclear maturity is made. Oocytes collected at a more advanced stage of maturation – metaphase II – present the polar body and provide the best chance of fertilization. Oocytes collected at the metaphase I stage require 5–15 hours of incubation to attain meiotic competence and mature and those collected at prophase I with incomplete germinal vesicle breakdown need more than 24 hours to mature (Veeck, 1990). Metaphase I oocytes demonstrate slightly lower rates of fertilization if the first polar body appears within 15 hours after harvesting. The remainder demonstrate a very marked reduction in fertilizing potential.

Microscopic determination of the oocyte maturity involves the morphological determination of the corona–cumulus complex. Metaphase II oocytes acquire a very expanded cumulus mass with stretching ability. The cells of the corona layer are bright and expanded. A polar body (PB) is clearly observed attached to the ooplasm. Lack of a PB defines a metaphase I oocyte.

Postmature oocytes acquire an expanded corona layer, a small cumulus mass with stained areas and darkened cells. Immature oocytes demonstrate a tightly packed cumulus mass, a compact corona, close to the zona pellucida.

Atretic oocytes are usually found with normal-looking oocyte corona–cumulus complexes (OCCC) but with abnormalities of the ooplasm and zona pellucida.

There are several reports on the relationship between the OCCC system, maturity and fertilizing capacity of the harvested oocyte (Cittadini and Palermo 1990).

Examination of the nuclear maturity is performed by cumulus spreading, and continues with an accurate insemination of each oocyte according to its maturity. It is very important in cases of a single oocyte harvest and in the gamete intrafallopian transfer (GIFT) procedure. It is a time-consuming procedure, needs separate incubation of each oocyte and laboratory personnel training, with only a slight increase in fertilization rates and a slight decrease in triploid fertilization rate.

The fertilizing capacity of the oocytes is not fully correlated to the maturity and some poor-quality oocytes can be found which produce two pronuclei. An analysis of the influence of oocyte quality can only be achieved by studying single embryo transfers. Even here there are conflicting results. Some have reported single embryo transfers with little prognostic value of oocyte evaluation whereas Sherrin *et al.,* (1991) reported that although some poor-quality oocytes did fertilize *in vitro*, none resulted in a pregnancy.

Timing of insemination in the IVF procedure is performed according to the maturity of the oocyte in order to avoid abnormal fertilization (1 or > 3 pronuclei).

Abnormal fertilization usually occurs when the oocytes are inseminated in an immature or postmature state. In immature oocytes the cortical granule numbers and response may be inadequate. In postmature oocytes, either cortical granule release after sperm penetration may be inhibited, or the zona reaction may function poorly (Trounson, 1982).

In our unit, oocytes diagnosed as metaphase II stage are inseminated 0–5 hours after harvesting, whereas oocytes diagnosed as metaphase I are inseminated 2–5 hours after the first PB extrusion. Oocytes diagnosed as having a germinal vesicle (GV) are inseminated at least 24 hours after harvesting, preferably after the first PB extrusion. In these cases, a second sample of semen is required 24 hours after the oocyte harvest. Despite this, we still have abnormal fertilization.

Oocyte maturity and micromanipulation

The assessment of the maturity of oocytes for micromanipulation is simple as the oocytes are denuded from surrounding cells by using hyaluronidase solution, hence the GV or PB are clearly identified. Intracytoplasmic sperm injection (ICSI) is performed in the metaphase II stage, 3–5 hours after harvesting and the other immature oocytes are not treated at that stage.

Partial zona drilling (PZD) or sub-zonal sperm injection (SZI) can be performed in the metaphase I oocytes as well as in metaphase II.

Oocyte morphology

Oocyte morphology assessed for surrounding OCCC can give a relatively accurate estimate of oocyte maturity but cannot predict the oocyte morphology. Atypical morphological appearances of the oocyte include granularity of the ooplasm, atypical characteristics of the first polar body (fragments, variations in size and shape), vacuoles within the ooplasm and many other atypical observations. A very granular ooplasm does not appear to affect the outcome of fertilization nor the pre-embryo appearance or pregnancy rate, whereas an overly large or small polar body may present less normal fertilizations and the presence of vacuoles or a 'refractile body' within the ooplasm provides a low possibility of fertilization of the oocytes (Veeck, 1985).

Oocyte chromosome anomalies

Several studies have shown a relatively high incidence of chromosome anomalies in inseminated-infertilized oocytes (Pellestor & Sele, 1988; Bongso *et al.,* 1988). Tarin *et al.,* (1991) have attempted to establish the actual importance of chromosome anomalies of human oocytes in IVF results. Although some oocytes did not fertilize because of the genomic constituent, no difference was demonstrated between pregnant and nonpregnant patients in the rate of chromosome anomalies in the oocytes. No increase in genomic abnormalities was observed as fertilization decreased. They concluded that fertilization rate and pregnancy outcome after IVF are not related to the incidence of oocyte chromosome anomalies.

Effect of age on oocyte quality

At approximately age 38–42 years, ovulation is clinically known to reduce in frequency. It has been suggested that the residual follicle units, now only a few thousand in number, are the least sensitive to gonadotrophin stimulation and hence, are less likely to achieve successful and complete maturation. As numbers of follicle units decrease, less oestrogen is produced from the surviving stimulated units. The associated, gradual increase in serum FSH concentrations at this time, due to negative oestrogen feed-back or release of inhibin inhibition, has thus been suggested as an indicator of a significant reduction in number and quality of the follicles remaining. This notion has been taken up and investigated in IVF programmes. Scott *et al.*, (1989) reported the association of FSH levels on cycle day 3 with the prediction of IVF outcome in 758 cycles. Ongoing pregnancy rate per attempt in patients with FSH levels that were low (<15 mIU/ml), moderate (15–25 mIU/ml) and high (>25 mIU/ml) were 17.0%, 9.3% and 3.6%, respectively ($P<0.01$). The three groups differed in the mean number of preovulatory oocytes obtained and peak oestradiol values. A further study (Toner *et al.*, 1991) concluded that basal FSH levels and age had independent contributions in predicting cancellation rate, peak oestradiol, number of oocytes retrieved, fertilized and transferred and total and ongoing pregnancy rates. Follicle stimulating hormone levels were found to be a significant and better predictor than age for all these outcome variables.

There is now little doubt that increasing maternal age has a deleterious effect on fertility potential. However, whether this age-related reproductive decline should be attributed to diminishing oocyte quality or to uterine/endometrial inadequacy, remains an unanswered question. Oocyte donation programmes have been utilized to try and solve this uncertainty but have, so far, produced conflicting results. Navot *et al.*, (1991*a*) studied 35 women aged >40 years who had failed to conceive with their own oocytes. With donated oocytes from younger individuals, a pregnancy rate of 56% and a 30% delivery rate was achieved. When oocyte quality was controlled with both donors and recipients receiving oocytes from the same induced cohort, rates for clinical pregnancy and delivery did not differ between donors and recipients. These data suggest that the age-related decline in female fertility is attributable to oocyte quality.

In contrast to these findings, Edwards *et al.*, (1991), examined age-related implantation and pregnancy rates in two large embryo transfer programmes and found that these rates were higher in previously amenorrhoeic women than in eugonadal women, irrespective of age and the number of embryos replaced. Oocyte quality, as determined by the age of the donor, *in vitro* growth of the embryo and proportion of defective embryos in culture, did not contribute to the difference. The insinuation of this study is that amenorrhoea maintains a favourable uterus and that it is the uterine environment, rather than oocyte quality, that accounts for the decline of fertility with age. Further data, from an oocyte donation programme, suggest that the independent function of the endometrium declines with age but, once implanted, the conceptus' risk of being aborted is dependent on the age of the oocyte and not the endometrium.

Cittadini & Palermo (1990), have suggested another possible influence of increasing age. Whereas they reported that various established protocols for controlled ovarian hyperstimulation had no influence on synchronized follicular growth, there was a wider asynchrony of oocytes of older ovaries and they suggested that this may account for the high rate of poor response in older women.

As Edwards et al., (1991) have suggested, the effects of quality of oocytes and of the recipient uterus can be differentiated only by transferring embryos arising from young oocyte donors into cyclic and acyclic women of comparable ages and doing the same with embryos from older oocyte donors.

Follicular microenvironment

Oocyte quality may be associated with the type of ovulation induction protocol. Administration of relatively small amounts of hMG is associated with fewer oocytes that are atretic and there is a tendency to a higher pregnancy rate. Higher doses of hMG leading to hyperstimulation may cause more oocytes to become atretic owing to higher follicular androstendione levels (Ben-Rafael et al., 1987: Romeu et al., 1988). A poor progesterone surge, together with high concentrations of FSH and reduced oestradiol levels, are correlated with luteal cyst formation, suggesting that this phenomenon is a produce of abnormal follicular metabolism and is therefore associated with a disturbance in the follicular microenvironment (Hamilton et al., 1990).

It appears that, when a good cohort of oocytes is harvested and inseminated with a fertilizing sperm sample, a few embryos with pregnancy potential are produced (Navot et al., 1991b; Levran et al., 1990). Can these few oocytes be detected for use in the IVF or zygote intra-fallopian transfer (ZIFT) procedures? The morphological appearance of the oocyte under the light microscope is not sufficiently predictive for the assessment of its maturity and fertilizability. Investigators therefore turned to an analysis of the endocrine environment in the follicular fluid (FF) in the search for a marker of the 'good' egg. Many assays have been performed, often with contradicting results.

Attempts to correlate angiotensin II and III, 17-β-oestradiol and progesterone concentrations in the individual FF with the ability of the oocyte to be fertilized, have failed (Jarry et al., 1988; Lindner et al., 1988). On the other hand, Zhang & Zhao (1990) reported that higher concentrations of FF oestradiol, progesterone, FSH, LH and lower testosterone concentrations were crucial for the maturation process of the oocyte and that the fertilization rate was significantly higher in mature rather than immature oocytes,

Facchinetti *et al.,* (1989) found no relation between FF steroid levels, oocyte maturity and subsequent fertilization but reported that oocyte fertilization was associated with high concentrations in the FF of immunoreactive β-endorphin. Lindner *et al.,* (1988) found that, when oocytes were fertilized, FF concentrations of prolactin were higher and those of cyclic adenosine monophosphate (cAMP) lower than in the FF of unfertilized oocytes. Significantly lower cAMP concentrations were also found by Pellicer *et al.,* (1987) in follicles whose oocytes were fertilized. Alpha-1 antitrypsin and fibrinogen were suggested as further possible markers. Both fibronectin and glycosaminoglycans appear to play a role in follicular maturity (Tsuiki, Preyer & Hung, 1988).

Several investigators seem to agree that a range of FF oestradiol/progesterone ratios define a stage of maturation that is compatible with successful subsequent implantation and pregnancy rates (Basuray *et al.,* 1988; Kreiner *et al.,* 1987; Franchimont *et al.,* 1989).

In order to answer the question of whether it is possible to select oocytes with the best pregnancy potential using the measurement of FF contents, it is clear that further prospective studies are needed

Endocrine factors affecting oocyte quality

Having described the state of maturation of the oocyte as an important factor in the assessment of oocyte quality, it is essential to know which factors may influence the state of oocyte maturity both in the physiologically normal ovulatory cycle and in pathological conditions. It is becoming increasingly clear that LH has a central role in the process of maturation of the oocyte and that abnormal secretion of this gonadotrophin may upset the intricate and delicate mechanisms involved.

Maturation of oocytes begins in late fetal life but the process is arrested at the diplotene (or dictyate) stage of the first meiotic division, in which stage the oocyte remains until shortly before ovulation (Tsafriri, 1988). Meiosis is then completed, the germinal vesicle breaks down and the mature oocyte is ovulated. The second meiotic division is completed only after fertilization. The arrest of oocyte maturation and its maintenance at the diplotene stage of meiosis depends upon its intra-follicular site and, since culture of the oocyte outside the follicle is associated with completion of meiosis, the concept of a follicle-derived oocyte maturation inhibitor has developed (Tsafriri, 1988). The notion is that inhibition of the production or antagonism of the action of this inhibitor of oocyte maturation occurs through the agency of the ovulatory stimulus, that is to say, through the action of LH. In this model, the events of the ovulation cycle are schematized thus: maturation of the dominant follicle results in increasing secretion of oestradiol which, via oestrogen-mediated positive feedback, results in the mid-cycle, preovulatory discharge of LH. Entry of LH into the preovulatory follicle results in completion of the first meiotic division of the oocyte contained within it; 36 hours or so later ovulation occurs with release of an oocyte of a maturity now appropriate for fertilization. The subsequent LH stimulation results in the formation of a corpus luteum, whose endocrine target is, of course, conversion of the oestrogen-stimulated proliferative endometrium into a secretory endometrium appropriate for implantation.

This scenario implies very precise timing of the various endocrine events described above. There is a species-specific interval between completion of the meiotic division of oocytes and their fertilization, during which conditions for producing a normal embryo are optimal (Baker, 1982). If the interval is extended, either by premature exposure to the ovulatory stimulus, as has been achieved in pigs by injections of hCG (Hunter, Cook & Baker, 1976) or by delaying insemination, as has been done in rats (Austin, 1982), poor rates of fertilization result and embryos that are produced survive poorly and are usually absorbed. In humans, Guerrero and Rojas (1975) found, in a study of the outcome of artificial insemination with donor semen, in which of course the timing of insemination is accurately known, that extension of the interval between ovulation and insemination was associated with a large increase in the rate of abortion of the ensuing pregnancies.

While the chemical nature of the putative oocyte maturation inhibitor is uncertain, work by Dekel (1986) and her group indicates that the presence of cAMP in the oocyte itself is essential to maintain it in its immature state. While the oocyte itself is unable to synthesize cAMP, intra-oocyte levels are maintained via the the cumulus granulosa cells, from which microfilamentous processes extend to make contact with the oocyte and serve as the conduits for this essential metabolite. Any process that disrupts physical contact between the cumulus granulosa cells and the oocyte therefore results in completion of oocyte maturation.

In a further series of elegant experiments in the rat, Dekel (1988) and her group (Sherizly, Galiani & Dekel, 1988) have shown that LH interrupts communication in the cumulus–oocyte complex prior to meiosis resumption and possible signals for oocyte maturation.

Thus, timely completion of the first meiotic division of the oocyte in the dominant follicle is induced by its exposure to LH at mid-cycle, the mechanism involving a reduction in the cAMP content of the oocyte through disruption of its microanatomical links with cumulus granulosa cells. This mechanism ensures ovulation of an oocyte of appropriate maturity. Extension of the interval between the completion of oocyte maturation and ovulation results in release of an egg that has become physiologically 'aged', less readily fertilizable and has lost, *inter alia,* its ability to block polyspermy (Austin, 1982); at fertilization it is therefore vulnerable to chromosomal disturbances, the most obvious of which is polyploidy. Whether other chromosomal disturbances that often have their origin at meiosis, for example, trisomy 21 (Bricarelli *et al.,* 1988), can be attributed to perturbations in the endocrine control of oocyte maturation is unknown, but is clearly an area for further study. In this model, the timing of the major endocrine signal in relation to ovulation and fertilization, that is the mid-cycle surge of LH, assumes a critical role. Premature exposure to LH, or exposure of the oocyte and follicular apparatus to agents that can minic its action, is seen in this model to be a potential cause for several clinical disorders of conception.

The hypothesis that inappropriate secretion of LH impairs oocyte quality and therefore fertility, first proposed by Jacobs *et al.* (1987), incorporates the notion of the crucial nature of the timing of oocyte maturation in relation to fertilization and the central role of mid-cycle LH surge in determining the duration of this interval. The hypothesis that widening of the interval between oocyte maturation and fertilization, and therefore prolonged exposure of the oocyte to LH, decreases the chance of a successful fertilization, may be extended to incriminate LH as a factor involved in an increased risk of miscarriage. A widening of the oocyte-maturation interval results in a loss of block to polyspermy and may result in chromosomal disturbances, both being factors which lead to miscarriage.

The working hypothesis before us is that hypersecretion of LH causes a premature maturation of the oocyte that becomes physiologically aged, is less readily fertilized and is more prone to miscarriage. How is this hypothesis born out by clinical experience? It implies that hypersecretion of LH may cause infertility and miscarriage independently of any impairment of the rate of ovulation and thus becomes a potential cause of 'unexplained' infertility in women with regular ovulatory cycles. Moreover, in patients with anovulatory infertility undergoing induction of ovulation, hypersecretion of LH may constitute a continuing adverse fertility factor, despite successful induction of ovulation.

There is now a growing body of clinical evidence to bear out this 'LH' hypothesis. In a study of 194 women with regular menstrual cycles, Regan, Owen & Jacobs (1990) found a striking association of raised follicular phase serum LH concentrations with infertility and miscarriage. In women with elevated serum LH concentrations (> 10 IU/l, RIA using MRC 68/40 IRP and polyclonal F87 anti-LH antiserum) the conception rate was 61% at 12 months, compared with 80% at 12 months in the women with normal LH levels ($P < 0.02$). In those who did conceive, the miscarriage rate in the women with normal LH concentrations was 12%, compared with 64% in those with elevated LH concentrations, a very highly significant difference. The impressive difference in miscarrige rates was

Table 1. *Mean (range) serum LH concentrations in relation to the outcome of therapy in 54 women with polycystic ovary syndrome who received treatment with LHRH* (From Homburg et al., 1988)

	Conception	Non-conception	Delivery	Miscarriage
Number of patients	27	27	18	9
Mean serum	12.4	19.0	9.6	17.9
LH (IU/l)	(1.3–29.0)	(3.5–50.0)	(1.3–29.0)	(7.0–29.0)
(range)		P = 0.02		P = 0.01

observed in both primigravid women and in those with recurrent abortion. This valuable study thus goes some way clinically to verify the hypothesis and provides us with a very powerful predictor of spontaneous miscarriage.

Women with polycystic ovary syndrome (PCOS) have an extremely high prevalence of high LH concentrations. Sagle *et al.* (1988) reported that ultrasonically diagnosed PCOS was present in some 80% of women with recurrent spontaneous abortions and the inference is that this very high rate of PCOS reflects raised concentrations of LH often associated with PCOS. It may be argued that the very presence of polycystic ovaries in some way determines the rates of infertility and miscarriage. However, there are two pieces of evidence suggesting that hypersecretion of LH is the true culprit, rather than the mere presence of polycystic ovaries. Conway, Honour & Jacobs (1989) published a series of more than 500 patients with PCOS in which those complaining of infertility had significantly higher LH concentrations than those whose fertility was proven (11.3 I.U./l vs 6.7 I.U./l; P = 0.0003). Of the subjects of this study, 44% had a serum LH concentration of >10 I.U./l and 37% of these complained of infertility, compared with 21% of those with normal concentrations of LH (P = 0.0004). In a study which measured serum LH concentrations and compared them to the outcome of therapy in 54 women with PCOS who received treatment with pulsatile luteinizing hormone-releasing hormone (LH-RH) (Homburg *et al.*, 1988), both failure to conceive despite ovulation and the occurrence of miscarriage rather than continuation of pregnancy were associated with elevated follicular-phase serum LH concentrations (Table 1). A summation of these two studies in which all the patients had PCOS leads us to conclude that it is the high follicular-phase LH concentrations rather than the presence of PCO, which predict the poor prognosis for fertility.

Stanger & Yovich (1985) were the first to report an association of a poor clinical outcome of fertility treatment to increase LH secretion. In an IVF programme they found that an endogenous high serum LH concentration on the day of administration of hCG was associated with a low rate of IVF and pregnancy. Howles *et al.*, (1986) confirmed these observations in a large series of patients undergoing IVF. They reported a poor outcome of the procedure in a patient who had a high excretion rate of LH in the days immediately preceding oocyte collection. Punnonen *et al.* (1988) reported similar findings and found that when an LH surge occurred more than 12 hours before the schedule time of hCG administration, embryo cleavage was significantly impaired.

A further clinical test of the proposed deleterious effect of high LH concentrations on oocyte quality would obviously be the use of superactive GnRH-a to block endogenous LH secretion followed by gonadotrophic stimulation of the ovaries. Results have so far proved disappointing. In a randomized, controlled clinical trial of the use of buserelin (Suprefact, Hoechst, UK) in induction of ovulation in patients with anovulation associated with PCOS (Homburg *et al.* 1990), results were compared with similar patients who received human menopausal gonadotrophin (hMG) or pure FSH alone. In this particularly difficult group of patients, buserelin failed to significantly increase pregnancy rates compared with hMG or FSH alone. The number of pregnancies obtained in this group of 46 patients over 122 treatment cycles was too small to assess the effect of buserelin on miscarriage rate. While others have reported improved pregnancy rates using buserelin, they have not achieved a decreased miscarriage rate. In our ongoing series employing Decapeptyl (DTRP6, slow release 3.75 mg, Ferring, Malmo, Sweden) in the treatment of anovulatory infertility associated with PCOS, 74 patients have so far been randomized to groups receiving GnRH-a + hMG, hMG alone, or pure FSH alone. So far, the cumulative conception rates of each group over six months are very similar (50–75%) and there is a trend towards a lower miscarriage rate in the GnRH-a group (22%) compared with those receiving hMG (42%). However, much larger numbers will be required to be of any statistical significance. An encouraging study of Johnson & Pearce (1990), in a group of women who had PCOS associated with recurrent spontaneous abortion, reported that 48% of women randomized to receive clomiphene had a repeat spontaneous miscarriage compared with 9% who received buserelin and FSH. Shoham *et al.* (1990) have reported a reduced fertility rate in patients receiving clomiphene citrate in whom LH concentrations were high in the follicular phase, compared with those with normal LH levels following clomiphene treatment.

While some of these results may appear to give some clinical weight to the hypothesis that high LH levels have a deleterious effect on the oocyte, the indirect evidence from the proposed treatment with GnRH-a is, as yet, far from convincing. Either the hypothesis is incorrect, or the treatment is unsuitable to prove the hypothesis. When considering the latter possibility, it should be noted that in the rat, GnRH can mimic LH action and induce oocyte maturation (Dekel, 1988). The rat oocyte contains receptors for GnRH. As Loumaye *et al.*, (1989) have demonstrated, using standard doses of buserelin, there was an accumulation of biologically active GnRH-a in FF. The desensitization with GnRH-a may not, therefore, provide the optimum context in which to test the 'LH hypothesis'.

In addition to LH and GnRH-a, other factors have been identified that accumulate in FF and experimentally cause oocyte maturation. These include clomiphene, tetrahydroxycannabinol and epidermal growth factor (Tsafriri & Pomerantz, 1986).

We have thus discussed the possible influence of endocrine factors on the oocyte rather than on the physiological process or induction of ovulation. It now appears obvious that their influence on the oocyte may be profound and may, when abnormal, cause disturbances in fertilization and the production of a normal embryo.

Summary

The advent of human IVF has given us the opportunity to approach the subject of oocyte quality and open up a field which previously had involved only guesswork. The determination of oocyte nuclear maturity has emerged as a most important factor in the assessment of oocyte quality and the normal 'fertilizability' of the oocyte. It is now also apparent that the environment of the oocyte influences its quality and that both endogenous imbalance and exogenously-given substances may have a deleterious effect.

References

Austin BR. The egg. In: Austin CR, Short RV, eds. *Reproduction in Mammals. Part 1. Germ Cells and Fertilization.* 2nd ed. Cambridge, UK: Cambridge University Press, 1982: 46–62.

Baker TG. Oogenesis and ovulation. In: Austin CR, Short RV, eds. *Reproduction in Mammals. Part 1. Germ Cells and Fertilization.* 2nd ed. Cambridge, UK: Cambridge University Press, 1982: 17–45.

Basuray R, Rawlins RG, Radwanska E, Henig I, Sachdeva S, Tummon I, Binor Z, Dmowski WP. High progesterone/estradiol ratio in follicular fluid at oocyte aspiration for *in vitro* fertilization as a predictor of possible pregnancy. *Fertil Steril* 1988; **49**: 1007–11.

Ben-Rafael Z, Benadiva CA, Ausmanas M, Barber B, Blasco L, Flickinger GL, Mastroianni L, Jr. Dose of human menopausal gonadotropin influences the outcome of an *in vitro* fertilization program. *Fertil Steril* 1987; **48**: 964–8.

Bongso A, Ng SC, Ratnam S, Sathananthan H, Wong PC. Chromosome anomalies in human oocytes failing to fertilize after insemination *in vitro. Hum Reprod* 1988; **3**: 645–9.

Bricarelli FD, Pierluigi M, Perroni L, Grasso M, Arslanian A, Sacchi N. High efficiency in the attribution of parental origin of non-disjunction in trisomy 21 by both cytogenetic and molecular polymorphisms. *Hum Genet* 1988; **79**: 124–7.

Cittadini E, Palermo R. Oocyte quality according to protocols for controlled ovarian hyperstimulation and patients' age. In: Mashiach S, Ben-rafael Z, Laufer N, Schenker JG, eds. *Advances in Assisted Reproductive Technologies.* New York and London: Plenum Press, 1990: 745–65.

Conway GS, Honour JW, Jacobs HS. Heterogeneity of polycystic ovary syndrome: clinical, endocrine and ultrasound features in 556 cases. *Clin Endocrinol* 1989; **30**: 459–70.

Dekel N. Hormonal control of ovulation. In: Litwack G, ed. *Biochemical Action of Hormones.* Vol. 13, Orlando, FL. USA: Academic Press, 1986: 67–90.

Dekel N, Lewysohn O, Ayalon D, Hazum E. Receptors for gonadotrophin releasing hormone are present in rat oocytes. *Endocrinology* 1988; **123**: 1205–7.

Edwards RG, Morcos S, Macnamee M, Balmaceda JP, Walters DE, Asch R. High fecundity of amenorrhoeic women in embryo-transfer programmes. *Lancet* 1991; **338**: 292–4.

Facchinetti F, Artini PG, Monaco M, Volpe A, Genazzani AR. Oocyte fertilization *in vitro* is associated with high follicular immunoreactive beta-endorphin levels. *J Endocrinol Invest* 1989; **12**: 693–8.

Franchimont P, Hazee-Hagelstein MT, Hazout A, Frydman R, Schatz B, Demerle F. Correlation between follicular fluid content and the results of *in vitro* fertilization and embryo transfer. I. Sex steroids *Fertil Steril* 1989; **52**: 1006–11.

Guerrero RJ, Rojas OI. Spontaneous abortion and ageing of human ova and spermatozoa. *New Engl J Med* 1975; **293**: 573–5.

Hamilton MP, Fleming R, Coutts JR, MacNaughton MC, Whitfield CR. Luteal phase deficiency: ultrasonic and biochemical insight into pathogenesis. *Br J Obstet Gynaecol* 1990; **97**: 569–75.

Homburg R, Armar NA, Eshel A, Adams JU, Jacobs HS. Influence of serum luteinising hormone concentrations on ovulation, conception and early pregnancy loss on polycystic ovary syndrome. *Br Med J* 1988; **297**: 1024–6.

Homburg R, Eshel A, Kilbourn J, Adams J, Jacobs HS. Combined luteinising hormone releasing hormone analogue and exogenous gonadotrophins for the treatment of infertility associated with polycystic ovaries. *Hum Reprod* 1990; **5**: 32–5.

Howles CM, MacNamee MC, Edwards RG, Goswamy R, Steptoe PC. Effect of high tonic levels of luteinising hormone on outcome of *in vitro* fertilisation. *Lancet* 1986; **ii**: 521–3.

Hunter RHF, Cook B, Baker TG. Dissociation of response to injected gonadotrophin between the Graafian follicle and oocyte in pigs. *Nature, London* 1976; **260**: 156–8.

Jacobs HS, Porter RN, Eshel ?, Craft I. Profertility uses of LHRH analogues. In: Vickery BH, Nestor Jr JJ, eds. *LHRH and its Analogues: Contraceptive and Therapeutic Applications,* part 2. Lancaster, UK: MTP Press, 1987: 303–22.

Jarry H, Meyer B, Holzzapfel G, Hinney B, Kuhn W, Wuttke W. Angiotensin II/III and substance P in human follicular fluid obtained during IVF: relation of the peptide content with follicular size. *Acta Endocrinol Copenh* 1988; **119**: 277–82.

Johnson P, Pearce JM. Recurrent spontaneous abortion and polycystic ovarian disease: comparison of two regimens to induce ovulation. *Br Med J* 1990; **301**: 154–6.

Kreiner D, Liu HC, Itskovitz J, Veeck L, Rosenwaks Z. Follicular fluid estradiol and progesterone are markers of preovulatory oocyte quality. *Fertil Steril* 1987; **48**: 991–4.

Levran D, Dor J, Rudak E *et al.* Pregnancy potential of human oocytes – the effect of cryopreservation. *N Engl J Med* 1990; **323**: 1153–6.

Lindner C, Lichtenberg V, Westhof G, Braendle W, Bettendorf G. Endocrine parameters of human follicular fluid and fertilization capacity. *Horm Metab Res* 1988; **20**: 243–6.

Loumaye E, Coen G, Pampfer S, Vankrieken L, Thomas K. Use of a gonadotropin-releasing hormone agonist during ovarian stimulation leads to significant concentrations of peptide in follicular fluids. *Fertil Steril* 1989; **52**: 256–63.

Navot D, Bergh PA, Williams MA, Garrisi GJ, Guzman I, Sandler B, Grunfeld L. Poor oocyte quality rather than implantation failure as a cause of age-related decline in female fertility. *Lancet* 1991*a*; **337**: 1375–7.

Navot D, Bergh PA, Williams M, Garrisi GJ, Guzman I, Sandler B, Fox J, Schriener-Engel P, Hofmann GE, Grunfeld L. An insight into early reproductive processes through the *in vivo* model of ovum donation. *J Clin Endocrinol Metab* 1991*b*; **72**: 408–14.

Pellestor F, Sele B. Assessment of aneuploidy in the human female by using cytogenetics of IVF failures. *Am J Hum Genet* 1988; **42**: 274–9.

Pellicer A, Diamond MP, DeCherney AH, Naftolin F. Intraovarian markers of follicular and oocyte maturation. *J in vitro Fert Embryo Transf* 1987; **4**: 205–17.

Punnonen R, Ashorn R, Vilja P, Heinonen PK, Kujansuu E, Tuohimaa P. Spontaneous luteinizing hormone surge and cleavage of *in vitro* fertilized embryos. *Fertil Steril* 1988; **49**: 479–82.

Regan L, Owen EJ, Jacobs HS. Hypersecretion of luteinising hormone, infertility and miscarriage. *Lancet* 1990; **336**: 1141–4.

Romeu A, Veeck LL, Oehninger S, Acosta AA. Significance of the recovery of fractured-zona oocytes in an *in vitro* fertilization program. *J In Vitro Fert Embryo Transf* 1988; **5**: 216–24.

Sagle M, Bishop K, Ridley N, Alexander FM, Michel M, Bonney RC, Beard RW, Franks S. Recurrent early miscarriage and polycystic ovaries. *Br Med J* 1988; **297**: 1027–8.

Scott RT, Toner JP, Muasher SJ, Oehninger S, Robinson S, Rosenwaks Z. Follicle-stimulating hormone levels on cycle day 3 are predictive of *in vitro* fertilization outcome. *Fertil Steril* 1989; **51**: 651–4.

Sherizly I, Galiani D, Dekel N. Regulation of oocyte maturation: communication in the rat cumulus–oocyte complex. *Hum Reprod* 1988; **3**: 761–6.

Sherrin D, Harrison K, Breen T, Wilson L, West G, Bell K. The prognosis value of grading oocyte and embryo quality. *(Abstract) Paris: 7th Congress of IVF*, 1991: 192.

Shoham (Schwartz) Z, Borenstein R, Lunenfeld B, Pariente C. Hormonal profiles following clomiphene citrate therapy in conception and non-conception cycles. *Clin Endocrinol* 1990; **33**: 271–8.

Stanger JD, Yovich JL. Reduced *in vitro* fertilisation of human oocytes from patients with raised basal luteinising hormone levels during the follicular phase. *Br J Obstet Gyn* 1985; **92**: 385–90.

Tarin JJ, Ruiz A, Miro F, Bonilla-Musoles F, Pellicer A. Failed *in vitro* fertilisation of human oocytes: a cytogenetic analysis. *Fertil Steril* 1991; **56**: 290–5.

Toner JP, Philput CB, Jones GS, Muasher SJ. Basal follicle-stimulating hormone level is a better predictor of *in vitro* fertilization performance than age. *Fertil Steril* 1991; **55**: 784–91.

Tsafriri A, Pomerantz SH. Oocyte maturation inhibitor. *Clinics in Endocrinology and Metabolism* 1986; **15**: 157–70.

Tsafriri A. Local nonsteroidal regulators of ovarian function. In: Knobil E, Neill J, eds. *The Physiology of Reproduction*. New York: Raven Press, 1988: 527–65.

Tsuiki A, Preyer J, Hung TT. Fibronectin and glycosaminoglycans in human preovulatory follicular fluid and their correlation to follicular maturation. *Hum Reprod* 1988; **3**: 425–9.

Trounson A. Risks of triploidy arising through polyspermy *in vitro*. In: Edwards RE *et al.*, eds. *Human Conception* in vitro. London: Academic Press, 1982: 227.

Veeck LL. Oocyte assessment and biological performance. *Ann NY Acad Sci* 1985; **541**: 259–273.

Veeck LL. Pregnancy rate and pregnancy outcome associated with laboratory evaluation of spermatozoa, oocytes and pre-embryos. In: Mashiach S, Ben-Rafael Z, Laufer N, Schenker JG, eds. *Advances in Assisted Reproductive Technologies*. New York and London: Plenum Press, 1990: 745–65.

Zhang LZ, Zhao WX. Follicular development, oocyte maturity and fertilization *in vitro*. *Chin Med J Engl* 1990; **103**: 186–91.

12

Clinical disorders affecting ovulation and oocyte quality

M. G. R. HULL

Introduction

This chapter is concerned with indirect epidemiological evidence for disturbances of oocyte quality that could play a part in the underlying cause of subfertility associated with conditions like polycystic ovarian disease, endometriosis, unexplained infertility, miscarriage and ageing. But first I would like to discuss briefly some factors shown to have direct influence on oocyte quality, which illustrate possible subtle mechanisms which might be important in clinical conditions.

Oocyte maturation and disturbing factors

Towards the end of follicle maturation when oestrogen levels are rising, but before the LH surge, the centrally placed nucleus of the oocyte appears as a vesicle (the germinal vesicle) and moves to the periphery of the cell. The onset of the LH surge signals (1) resumption of meiosis, which is indicated after about 24 hours by germinal vesicle breakdown, and by 36 hours extrusion of the first polar body shortly before ovulation; (2) dissociation, mucification and expansion of the previously tightly packed cumulus and corona cells surrounding the oocyte. These are the characteristic features of a mature oocyte.

Meiosis was previously inhibited by factors in follicular fluid, the inhibition being overcome by the LH surge or by removal of the immature oocyte from the follicle prematurely. It is thought that dissociation of the cumulus and corona cells is accompanied by disruption of their fine processes which had penetrated the zona pellucida and made direct contact with the oocyte, conveying the inhibitory message. Furthermore, experimental studies in rabbits employing varying doses of HCG to mimic abnormal timing and amplitude of the LH surge show that whilst a low dose *starts* resumption of meiosis, progressively larger

292

doses are required to complete the process of meiosis, then to induce luteinisation of the granulosa cells, and finally high dosage to achieve follicular rupture (Bomsel-Helmreich *et al.*, 1989). Thus inappropriate rise in LH before the surge, or attenuation of the surge or an inadequate dose of HCG could disrupt oocyte maturation and release.

When the first sperm to penetrate the zona pellucida makes contact with the oolemma it triggers the distinctive cortical granule reaction, i.e. exocytosis of cortical secretory granules releasing enzymes which act on the zona pellucida to block entry of any more spermatozoa. However, the cortical granule reaction and consequent action on the zona pellucida can be disrupted by ageing, maturation of the oocyte *in vitro,* and cooling, leading to disturbances of fertilization and competence of the embryo.

The occurrence of fertilization (the formation of oocyte and sperm pronuclei followed by syngamy) does not necessarily imply normality of either the gametes or of the embryo. For example, fertilization and rates of fertilization and cleavage appear to be normal in women over 40 years old but implanting ability of the embryos is reduced and risk of miscarriage increased. That is now clearly known to be due to impaired quality of the oocyte in the first place, though appearing normal (see section later on ageing).

There is certainly crude evidence of impaired fertilizing ability of the oocyte when the oocyte–cumulus complex is obviously immature (Hill *et al.*, 1989). However, when mature-looking oocytes are fertilized and cleaving it is not until beyond the 6–8 cell stage that the rate and pattern of cleavage become indicative of subsequent success (Morgan, Boatman & Bavister, 1990), but that is too late for the stage at which embryos are transferred to the uterus in clinical practice.

The steroid environment of the oocyte in follicular fluid is an important determinant of both fertilizing ability of the oocyte, healthy rapid cleavage, and implantation. Differences are evident even when the oocyte appears normal. Most important are relatively low intrafollicular levels of oestradiol (Andersen, 1990) and high levels of progesterone (Morgan *et al.*, 1990) and particularly 20 α-dihydroprogesterone (Vanluchene *et al.*, 1991). Such measurements are not helpful in clinical practice, however.

Follicular steroidogenesis in response to LH can be directly inhibited by cortisol, but this seems to be beneficial in the preovulatory phase and the reverse in the luteal phase. The differential regulation of cortisol in the follicle by conversion to inactive cortisone depends on the presence of the enzyme 11β-hydroxysteroid dehydrogenase in the granulosa cells. Absence of this enzyme in preovulatory granulosa cells has been found to be highly favourable for implantation of the fertilized oocyte (Michael *et al.*, 1993), suggesting that high intrafollicular cortisol is necessary for complete maturation of the oocyte though not affecting fertilizing capacity. This observation offers the prospect of developing a quick qualitative test for the enzyme on granulosa cells collected with the eggs to decide which to transfer when fertilized.

Other experimental animal evidence concerning the cleaving embryo itself, such as alterations in dry mass weight indicating the balance between synthesis and breakdown of cellular material (Turner, Goldstein & Rogers, 1992), serves to illustrate how subtle are the features of healthy embryonic development.

Clinical study of oocyte quality

The present difficulties in assessing individual oocyte and embryo quality make it necessary to turn to epidemiological methods of studying the possible contributions of impaired gamete and embryo quality to different causes of infertility indirectly. For example, the chance of an individual embryo implanting is higher (e.g. FIVNAT, 1993), and the risk of subsequent miscarriage lower (Liu *et al.*, 1992; Balen, MacDougall & Tan, 1993), when the *proportion* of oocytes fertilized is high, which therefore seems to reflect gamete and consequent embryo quality. On the other hand, lower miscarriage rates with greater numbers of embryos transferred may be misleading, owing to masking of the loss of one fetal sac by successful continuation of another. Thus *rates* of fertilization, cleavage, implantation and miscarriage must be studied comparatively in well-defined diagnostic *groups* of patients and in *properly controlled* conditions. That is the approach I will now take in this chapter.

There are important constraints on this method, however, which involve considerable potential for bias, and requires strict standardization of diagnostic selection and therapeutic conditions as mentioned, and other factors such as age and parity (e.g. FIVNAT, 1993). The less well defined is a group for study, the greater is the likelihood of individual variation, which may invalidate comparison of pooled group data and necessitate comparison of medians of individual rates, to account for unrepresentative extreme cases (Walters, 1993).

In the first place, what should be the reference group for functional normality? Women with tubal occlusion as the sole cause of their infertility are the obvious choice. Yet ovarian responsiveness might be impaired, perhaps due to effects of periovarian adhesions on blood flow, and the capacity for implantation reduced (FIVNAT, 1992), possibly due to effects of organisms still present like *Chlamydia trachomatis*. Certainly, fluid from a hydrosalpinx can be expelled into the uterus in amounts easily seen on ultrasonography, and so disturb implantation. Furthermore, embryos transferred to the uterus can find their way into functionally incompetent Fallopian tubes as shown by the increased frequency of tubal pregnancy after IVF. Thus, whilst in conditions like endometriosis and unexplained infertility fertilization rates may be reduced, pregnancy and birth rate by IVF treatment are often higher than in tubal infertility (see later). Of fertilization, implantation or livebirth, which is the best index of oocyte quality?

In employing such indices, the data are usually derived from IVF results obtained after ovarian stimulation, which could be misleading in trying to discover the mechanisms involved in the reduction of *natural* fertility. There is no doubt that follicular function is perturbed by stimulation and oocyte quality is therefore often likely to be impaired. The success of IVF treatment and other assisted conception methods like GIFT depends mainly on the greater number of oocytes made available and on facilitating sperm access to the oocytes. On the other hand, there is evidence of subtle impairment of follicular function and fertilizing ability of the oocyte in endometriosis and unexplained infertility (see later), which may be masked by the stimulation involved in IVF and GIFT treatment.

Therefore the degree of stimulation should be standardized if the results of IVF are to be properly compared between diagnostic groups, and combination with pituitary desensitization to suppress endogenous gonadotrophin secretion should also be taken into account. Such combination, particularly with the 'long' desensitization protocol, leads to greater success (Hughes *et al.,* 1992), not only by yielding larger numbers of oocytes but probably also oocytes of better quality and implanting ability (FIVNAT, 1993). The preferable ideal, however, would be to study cycles that are wholly unperturbed by hormonal treatment. That is technically difficult because of the fine timing required and close monitoring to detect accurately the onset of the LH surge; even the use of HCG should be avoided. In addition, the availability of only one mature oocyte each cycle severely undermines the statistical conclusiveness of results.

A comparative study of fertilization and implantation rates in different diagnostic classes of infertility

The following study analysing data from my own centre (Ray *et al.,* unpublished data) provides a useful demonstration exposing possible differences between the main diagnostic classes of subfertility, as a background to more detailed discussion later.

The women were all under 40 years old with apparently normal ovulatory cycles. They received a standard treatment regimen of pituitary desensitization followed by ovarian stimulation using FSH alone (Metrodin, Serono). Only those with an isolated cause of infertility were included. Sperm function testing was used to distinguish male infertility from unexplained, and antisperm antibodies were diagnosed as significant only in seminal plasma and if there was failure of cervical mucus penetration in a controlled test. Fertilization was counted only

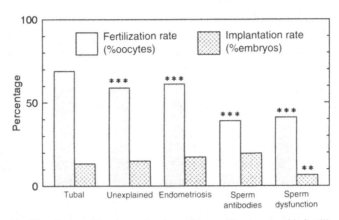

Fig. 1. Fertilization and implantation rates in specific classes of infertility treated by IVF, using standardized regimen of pituitary desensitization followed by ovarian stimulation in ovulatory women under 40 years old (Fleming *et al.,* unpublished data from University of Bristol IVF Unit). (**p < 0.025, ***p < 0.0001, compared with tubal group.)

if normal as defined by timely two-pronucleate formation and cleavage; and the fertilization rate was based on only mature oocytes as indicated by a fully developed oocyte–cumulus complex. Implantation was defined by ultrasound evidence of a pregnancy sac; and the rate was of individual sacs based on the number of individual embryos transferred to the uterus.

The results are shown in Fig. 1. Compared with the tubal group (fertilization and cleavage 69%, implantation 13%) there was the expected reduction in fertilization in cases of male infertility (39% with and 41% without antibodies but significantly better implantation rates when the cause was antibodies (19%) than inherent sperm dysfunction (7%). That suggests that when sperm function is hindered only by antibodies the spermatozoa are inherently healthy, and once fertilization is achieved a particularly healthy embryo is obtained. By contrast, sperm that are inherently dysfunctional – indicated primarily by poor motility – appear to give rise to substandard embryos. That conclusion is appealing but must be questioned in the light of the remarkably favourable outcome of direct intracytoplasmic injection of a single sperm from often severely defective populations (of sperm) as recently reported by Van Steirteghem *et al.* (1993).

Of greater relevance to this chapter, however, is the possibility of oocyte dysfunction contributing to unexplained infertility and endometriosis. Fertilization rates were significantly reduced in unexplained infertility (59%) and endometriosis (61%) but implantation rates, though apparently better, were not significantly greater (15% and 17%, respectively). Possible conclusions are impaired oocyte quality but more favourable uterine receptivity than in tubal infertility, but there is also a possible contribution of subtle impairment of sperm quality that cannot be recognized by the best tests of function other than fertilization. Basic physiological studies of the oocyte and follicle will be needed to elucidate possible contributions from those sources to the subfertility associated with endometriosis and unexplained infertility, as will be discussed later.

Assessing oocyte quality in individuals

In clinical practice, defining the contribution of unsuspected defective oocyte, or sperm, function to subfertility in individual cases presents a special problem. How can unexpected failure of fertilization be interpreted for a particular couple?

First, defects of sperm function are much more likely than defects of the oocyte. The main question concerning 'unexpected' fertilization failure in couples with 'unexplained' infertility is how sperm function was assessed initially. That will be discussed later, suffice to say that assessment of the sperm is often limited to microscopy in whole semen and outdated criteria are based on such sperm 'counts' which are of little functional and prognostic relevance.

If sperm function is properly assessed as favourable, then the most likely cause of unexpected fertilization failure is simply random variation. There may have been real though unsuspected factors causing the failure on that occasion, such as impaired stimulation of the follicles, timing of egg collection, or impaired culture conditions; but all as random events. It is clear that after unexpected complete failure of fertilization it is most likely that fertilization will occur on another occasion (see unexplained infertility). Indeed fertilization is also likely to occur in most cases of previous failure owing to sperm dysfunction, though reduced rates can be expected.

Natural cycle IVF has been advocated as a clinically useful means of assessing oocyte and sperm function (Lenton *et al.*, 1992), but the single oocyte offers no reliable conclusion whether it fertilizes or not. It is the *chance* of fertilization that matters, which must be based on the performance of *several* oocytes.

In the end, what can be done if there is *repeated* complete or severe reduction in fertilization given apparently favourable sperm? Controlled assessment of the sperm can be done, relatively easily, even after only one failure, by testing zona-free hamster egg penetration by comparison with normal sperm of proven fertilizing ability (Chan & Tucker, 1991; Liu & Gordon Baker, 1992). This test has the attractiveness of quantitative power: not only because of large numbers of oocytes, but each oocyte should normally be penetrated by numerous sperm. It lacks specificity, however, because zona pellucida penetration is not tested and because of species difference, though *failure* of penetration by sperm that have previously failed in IVF treatment is very persuasive.

The capacity of sperm to bind to human zona pellucida can be tested using salt-stored unfertilized oocytes. The storage method destroys the cytoplasm but the zona pellucida is preserved. The zonae can be divided into halves and sperm binding compared semi-quantitatively using normal donor sperm (Chan & Tucker, 1991; Liu & Gordon Baker, 1992).

Retrospective study in cases of complete fertilization failure has suggested the likelihood of an oocyte defect when sperm penetration of the zona pellucida has been obstructed only at the deepest layer in association with cryptic cytoplasmic anomalies (Bedford & Kim, 1993). The question remains, however, whether such oocyte defects would be a persistent feature. To test fertilizing ability of the *oocyte* in a prospective controlled way, there are the possibilities of using the partner's sperm and normal sperm with different sibling oocytes collected in the same cycle of IVF treatment and with donor oocytes. However, there are ethical and emotional difficulties, and a relatively large yield of sibling oocytes is needed. Alternatively, donor sperm may be chosen empirically in complete place of the husband's sperm. When this has been done after repeated fertilization failure, a very favourable pregnancy rate has been achieved apparently (though numbers are small), strongly suggesting that true, persistent fertilization is much more likely to be due to dysfunction of sperm than oocyte (Molloy *et al.,* 1991).

In clinical practice it remains impossible to reach a reliable conclusion about the functional competence of normal-looking oocytes. If the sperm appear functionally favourable all that a couple can do is try IVF treatment again if they still feel determined to do so. The decision to try again or give up, or later use donor sperm, remains a personal empirical one.

Ovulatory disorders

Ovulatory disorders, presenting typically with oligomenorrhoea or amenorrhoea, seem to be an obvious example of oocyte defectiveness. This is not so, however, in the causes of ovulatory failure presenting with amenorrhoea due to gonadotrophin deficiency. In such cases the failure of ovarian function is secondary to hypothalamic or pituitary failure or dysfunction, and there is good clinical evidence that induced ovulatory function is completely normal.

Hypothalamic–pituitary dysfunction

In all cases of gonadotrophin deficiency the ovaries can be stimulated directly using exogenous gonadotrophins, resulting in pregnancy rates per cycle that are as good as in normal fertile couples. However, that is not an appropriate index of potential follicular function and oocyte quality, because of the advantage gained by multiple ovulation. The appropriate use of pregnancy rates as an index is when mono-ovulation can be induced by restoring normal pituitary–ovarian endocrine control, by restoring or mimicking the normal hypothalamic pulsatile secretion of gonadotrophine-releasing hormone (GnRH).

The classic example of hypothalamic failure of GnRH secretion is Kallman's syndrome, presenting with primary amenorrhoea, lack of secondary sexual development and hyposmia. Much more common impairment of hypothalamic secretion of GnRH is due to weight loss and the psychological disorder of anorexia nervosa. Employing pulsatile GnRH treatment in these conditions results in normal mono-ovulation and normal conception rates (Shoham, Homburg & Jacobs, 1990; Braat, Schoemaker & Schoemaker, 1991). Hyperprolactinaemia induces gonadotrophin deficiency by suppression of hypothalmic GnRH secretion, and suppression of prolactin to normal using bromocriptine also results in normal mono-ovulation and conception rates (Crosignani & Ferrari, 1990).

The term 'hypothalamic-pituitary dysfunction' is used here in the sense of impaired secretion of GnRH resulting in gonadotrophin deficiency, which is reversible and due to correctable extraneous influences on the hypothalamus such as psychological disorder or pituitary hyperprolactinaemia. The term 'failure' is used in inherent permanent failure of hypothalamic (e.g. Kallman's syndrome) or pituitary (e.g. therapeutic ablation or infarction) function. By contrast, the now out-dated WHO classification applies 'failure' to all the foregoing conditions, and applies 'hypothalamic-pituitary dysfunction' *presumptively* to all menstrual cycle disturbances including amenorrhoea which present with evidence of oestrogenization as an index of ovarian activity (originally called WHO Group II). However, nearly all these cases are due to a primary disorder of ovarian function associated with polycystic disease (PCOD). Perhaps the simplest evidence that the hypersecretion of LH by the pituitary associated with PCOD is a secondary, not primary, disorder is its correction which often follows wedge resection or laparoscopic multiple cautery of the ovaries.

Polycystic ovarian disease

In many women with oligo- or amenorrhoea the cause is polycystic ovaries (PCO) even without the classical features of the Stein–Leventhal syndrome (PCOS) of obesity and hirsutism. PCO accounts for about one-third of women with amenorrhoea and 90% with oligomenorrhoea (Adams, Polson & Franks, 1986; Hull, 1987). Furthermore PCO accounts for about 95% of women who consider themselves to have normal menstrual cycles but which are in fact slightly irregular (Polson *et al.*, 1988), whereas in women with very regular cycles the

Table 1. *The main distinctive hormonal findings in oligomenorrhoeic and amenorrhoeic women with and without polycystic ovaries (PCO) defined by ultrasonography related to the presence or absence of hirsutism. The patients with normal ovaries typically have gonadotrophin deficiency due to hypothalamic–pituitary failure or disorder.* (Fox et al., 1991)

	PCO		Normal ovaries
	Hirsute	Non-hirsute	
Serum LH (I.U./l, mean)	12.0	11.9	5.7
Serum free testosterone index (mean)	19.4	8.0	2.8
Oestrogenized state*	88%	94%	12%

* menstrual bleeding in response to progestogen challenge test.

frequency is less than 10%–still not zero! It appears that the development of PCO is genetically determined and its full expression depends on the separate genetically determined condition of insulin resistance and consequent hyper-insulinaemia. The latter is thought to be responsible for stimulating excessive secretion of LH, amplifying LH effects on ovarian thecal and stromal production of androgens, and suppressing hepatic production of SHBG (sex hormone binding globulin) resulting in excessive free testosterone (see Tolis, Bringer & Chrousos, 1993). Clinical expression of the hyperandrogen*aemia* as hirsutism and sometimes other features of hyperandrogen*ism* is, however, dependent on peripheral enzymic utilization of circulating testosterone in the responsive end-organs (hair follicles, etc), which varies between individuals and races. Raised androgen levels in blood are a feature of non-hirsute as well as hirsute women with PCO, though to a lesser degree.

Table 1 summarizes the key hormonal findings in women presenting with oligo-amenorrhoea comparing those with ultrasound evidence of PCO or normal ovaries, and with or without hirsutism as an index of PCOD (Fox et al., 1991). Women with PCOD but without hirsutism have substantially increased free testosterone blood levels, though not as high as those with hirsutism. Oestrogenization, indicated by menstruation in response to a progestogen challenge test, is a characteristic of women with PCO, in contrast to the others whose oligo-amenorrhoea is usually due to gonadotrophin deficiency. Though the *individual* follicles in PCO are hypo-oestrogenetic, there are so many of them, a minimum of 15 in each ovary, usually many more, up to 100, that the *combined* output of oestrogen by the ovaries is substantial (Fox et al., 1991).

Basal LH levels are on average equally raised in women with PCO, with or without hirsutism (Table 1). However, nearly half the women with PCO or PCOD do *not* have evidently raised LH levels (i.e. > 10 I.U./l). On the other hand, due to fluctuation in levels of LH and excessive nocturnal secretion, elevation may often be missed in random samples. Watson *et al.,* (1993) have shown that urinary LH excretion is substantially increased in most women with PCO.

Apart from the relevance of raised LH levels in the endocrine diagnosis of PCO, they appear to be an increasingly important issue in determining oocyte quality and consequent chance of conception, miscarriage and ultimately livebirth (see below). Though excessive androgen levels within the follicle are known to cause atresia of both oocyte and granulosa cells, there is no clear evidence that in PCO they are the cause of the associated subfertility and increased miscarriage rates (see below).

Oocyte quality and PCO

Women with PCO who have failed to conceive despite apparently favourable induction of ovulation may often proceed to IVF treatment. Fertilization and cleavage rates are substantially reduced compared to controls with normal ovaries, from 66–75% to 34–55% in several reports (Dor *et al.,* 1990; Urman *et al.,* 1992; MacDougall *et al.,* 1993). However, pregnancy rates are very similar.

The reduced fertilization rates strongly suggest, at first sight, impaired oocyte quality; but this may be a misleading statistic. The same reports all show that PCO gives rise to much greater numbers of oocytes and much higher oestrogen levels. However, the criteria of the *leading* follicles required to administer HCG to induce final maturation for egg collection were the same with PCO and with normal ovaries. Therefore the excess follicles are likely to be relatively immature, which could account for the reduced overall fertilization rate. By contrast, the similar pregnancy rates, arising from transfer of similar numbers of embryos, indicate that the implanting ability of the best embryos, and therefore the original quality of the leading oocytes, is favourable, in accord with the hypothesis that follicular function in PCO was similar to normal follicles of the same size. However, a recent study by Erickson *et al.* (1992) of granulosa cells from PCO follicles found marked impairment of their capacity to produce progesterone – in striking contrast to oestrogen – and relative insensitivity to bioactive FSH. Such granulosa cell dysfunction is, in turn, likely to affect oocyte quality adversely.

Indirect evidence to suggest impaired oocyte quality is the high rate of miscarriage associated with PCO. A review comparing the results of standard and low-dose gonadotrophin therapy from several reports (Hull, 1991), shows that low-dose therapy has achieved the objective of reducing the risk of multiple pregnancy though at the price of reducing the chance of any pregnancy. However, the risk of miscarriage was not reduced by the lower dosage (39%), suggesting that gonadotrophin therapy is not itself the cause. Also, the use of pulsed GnRH therapy to induce ovulation, resulting in an even lower multiple pregnancy rate (7%), failed to reduce the miscarriage rate (also 39%) (Shoham, Homburg & Jacobs, 1990). Indeed, the risk of miscarriage remains high even in women with PCO who are ovulating spontaneously. Sagle *et al.* (1988) found PCO in 82% of women with recurrent early miscarriage, compared with 2 out of 11 (18%) normal parous women. None of the women with PCO had raised LH levels on random testing, but 41% had hirsutism or acne, suggesting that excess androgen rather than LH (see below) may account for the miscarriages, though whether by influence on the oocyte, the endometrium or implanted conceptus is open to speculation. Conversely, repeated measurement of LH may have revealed raised levels (Watson *et al.*, 1993), but that too is speculation. Nevertheless, the implication of LH hypersecretion in the causation of miscarriage directly or indirectly is clearly supported.

LH Hypersecretion

There is extensive evidence that excessive levels of LH are associated with impaired chance of conception and increased risk of miscarriage, and are the likely cause by both direct actions on the oocyte and indirect actions mediated by disturbance of follicular steroid production (Jacobs & Homburg, 1990; Shoham, Jacobs & Insler, 1993). The evidence relates mainly to hypersecretion of LH during the mid-follicular phase of the ovarian cycle, also in the periovulatory period including the occurrence of a premature LH surge. The first evidence of a deleterious effect of hypersecretion during the mid-follicular phase came in 1985 from IVF studies which showed reduced fertilization rates, asymmetrical cleavage and fragmentation of the blastomeres. Soon similar effects were shown in other IVF studies when there was evidence of an excessive 'tonic' rise in LH levels or exposure to HCG before the occurrence of a spontaneous LH surge. Those findings, and evidence of increased miscarriage after delayed donor insemination in ovulating women, suggest that over-prolonged exposure of the maturing oocyte to LH has an effect of either premature maturation and/or ageing of the oocyte.

Studies in anovulatory women in whom ovulation was apparently successfully induced using clomiphene – and who were therefore likely to have had PCO – or using pulsed GnRH in women with known PCO have shown that mid-follicular LH levels were higher in those who failed to conceive. Furthermore, in those with raised LH levels who conceived there was a high miscarriage rate.

In spontaneously ovulating women with elevated LH levels trying to conceive conception rates were seen to be reduced proportionately by 13% over the course of 2 years. Furthermore two-thirds of the women who conceived with high LH miscarried, a rate which was five times greater than the rate in women with normal LH.

Women with PCO but ovulating spontaneously were also found to have a high risk of miscarriage, and PCO has been found to account for about 80% of women suffering recurrent miscarriage. The association seemed at first to be independent of LH, but subsequent study has found that most women with PCO and a normal random serum LH level have evidence of hypersecretion when detailed patterns of secretion are examined. Watson *et al.* (1993) have recently shown that the hypersecretion may occur principally during sleep, and urinary LH excretion, which integrates the effects of pulsatile and diurnal variation, is significantly increased in women with recurrent miscarriage, *with or without* evident PCO. Raised LH levels were associated with significantly higher levels of serum testosterone during the follicular phase. The difference in LH levels was most marked during the early luteal phase and there was associated excessive secretion of oestrogen (measured in urine) though normal protesterone.

Mechanisms of action

Several mechanisms of action have been hypothesized for the effect, or effects, of LH hypersecretion in reducing fecundity and increasing miscarriage. The action may be mediated by excessive thecal androgen production in response to LH, perhaps amplified by excessive insulin. Excess androgens are known to induce atresia in both the oocyte and granulosa cells (McNatty *et al.*, 1979; DeSutter *et al.*, 1991) and the chance of pregnancy in IVF treatment has been linked to lower circulating free (unbound) androgens and oestradiol throughout the follicular phase (Andersen & Ziebe, 1992).

The conversion of thecal androgens to oestrogen by granulosa cells may simply explain the oestrogen hypersecretion during the early luteal phase observed by Watson *et al.* (1993). On the other hand, excessive oestrogen levels at that time, coupled with excess androgen, may disturb endometrial development in preparation for implantation. LH may also have a direct effect on the endometrium because it contains LH receptors, though any functional relevance of the receptors remains obscure.

Apart from possible androgen-mediated atresia of the oocyte, excess LH may instead induce premature maturation of the oocyte leading to impaired and abnormal fertilization, an attractive hypothesis originally proposed by Jacobs (Jacobs & Homburg, 1990). Rising LH levels normally associated with the preovulatory surge induce resumption of meiosis by releasing the oocyte from the effect of inhibitory factors (originally referred to as oocyte maturation inhibitor, though it now appears there may be several) present in follicular fluid. The inhibitory factors are probably produced by granulosa cells and conveyed to the oocyte by fine processes extending from the cumulus oophorus through the zona pellucida to the cytoplasmic membrane of the oocyte. Expansion and dissociation of the cumulus cells induced by the onset of the LH surge may disrupt the connections conveying the inhibitory message. Thus premature exposure to excessive LH can lead to changes in the oocyte that can interfere with fertilization and the normal block to polyspermy, and consequently disturb the capacity for normal cleavage and implantation.

Treatment of LH hypersecretion and PCO

If hypersecretion of LH is the primary cause of all those disturbances affecting ultimate successful fertility, suppressing secretion to normal should improve the outcome.

Suppression sometimes occurs, inexplicably, when ovulation is successfully induced by stimulation using gonadotrophins. By contrast, ovarian wedge resection or multiple injury to the ovary by cauterization lead principally to reduction in circulating androgen levels, with little or no effect on LH but usually a rise in FSH (Campo et al., 1993). Those examples suggest that intra-ovarian factors are of primary importance in the disorders associated with PCO. Possibilities include disturbances of granulosa cell secretion of inhibin affecting FSH secretion, and of a non-steroidal hormone or hormones called gonadotrophin surge-attenuating factor affecting LH (Shoham, Jacobs & Insler, 1993).

Pituitary desensitization using superactive GnRH analogues provides the obvious means of testing the LH hypothesis, but there have been few studies so far: (1) in anovulatory infertile women who had also suffered recurrent miscarriage (Johnson & Pearce, 1990); (2) in anovulatory infertile women with PCO syndrome (Homburg et al., 1993); (3) ovulatory infertile women with ultrasound evidence of PCO undergoing IVF treatment for other causes of infertility (Balen et al., 1993).

Johnson & Pearce (1990) studied anovulatory women with PCO and LH hypersecretion who had required clomiphene treatment to induce ovulation and suffered recurrent miscarriage. Prospective randomized comparison of further treatment by clomiphene or by buserelin followed by FSH resulted in significant reduction in the miscarriage rate from 55% to 10% using buserelin. It was also noted that in the clomiphene-treated patients who miscarried almost all had higher LH levels at the preovulatory stage when related to the size of the leading follicle.

Homburg et al. (1993) studied women with the polycystic ovary syndrome indicated by oligo-amenorrhoea and/or hirsutism but without information on

LH levels, though hypersecretion of LH can be assumed. They included women having ovulation induction or IVF treatment, together because their outcomes were similar. Retrospective analysis of the results of concurrent gonadotrophin therapy (HMG and FSH) alone or following pituitary desensitization using decapeptyl showed significant reduction in the miscarriage rate from 39% to 18% using decapeptyl. They also recorded a significant improvement in the cumulative livebirth rate after 4 cycles from 26% to 64%.

It is perhaps important to note that those two studies both employed a 'long' protocol to achieve pituitary desensitization before starting gonadotrophin therapy. Balen *et al.* (1993) compared 'short' (coincidental) and 'long' protocols of pituitary desensitization using buserelin and gonadotrophins, and a combination of clomiphene and gonadotrophins. The study was large but retrospective and the treatments may not have been employed concurrently. However, they found significant benefit only from the 'long' protocol of pituitary desensitization, which when compared with clomiphene reduced the miscarriage rate in women with ultrasound evidence of PCO from 47% to 20%. By contrast, there was no significant difference in women with normal ovaries (20% with clomiphene and 26% with pituitary desensitization), presumably because the increased risk with clomiphene in PCO is due to the ovarian disorder and LH hypersecretion, and not to clomiphene. Furthermore, there was no difference between the types of gonadotrophin preparation, whether FSH alone or in combination with LH (HMG) (overall miscarriage rates 17% and 21%, respectively, when combined with the 'long' buserelin protocol).

In comparing hormone treatments it is important to distinguish between their use in women with and without PCO and/or LH hypersecretion. Several comparisons of FSH and HMG with or without pituitary desensitization have shown no differences in conception or miscarriage rates, for either ovulation induction or IVF treatment. The lack of benefit of FSH alone in PCO seemed at first surprising, but it is now clear that the slight rise in LH levels achieved by HMG treatment is negligible in relation to the already raised endogenous levels.

Treatment of normal ovulatory women

By contrast, some benefit from FSH therapy compared with HMG might be expected in women with normal LH levels, in whom HMG treatment leads to distinct elevation of circulating LH and in turn higher follicular levels of testosterone (Polan *et al.*, 1986; Porter *et al.*, 1986). However, clinical studies of fertility outcome have so far shown no significant benefit, though they have been inadequately designed to reach a reliable negative conclusion.

There is now, however, clear evidence that routine use of a 'long' protocol of pituitary desensitization before gonadotrophin therapy for IVF or GIFT, in women most of whom must have normal ovaries, is of significant benefit. Meta-analysis by Hughes *et al.* (1992) of numerous comparative studies shows pregnancy rates about doubled per cycle of treatment started. This is partly because the failure rate to complete treatment cycles was 3-fold greater without GnRH, and due to untimely occurrence of an LH surge. In addition there is a greater yield of oocytes (by nearly one-third). However, the pregnancy rate per embryo transfer was also significantly greater (by 40%), suggesting more favourable conditions for implantation, though miscarriage rates were not different as observed in the study by Balen *et al.* (1993) when they focused on women with defined normal ovaries in contrast to PCO.

Those findings suggest that suppressing LH to low levels improves either oocyte quality or endometrial receptivity, or both, but the distinction cannot be made. Liu *et al.* (1992) have, however, questioned any improvement in implanting ability, claiming that improved pregnancy rates are due to the greater yield of oocytes and consequently more embryos to transfer. When they controlled for the number of embryos transferred they could find no benefit of GnRHa therapy. Any effect on oocyte quality of suppressing normal LH levels in women with normal ovaries remains doubtful.

Premature luteinization may have a direct adverse effect independent of LH. In cycles stimulated without pituitary desensitization progesterone will of course rise along with LH, but can rise in the absence of any elevation of LH before administration of HCG and has been associated with impaired fertilization and pregnancy rates following stimulation with a combination of clomiphene and gonadotrophins (Kagawa *et al.*, 1992; Mio *et al.*, 1992). Increase in progesterone was associated with higher oestrogen levels and greater number of follicles but fewer mature oocytes, suggesting an element of follicular dysfunction, perhaps induced by the stimulation (Mio *et al.*, 1992).

Premature luteinization can also occur after ovarian stimulation in pituitary desensitized women and has been associated with lower pregnancy rates by IVF treatment (Schoolcraft *et al.*, 1991; Silverberg *et al.*, 1991). In unperturbed ovulatory cycles progesterone normally rises shortly before the onset of the LH surge (Hoff, Quigley & Yen, 1983) and is probably the trigger for the surge. The luteinization may occur in response to the slight rise in 'tonic' LH levels that normally precedes the surge (Hoff *et al.*, 1983), or as a spontaneous event in fully mature follicles thus normally ensuring perfect coordination of follicular requirements. These effects may be exaggerated in stimulated cycles, leading to premature dissociation of cumulus cells and interruption of the maturation inhibitor signal to the oocyte. Spontaneous luteinization might be considered more likely to occur in pituitary desensitized women because administration of

HCG can be delayed without fear of an untimely LH surge, but adverse effects on the oocyte do not seem to be born out in practice. A study of pituitary-suppressed egg donors showed that premature luteinization had no adverse effect on implanting ability in steroid-prepared recipients (Legro *et al.,* 1993). Higher progesterone levels were associated with higher oestradiol levels and more oocytes, suggesting a simple effect of summation of no functional importance, except possibly on the endometrium, though unlikely.

Effect of drugs used to stimulate ovulation

Gonadotrophins

FSH acts only on granulosa cells, to induce aromatizing enzymes and later LH receptors, thus enabling LH in the late follicular phase to maintain aromatizing activity (prior to the specific effects associated with the LH surge). LH acts on theca cells to stimulate steroidogenesis, principally androgen production; later on mature granulosa cells when LH receptors have developed; and directly and indirectly on the oocyte to induce resumption of meiosis as described earlier.

It is important to recognize that minimal LH is required to provide sufficient androgen precursors for oestrogen production by granulosa-cells, and furthermore paracrine signals, like inhibin from the granulosa cells, amplify the effects of LH on the theca (Bergh *et al.,* 1993). However, excessive LH stimulates increased thecal androgen production in a dose-related manner (Bergh *et al.,* 1993) which may induce follicular and oocyte atresia (McNatty *et al.,* 1979; DeSutter *et al.,* 1991), and LH treatment combined with FSH leads to increased circulating levels of LH and intrafollicular levels of testosterone (Polan *et al.,* 1986; Porter *et al.,* 1986), as discussed earlier. Nevertheless, at dosages employed in clinical practice there are no demonstrable adverse effects of gonadotrophins on outcome in terms of pregnancy, miscarriage (except due to PCO) or congenital abnormality rates (Lunenfeld *et al.,* 1986).

Gonadotrophin-releasing hormone agonists (GnRHa)

When gonadotrophin therapy is combined with 'short' or 'ultra-short' regimens of GnRHa, there is the added rise in endogenous gonadotrophin levels owing to the initial agonist action of GnRHa before the pituitary becomes desensitized. It is therefore difficult, in considering possible adverse effects of GnRHa, to distinguish them from those of LH. The initial agonist effect on LH secretion using 'short' regimens of GnRH may, however, explain the now consistently demonstrated benefits of 'long' protocols which establish pituitary desensitization before ovarian stimulation begins (Hughes *et al.*, 1992; Balen *et al.*, 1993; FIVNAT, 1993). Nevertheless, it remain unclear whether the benefits are due to improved quality of the oocytes or endometrium, or simply due to the greater numbers of oocytes available.

GnRH and its agonists can act directly via receptors that have been demonstrated to be present on granulosa, granulosa-lutein cells and the oocyte, and gain entry to follicular fluid. The subject including animal experimental evidence has been reviewed by Testart, Lefevre & Gougeon (1993).

GnRHa induces resumption of oocyte meiosis in intact follicles, and the response is quicker than to LH. Maturation has also been associated with increasing degeneration of the oocyte and granulosa cells, and failure of dissociation of the cumulus, in experimental conditions. There have also been clinical reports that, though greater numbers of oocytes are yielded using GnRHa, the proportion that is fully mature is reduced. Effects on follicular steroidogenesis have been very variable. However, all these effects can also be induced by excessive exposure to gonadotrophins, which cannot be distinguished.

Increased triploidy of human embryos has also been found, and a tendency to increased chromosomal abnormalities in the oocyte. However, there appear to be no teratogenic effects on embryos and fetuses, or adverse effects on pregnancy outcome for mother or newborn. In the final analysis, the practical benefits of a 'long' GnRHa protocol for IVF in normal ovulatory women, and to suppress LH to normal in cases of LH hypersecretion causing recurrent miscarriage, are now well established.

Clomiphene

Clomiphene acts not only on the pituitary but also directly on the ovary and on oestrogen-dependent end-organs like the endometrium and endocervical mucosa. The subject including animal experimental evidence has been reviewed by Birkenfeld, Beier & Schenker (1986). Glasier (1990) and Saunders, Lancaster & Peidisch (1992). In women, clomiphene has been shown to enter the follicle, decrease progesterone production by granulosa–lutein cells, induce chromosomal abnormalities in oocytes, induce blastocyst degeneration, and have possible deleterious effects on endometrium. In animals, clomiphene has been found to reduce fertilization and implantation.

In clinical practice clomiphene has been specifically implicated in the greater risk of both miscarriage and ectopic pregnancy observed in the national Australian and New Zealand results reported by Saunders, Lancaster & Pedisch (1992) compared with pituitary desensitized women. By contrast, Balen *et al.* (1993)

observed no increased risk with clomiphene except in women with PCO, in a large series. Extensive experience has shown no greater miscarriage rate than occurs generally in infertile women, and no increased congenital abnormality rates (Lunenfeld *et al.*, 1986; Glasier, 1990).

Conclusions

In summary, there is no consistent evidence that any particular methods of ovarian stimulation directly perturb follicular function and oocyte maturation to a clinically relevant degree. However, multiple follicular development is the probable cause of periovulatory hypersecretion of LH leading to perturbation of oocyte maturation. As yet there is no controlled study of pituitary desensitization specifically to prevent the periovulatory perturbation, and it would be difficult to undertake, but the general lack of benefit from 'short' protocols which would become effective only in the late follicular phase suggests that it is mainly basal hypersecretion that really matters.

Nevertheless, even in women with normal basal secretion of LH, pituitary desensitization in undoubtedly beneficial in preventing untimely occurrence of an LH surge, and consequently enables more cycles of IVF or GIFT treatment to be completed, and it yields larger numbers of mature oocytes and consequently more embryos to transfer. Whether it improves the quality of the oocytes, except in women with PCO and basal hypersecretion of LH, or of the endometrium remains unproven.

By contrast, the beneficial effects of pituitary desensitization to suppress basal *hypersecretion* of LH to normal are now clearly established, improving fertilization and implantation and reducing the risk of miscarriage. The effects on the oocyte are presumptive but the hypothesis is sound.

Endometriosis

Fertilization rates in women with endometriosis are significantly reduced but the rate of implantation is normal (Fig. 1). These findings in women who received standardized hormonal preparation by pituitary desensitization followed by stimulation using FSH alone (rather than HMG), are consistent with observations in women receiving clomiphene and HMG (Wardle *et al.*, 1985) and various regimens (Mills *et al.*, 1992).

In most cases endometriosis is present without major structural damage, and the cause of associated infertility remains largely unexplained. Other associated causes are more likely to occur with endometriosis than with distinct causes like tubal damage due to infection or ovulatory failure. The most likely association is sperm dysfunction, as is so often seen in 'unexplained' infertility. In our studies, the 'male factor' was also defined by tests of sperm function rather than traditional seminal microscopy, and cases of sperm dysfunction excluded from study. There remains the possibility of indistinguishable subtle sperm dysfunction being present, contributing to the subfertility associated with endometriosis but mean sperm measurements were similar to the tubal group.

Attention can therefore be focused on the possibilites of follicular and oocyte dysfunction. Preliminary studies in cycles stimulated for IVF treatment indicate significant perturbation of follicular steroid concentrations at the time of oocyte recovery, but what happens in unstimulated 'natural' cycles is more relevant to the study of endometriosis-associated subfertility.

Mahmood, Arumugam & Templeton (1991) studied 20 patients and 10 controls, aspirated the follicles about 32 hours after the onset of a spontaneous LH surge and found no significant differences in follicular fluid concentrations of oestradiol, protesterone or androstenedione. They also failed to find a significant difference in fertilization rates though oocyte numbers were small and the observed rate with endometriosis (10/19 = 53%) was lower than in the controls (5/8 = 63%) (it was not possible to collect an oocyte every time).

Our own on-going studies have resulted in fertilization rates of 53% (9/17) and 73% (22/30), respectively, which are also not significantly different though consistent with previous findings. We could not find significant differences between follicular fluid concentrations of oestradiol or progesterone, but dynamic studies *in vitro* have demonstrated significantly reduced capacity of granulosa cells to produce oestradiol and progesterone (Pettigrew *et al.*, 1993). In addition, we have found reduced concentrations of LH in follicular fluid and reduction in peak serum LH levels during the preovulatory surge.

Those findings are consistent with reports of impaired preovulatory LH secretion and action and progesterone metabolism associated with endometriosis (Wardle *et al.*, 1985), suggesting that disordered preovulatory secretion of LH could be a primary factor causing the evident follicular dysfunction. On the other hand, it is possible that attenuation of the LH surge is related to impairment of preovulatory follicular maturation, resulting in disturbed signalling to the pituitary. The apparent fact that impairment of oocyte and follicular function can be demonstrated even in women undergoing follicular stimulation, including an ample dose of HCG, strongly suggests that there is an inherent disorder of follicular function affecting oocyte quality associated with endometriosis.

In practice, that could reduce the chance of natural conception substantially, whereas in assisted conception treatments it seems to be overcome by making available more than enough oocytes.

Unexplained infertility

Aitken (1982) demonstrated that one-third of couples with prolonged unexplained infertility had demonstrable failure of fertilizing ability of the sperm tested with hamster oocytes despite normal finding by traditional seminal microscopy (Aitken, Irvine & Wu, 1991). Since then fertilizing ability has been correlated with numerous other tests of function ranging from complex (see Chan & Tucker, 1991; Liu & Gordon Baker, 1992) to simple penetration of (normal) cervical mucus or mucus substitutes (see Hull *et al.*, 1984; Glazener *et al.*, 1987; Aitken, Irvine & Wu, 1991). Prospective studies of both IVF and natural fertility have demonstrated strong predictive power of various tests of function (mucus penetration, seminal reactive oxygen species generation, and hamster oocyte penetration) (see Hull *et al.*, 1984; Glazener *et al.*, 1987; Aitken, Irvine & Wu, 1991), by contrast with standard seminal microscopy which has been of little or no predictive value. These findings emphasize that some reliable test of sperm function must be included in any proper definition of unexplained infertility. Then the main factor determining the chance of natural conception is simply the duration of infertility at the time the couple present for investigation (Hull *et al.*, 1985). Most couples with less than 3 years unexplained infertility have a good chance, within the normal range, of conceiving without help and can be considered to be essentially normal and simply unlucky. After more than 3 years, however, the chance of natural conception falls to about 1–2% each cycle. Therefore, any study of possible mechanisms should focus on *prolonged* unexplained infertility.

It is important to recognize that abnormalities found in one or two cycles are unlikely to be persistent enough to cause *prolonged* infertility and are usually found to occur equally frequently in normal women, demonstrating that variability between cycles is a normal phenomenon. *Prospective* studies of pituitary–ovarian–endometrial function have found that the only significant predictor of natural conception is the pattern of salivary progesterone relative to serum oestradiol measured daily during the early luteal phase (Dunphy *et al.*, 1990). Such an abnormality is too subtle and elusive to have any diagnostic application in clinical practice, but it suggests the possibility of (relatively frequent) inherent dysfunction of the ovarian follicle and oocyte as mechanisms for the subfertility. On the other hand, ovarian stimulation using clomiphene or gonadotrophins leads to only slight improvements in the chance of conception, despite the advantage of multiple ovulation. It is not until multiple ovulation is combined with delivery of prepared motile sperm to the oocytes by IVF, GIFT or IUI that the chance of conception is substantially increased.

Fig. 1 shows that the fertilization and cleavage rate is significantly reduced in unexplained infertility compared with the tubal reference group, the proportionate reduction being by 14%. However, the chance of implantation is normal. Other studies of IVF treatment for unexplained infertility have shown greater reductions in fertilization rates, for example by as much as 31% (Mackenna *et al.*, 1992), but based sperm assessment on semen microscopy. The extensive French national data (FIVNAT, 1992) have shown a proportional reduction in fertilization rate by 19%, but seminal sperm counts and sperm migration rates and survival in culture medium were on average significantly impaired.

Incidentally, the French data also showed that in *tubal* infertility ovarian responsiveness to stimulation is reduced (in terms of dosage required, peak oestradiol levels and number of oocytes yielded) and implantation rate per embryo and pregnancy rate per cycle are reduced. Those findings suggest the possible effects of periovarian adhesions and the continuing presence of organisms like *C. trachomatis*.

Possible definable factors recently described that could interfere with fertilization or implantation in unexplained infertility include antisperm antibodies, sperm acrosome defects, and human leucocyte antigen (HLA) homozygosity, but none of these affects oocyte quality.

Coulam, Moore and O'Fallon (1988) found HLA-B locus homozygosity in the two partners to be three times more common in unexplained infertility than in fertile couples. That could only be implicated, however, in implantation failure as in recurrent miscarriage. Yet *generally* implantation occurs favourably in unexplained infertility.

Witkin *et al.* (1992) have demonstrated significantly impaired fertilization due to the presence of antisperm antibodies directed against the sperm tail in either seminal plasma or the woman's serum, but not in the man's serum. However, the finding of seminal antisperm antibodies interfering with sperm motility is a common specific cause which should be excluded by routine testing from any diagnosis of unexplained infertility, and the woman's serum should not be used for embryo culture when antibodies are present. Those factors were specifically excluded from our data illustrated in Fig. 1.

Albert *et al.* (1992) have demonstrated defects of the sperm acrosomal cap and acrosomal reaction in 25–40% of men with unexplained failure of fertilization, compared with 0–4% of controls. Such testing is not a common routine and highlights the frequent finding of sperm disfunction that comes to light after unexpected failure of fertilization.

By contrast, demonstration of an oocyte defect is rare though it may be difficult. In a *retrospective* study of fertilization failure Bedford and Kim (1993) have described blockage of sperm penetration at the deepest layer of the zona pellucida (despite normal surface binding and partial penetration) and various cryptic cytoplasmic abnormalities suggesting defectiveness of the oocytes. However, while such oocyte defects could well explain fertilization failure on that occasion, the key issue is whether such defects are a consistent feature leading to *repetitive* failure. The weight of evidence is against that.

There have been three recent reports (and other earlier reports) of outcome of IVF treatment following previous complete fertilization failure. Lipitz *et al.* (1993) found relatively low oocyte fertilization rates in further cycles (average 27%) though 81% of couples achieved fertilization and several conceived both by IVF and spontaneously. It is perhaps relevant that in their couples with apparently unexplained infertility the average oocyte fertilization rate is reduced by a relatively large margin, proportionately by 32%. There was no further information to suggest the finding of a likely cause. Sperm assessment was, however, by traditional seminal microscopy.

Molloy *et al.* (1991) reported oocyte fertilization rates of 51–66% in subsequent cycles, and cycle and cumulative pregnancy rates that were 'similar' to their overall results. Interestingly, six couples opted empirically to employ donor sperm and three conceived. Original sperm assessment had been only by traditional seminal microscopy. It was also notable that a relatively high proportion of the couples had produced only 1–2 oocytes in the first cycle, therefore the initial failure of fertilization may often have been due simply to chance.

In my own centre, Rowlands, McDermott & Hull (1994) found in further cycles oocyte fertilization rates of 40–100% and a cycle pregnancy rate of 27%, though lower than in couples undergoing further cycles after initial oocyte fertilization rates of at least 25%. In our practice, sperm function testing was the diagnostic criterion for the male rather than semen microscopy.

Though not yet fully defined, any evidence that has emerged to explain previously unexplained fertilization failure has pointed to hidden dysfunction of sperm. Indeed, the main factor is simply chance failure. There is no real evidence of any persistent defect of oocytes, though individual cases are sometimes strongly suspected, but rarely.

In practice, unexplained failure of fertilization is unlikely to recur and couples can be encouraged to try again, though a moderately reduced oocyte fertilization rate can be expected. There is no reliable means of distinguishing a recurring defect.

Ageing

There is a well-recognized decline in female fertility, which accelerates some time between 35 and 40 years of age and reaches almost zero by 45. Yet as long as menstrual regularity is maintained, ovulation, follicular hormone production and fertilizing ability remain apparently normal. It is not until the number of follicles in each ovary falls below 1000 that menstrual regularity and ovulatory frequency

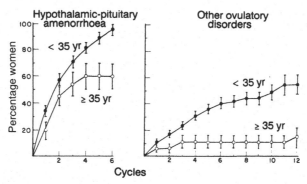

Fig. 2. Cumulative pregnancy rates resulting from gonadotrophin therapy to induce ovulation according to the cause of ovulation failure ('other' disorders being mainly due to PCO) and age of the woman (from Dor *et al.*, 1980.)

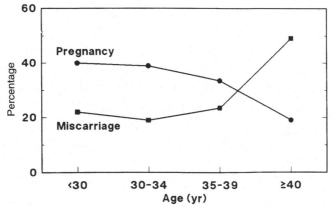

Fig. 3. Pregnancy per cycle and miscarriage rates resulting from GIFT treatment related to the woman's age (from Craft *et al.*, 1988.)

decline indicating the premenopausal transition (see Richardson & Nelson, 1990). So why the earlier decline in fecundity?

In attempting to study the age-related decline in female fecundity there are several confounding factors which can all be interrelated including falling coital frequency and the spouse's age (Wood, 1989). Calculations based on societies practising celibacy until marriage suggest that male fertility declines little until after 55 yr. The best clinical evidence of the true decline in female fecundity comes from donor insemination studies, which completely control for coital frequency and the spouse's age (Federation CECOS, 1982). Treatments like gonadotrophin therapy to induce ovulation (Dor *et al.*, 1980) and GIFT (Craft *et al.*, 1988) should largely control for coital timing and the results, illustrated in Figs 2 and 3, demonstrate the great importance of the woman's age in determining therapeutic

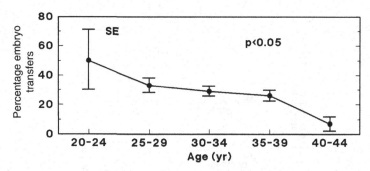

Fig. 4. Implantation rates of individual embryos after IVF treatment related to the woman's age, limited to ovulatory women with normal uterus and men with normal sperm, and only triple-embryo transfers (Hull *et al.*, unpublished data from University of Bristol IVF Unit) (probability by chi-square test for trend; SE = standard error.)

outcome and therefore choices. Fig. 3 further emphasizes that the declining chance of pregnancy is compounded by an exponential rise in the risk of miscarriage in reducing the ultimate hope of successfully having a baby. But what are the underlying mechanisms?

IVF and embryo transfer offer a model for specific study. Every reported analysis of clinical outcome demonstrates the age-related decline in pregnancy and birth rates, associated with declining numbers of oocytes and consequently embryos to transfer, but oocyte fertilization rates remain normal. Indirect statistical analysis of the French national data has indicated an independent effect of age on the implanting ability of individual embryos (FIVNAT, 1993). A specific study standardizing the number of embryos transferred – three in every case – illustrated in Fig. 4 shows the quantitative decline in implanting ability. The remarkable success of egg donation to postmenopausal women (e.g. Sauer, Paulson & Lobo, 1993) strongly suggests that oocyte quality is the main factor. Furthermore, egg donation studies in women (donors and recipients of all ages) show that the age-related increase in miscarriage is determined largely by oocyte quality (Abdalla *et al.*, 1993).

Endometrial and uterine receptivity should not be entirely dismissed as causes, however. There is animal experimental evidence showing declining receptivity with age, but, on the other hand, enhanced receptivity after prolonged lack of oestrogen, which is echoed by enhanced success rates in women receiving donated eggs if they have postmenopausal amenorrhoea rather than if still menstruating (Edwards *et al.*, 1991).

There is also evidence from ultrasonography that endometrial development is frequently impaired in women over 40 yr, though in most cases there was also

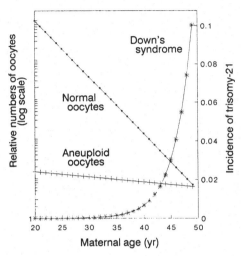

Fig. 5. Incidence of Down's syndrome (trisomy-21) compared with the relative numbers of normal and abnormal oocytes remaining in the ovary (and therefore relative numbers to be released) according to the woman's age (from Zheng & Byers, 1992.)

obvious uterine pathology like multiple fibroids or severe synechiae (Sher *et al.*, 1991).

Declining oocyte quality seems to be the main cause of impaired implantation, despite normal appearances. The declining potential for fertility seems to be accompanied by increasingly frequent chromosomal abnormalities (Richardson & Nelson, 1990). The decline in fertility and rise in chromosomal abnormalities occur exponentially and seem to be linked to acceleration in the rate of depletion of oocytes in the ovaries. The acceleration seems to occur when the complement of follicles remaining in each ovary has fallen to about 10 000, at around 37 yr of age on average.

The possible causes of the accelerated follicular atresia include rising FSH levels (see below) and emergence of a relative preponderance of genetically defective oocytes, which would also explain the reduced implanting ability, and increased risks of miscarriage and genetic abnormality in the child. The classical explanation is prolonged meiotic arrest of the oocyte making it vulnerable to ageing and environmental influences. However, a leading current hypothesis is that the defective oocytes were defective from the start, and due to their defectiveness were also less readily recruited for ovulation than healthy oocytes. This model, proposed by Zheng & Byers (1992) and illustrated in Fig. 5, would explain the exponential rise in genetic abnormalities affecting the pregnancies of women over 37.

In clinical practice, the genetic risks associated with ageing oocytes are unavoidable, except by women not delaying their attempts at childbearing too long, and by doctors minimizing delays in the process of diagnosis and treatment of infertility. However, young women faced with pelvic surgery need careful consideration to protect their future fertility. Loss or damage of large numbers of oocytes (by surgery or cytotoxic treatment) will lead to early menopause and possibly earlier increase in genetic risks for pregnancy. Experimental evidence in mice shows that unilateral ovariectomy leads to shortening of reproductive life and earlier rise in aneuploidy (Brook, Gosden & Chandley, 1984).

In women, removing an ovary in early adult life would not halve the reproduction span because oocyte depletion occurs exponentially, but expectation would be advancement of the menopause by 7 years. Large-scale reduction of ovarian mass, as can occur in surgical excision of endometriosis for example, can be disastrous. Ovarian conservation should be a dominating priority of surgery – and if it were possible, radiotherapy and chemotherapy – in young women. In surgery for ovarian endometriosis internal ablation of cysts should probably be preferred to attempting excision.

Ovarian responsiveness and FSH levels

The typical gross elevation of FSH and LH that marks the menopause is preceded by a gradual rise in FSH levels for at least 5–6 years before the menopause, though LH for only about one year before, despite continuation of apparently normal ovulatory cycles (Lenton et al., 1988). The rise in FSH is still within the normal range at first but in most cases is clearly abnormal 3–4 years before reaching the menopause. The presumed explanation is falling inhibin levels due to diminishing numbers of follicles recruitable for maturation.

As FSH levels rise, in women apparently still ovulating normally, ovarian responsiveness to stimulation declines. This results in progressively fewer oocytes being yielded for IVF treatment, and as Fig. 6 shows, increasing cancellations owing to inadequate responses and diminishing pregnancy rates (Toner et al., 1991). The pregnancy rate decreased substantially when the FSH level reached the upper limit of normal (22 I.U./l) and reached zero when only slightly higher. The decline seemed to be more sharply related to FSH than age, but the distinction was not analysed.

Our own studies have demonstrated significant reduction in ovarian responsiveness even when FSH levels have risen into the upper half of the normal range, and of course further reduced when above the normal limit (9 I.U./l by our assay). In particular, analysis of variance showed the FSH level to be a more important independent determinant of ovarian responsiveness than age (Cahill

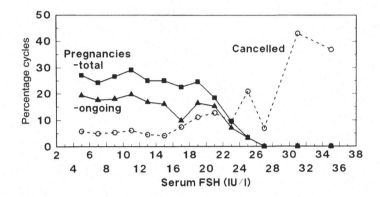

Fig. 6. Results of IVF treatment per cycle started (for the cancellation rate) or attempted egg recovery, related to the basal (day 3) serum FSH concentration (upper normal limit in this assay 22 iu/l) (from Toner *et al.*, 1991.)

et al., 1994). In other words, biological age of the ovary appears to be more important that chronological age. Whether that is also reflected in oocyte quality, as well as quantity, remains to be shown.

In practice, it is important to appreciate the wide variation between FSH assays, as indicated above. A raised FSH concentration is a valuable prognostic index but the normal range must be properly determined by each laboratory.

Irradiation and cancer chemotherapy

Gonadal failure is well known to occur after irradiation or chemotherapy, whether received for gonadal or other cancer, commonly lymphoma in young adults. Bone marrow transplantation following whole-body irradiation for leukaemia will become increasingly frequent. The exact nature of the damage, and relation to particular therapeutic agents and dosage, are not well defined, and the effects of particular treatments are usually obscured by combination therapy (Shalet, 1980; Scialli, 1992). It is clear, however, that the damaging effects on the ovary are related to both dose and age. The greater the dose, the greater is the proportion of women who develop oligo- or amenorrhoea due to ovarian failure, and the earlier it develops. Amenorrhoea develops in women aged in their 40s with half the dose that affects women in their 30s, and a quarter of the dose in their 20s.

In general, 3 years after chemotherapy for Hodgkin's disease as an example, barely 10% of women have regular menstrual cycles, a quarter have oligomenorrhoea and two-thirds have amenorrhoea. One feature which is difficult to explain is the return of menstruation in up to a quarter of women who develop amenorrhoea initially. However, even if menstruation returns ovarian function usually deteriorates subsequently, and pregnancies are rare in women with previous evidence of impaired ovarian function following chemotherapy. There is no evidence that suppressing gonadotrophin secretion, to reduce follicular recruitment and hopefully reduce the rate of atresia, offers any protection against the cytotoxic effects.

The evident ovarian changes are reduction in number and size of antral follicles and depletion of primordial follicles. It is usually assumed that the cytotoxic damage affects the oocytes primarily, but it is also likely that theca and granulosa cells are damaged, and of course oocytes cannot survive without the support of those follicle cells. Impairment of the steroidogenic capacity of human granulosa cells exposed to cytoxic agents *in vitro* has been demonstrated. Serum FSH levels are related (inversely), not so much to the number of remaining follicles as to their size, indicative of the quantity of granulosa cells.

There is also the possibility of adverse effects on uterine vasculature, which may contribute to the (rather inconsistently observed) high pregnancy wastage rate after radiotherapy. That could be relevant in egg donation treatment.

Autoimmune ovarian failure

Autoimmune ovarian failure is characterized by the typical menopausal features of raised FSH levels and oestrogen deficiency, and serological evidence of antibodies to steroid-producing cells. These antibodies also affect the adrenal glands and autoimmune ovarian failure is often associated with Addison's hypoadrenalism or future disposition to it and vice versa. Other autoimmune disorders such as hypothyroidism and atrophic gastritis are sometimes associated, or asymptomatic thyro-gastric antibodies may be found (Betterle *et al.*, 1993).

Histology shows abundant follicles. Antibodies of IgG type are localized to hilar cells and theca cells, and there is evidence of complement-dependent cytotoxicity to granulosa cells *in vitro*. There is mononuclear chronic inflammatory cell infiltration around developing and atretic follicles, but sparing of primordial follicles. The theca layer is also infiltrated, and later the granulosa cells, which become degenerative (Fox, 1992). Ovarian biopsy is sometimes advocated to make the diagnosis and prognosticate the possibility of functional recovery, but the prognosis is unreliable whatever the findings, and the diagnosis rests principally on serological findings.

There is no effective treatment to restore ovarian function. There are anecdotal reports of recovery following immunosuppressive therapy, but equally there has been complete lack of response to high dosage with glucocorticoids, and more frequently recovery occurs spontaneously. Recovery can be intermittent, with alternating episodes of typical symptomatic ovarian failure and normal fertile cycles. The explanation remains obscure.

The issue in this chapter is the functional state of the oocytes. There is too little information to judge reliably, but the remarkable fertility displayed by some women during episodes of recovery suggests that only the follicular cells are affected by antibody blockade and if atresia does not occur the oocytes remain inherently healthy.

Smoking and other environmental toxins

Of the vast number of possible environmental toxins, many are confined to industrial sites by regulation. The main general interest lies in ubiquitous pollutants like the polycyclic aromatic hydrocarbons produced by combustion of fossil fuels (and tobacco) and social drugs like caffeine and nicotine, though, in addition to nicotine, tobacco smoking produces a vast range of substances, the effects of which are difficult to distinguish. Phyto-oestrogens are potential toxins present in many plant foods consumed by people and livestock, and in coffee and marijuana, though the everyday risks to reproduction suggested by experimental evidence are not clear. Caffeine and smoking will be discussed here, including reference to polycyclic aromatic hydrocarbons. The subject has been reviewed (Mattison *et al.*, 1989; Scialli, 1992).

Caffeine

Caffeine is a plant alkaloid with stimulant effects and is rapidly absorbed and diffused to all tissue compartments including the preimplantation blastocyst. It is found in coffee, tea, cocoa, cola beverages and eating chocolate. Compared with brewed coffee, instant coffee contains about two-thirds the amount of caffeine, tea and cola drinks about half.

Heavy coffee drinking is often associated with smoking, and independent effects of caffeine are difficult to distinguish. It appears that caffeine intake from only two or more cups of coffee a day in non-smokers reduces fertility significantly, and the effect increases with greater intake; and heavy intake further reduces fertility in smokers. However, it remains impossible to distinguish the effects of caffeine consumption from other aspects of life-style, and no mechanism has been found to explain reproductive toxicity, if it is real.

Smoking

By contrast, several direct effects on the reproductive process have been found for both polycyclic aromatic hydrocarbons (produced also from combustion of fossil fuels) and nicotine released in cigarette smoke.

The effects of polycyclic aromatic hydrocarbons vary by species, age, dose and metabolism, but animal experiments consistently demonstrate destruction of oocytes and errors in meiosis resulting from induced enzymic metabolism in the ovary (as occurs in other tissues), and reduced fertility.

Nicotine has powerful actions on smooth muscle and has been shown in women to increase the amplitude of utero-tubal contractions, and animal studies have shown delay of the LH surge and prevention of the cortical granule reaction in the oocyte which normally induces the post-fertilization block to polyspermy.

The clinical effects of smoking, though not attributable to specific constituents, include increased frequency of menstrual irregularity and amenorrhoea (suggesting hypothalamic-pituitary actions), infertility, miscarriage of chromosomally normal conceptuses, fetal growth retardation and premature birth. The menopause is brought forward by 2–3 years on average, the advance related to the amount of smoking, and the onset of osteoporosis occurs earlier, possibly due to alterations in hepatic metabolism of oestrogens to catechol oestrogens and increased excretion.

Fecundity per cycle is reduced by about a quarter, from 38% to 28% in one study of *couples of eventually proven fertility,* the reduction being related to the amount of smoking. The smokers of course caught up with the non-smokers in the fertile population but the average delay to conception was about 3 months. In the general population, prolonged infertility affects about 5% more couples who smoke than non-smokers. Childhood exposure to smoking parents reduces later fertility.

The causes are not clear. No consistent effects have been found on sperm production, morphology or motility. Nicotine and anabasine (another constituent of cigarette smoke) inhibit granulosa cell aromatase activity. However, a detailed study of the pituitary–ovarian hormone cycle has revealed no significant abnormality of LH pulsatility, follicular or luteal phase lengths, or oestrogen, progesterone or androgen levels in circulation or excreted in urine (Thomas *et al.*, 1993). These findings suggest that the known anti-oestrogenic effect of smoking does not work through alterations of pituitary or follicular endocrine function or metabolism of oestrogens. On the other hand, Elenbogen *et al.* (1991) found follicular fluid levels of oestradiol were significantly reduced in women smokers undergoing ovarian stimulation for IVF, despite reaching similar peak serum oestradiol levels.

There is also consistent finding of reduced fertilization rates. Studies of smokers undergoing IVF treatment have generally shown reduced success rates at every stage, though differences were often not significant in individual studies, which were sometimes fairly small in size. Lower rates were observed in smokers than non-smokers for fertilization and/or cleavage (Trapp, Kemeter & Feichtinger, 1986; Elenbogen *et al.*, 1991; Pattinson, Taylor & Pattinson, 1991; Hughes,

YoungLai & Ward, 1992; Rosevear *et al.*, 1992; Rowlands, McDermott & Hull, 1992), implantation (Pattinson *et al.*, 1991), pregnancy (Trapp *et al.*, 1986; Rowlands *et al.*, 1992) and birth (Pattinson *et al.*, 1991; Hughes *et al.*, 1992; Rowlands *et al.*, 1992), and increased rates of miscarriage (Pattinson *et al.*, 1991; Hughes *et al.*, 1992).

It is clear that smoking products reach the follicle and oocyte. Trapp *et al.* (1986) measured rhodanide, a product of cigarette-smoke cyanide, in blood and follicular fluid, but it was often present in non-smokers and levels were only 20–30% lower on average than in smokers. Rosevear *et al.* (1992) measured cotinine, a product of nicotine but with a much longer life and therefore a reliable marker of smoking, in follicular fluid and found significant reduction in oocyte fertilization and cleavage rates in the presence of cotinine. The proportional reduction was by about one-third.

The possible contribution of the male partner's smoking to reduced fertilization has been explored in Bristol by studying the results of IVF treatment using donor sperm. Smoking donors were excluded both by history and detection of cotinine in seminal plasma, which in some cases could have been present due to passive smoking. Follicular fluid cotinine measurements were not available, but fertilization rates were equally and significantly reduced in non-smoking women whose partner smoked as in women who themselves smoked. There seems to be the clearest evidence that not only does smoking directly damage the fertilizing ability of the oocyte, but simply living with a smoker has the same direct effect on oocytes.

References

Abdalla HI, Burton G, Kirkland A, Johnson MR, Leonard R, Brooks AA, Studd JWW. Age, pregnancy and miscarriage: uterine versus ovarian factors. *Hum Reprod* 1993; **8**: 1512–7.

Adams J, Polson DW, Franks S. Prevalence of polycystic ovaries in women with an ovulation and idiopathic hirsutism. *Br Med J* 1986; **293**: 355–9.

Aitken RJ, Irvine DS, Wu FC. Prospective analysis of sperm–oocyte fusion and reactive oxygen species generation as criteria for the diagnosis of infertility. *Am J Obstet Gynecol* 1991; **164**: 542–51.

Albert M, Gallo JM, Escalier D, parseghian N, Jouannet P, Schrevel J, David G. Unexplained *in vitro* fertilization failure: implication of acrosomes with a small reacting region, as revealed by a monoclonal antibody. *Hum Reprod* 1992; **7**: 1249–56.

Andersen CY. Levels of steroid-binding proteins and steroids in human preovulatory follicle fluid and serum as predictors of success in *in vitro* fertilization–embryo transfer treatment. *J Clin Endocr Metab* 1990; **71**: 1375–81.

Andersen CY, Ziebe S. Serum levels of free androstenedione, testosterone and oestradiol are lower in the follicular phase of conceptual than of non-conceptual cycles after ovarian stimulation with a gonadotrophin-releasing hormone agonist protocol. *Hum Reprod* 1992; **7**: 1365–70.

Balen AH, MacDougall J, Tan SL. The influence of the number of embryos transferred in 1060 *in vitro* fertilization pregnancies on miscarriage rates and pregnancy outcome. *Hum Reprod* 1993; **8**: 1324–8.

Balen AH, Tan SL, MacDougall J, Jacobs HS. Miscarriage rates following *in vitro* fertilization are increased in women with polycystic ovaries and reduced by pituitary desensitization with buserelin. *Hum Reprod* 1993; **8**: 959–64.

Basuray R, Rawlins RG, Radwanska E, Henig I, Sachdeva S, Tummon I, Binor Z, Dmowski WP. High progesterone/estradiol ratio in follicular fluid at oocyte aspiration for *in vitro* fertilization as a predictor of possible pregnancy. *Fertil Steril* 1988; **49**: 1007–11.

Bedford JM, Kim HH. Sperm/egg binding patterns and oocyte cytology in retrospective analysis of fertilization failure. *in vitro. Hum Reprod* 1993; **8**: 453–63.

Bergh C, Olsson JH, Selleskog U, Hillensjo T. Steroid production in cultured thecal cells obtained from human ovarian follicles. *Hum Reprod* 1993; **8**: 519–24.

Betterle C, Rossi A, Dalla Pria S, Artifoni A, Pedini B, Gavasso S, Caretto A. Premature ovarian failure: autoimmunity and natural history. *Clin Endocr* 1993; **39**: 35–43.

Birkenfeld A, Beier HM, Schenker JG. The effect of clomiphene citrate on early embryonic development, endometrium and implantation. *Hum Reprod* 1986; **1**: 387–95.

Bomsel-Helmreich O, Vu L, Huyen N, Durand-Gasselin I. Effects of varying doses of HCG on the evolution of preovulatory rabbit follicles and oocytes. *Hum Reprod* 1989; **4**: 636–42.

Braat DDM, Schoemaker R, Schoemaker J. Life table analysis of fecundity in intravenously gonadotropin-releasing hormone-treated patients with normogonadotropic and hypogonadotropic amenorrhoea. *Fertil Steril* 1991; **55**: 266–71.

Brook JD, Gosden RG, Chandley AC. Maternal ageing and aneuploid embryos – evidence from the mouse that biological and not chronological age is the important influence. *Hum Genet* 1984; **66**: 41–5.

Cahill DJ, Prosser CJ, Wardle PG, Ford WCL, Hull MGR. Relative influence of serum follicle stimulating hormone, age and other factors on ovarian response to gonadotrophin stimulation. *Br J Obstet Gynaecol* 1994; **101**: 999–1002.

Campo S, Felli A, Lamanna MA, Barini A, Garcea N. Endocrine changes and clinical outcome after laparoscopic ovarian resection in women with polycystic ovaries. *Hum Reprod* 1993; **8**: 359–63.

Chan SYW, Tucker MJ. Fertilization failure and dysfunctions as possible causes for human idiopathic infertility. *Andrologia* 1991; **23**: 399–414.

Coulam CB, Moore SB, O'Fallon W. Investigating unexplained infertility. *Am J Obstet Gynecol* 1988; **158**: 1374–81.

Craft I, Al-Shawaf R, Kewis P, Serhal P, Simons E, Ah-Moye M, Fiamanya W, Robertson D, Shrivastav P, Brinsden P. Analysis of 1071 GIFT procedures – the case for a flexible approach to treatment. *Lancet* 1988: **i**: 1094–8.

Crosignani PG, Ferrari C. Dopaminergic treatments for hyperprolactinaemia. *Baillère's Clin Obstet Gynaecol* 1990; **4**: 441–55.

DeSutter P, Dhont M, Vanluchene E, Vanderkerckove D. Correlations between follicular fluid steroid analysis and maturity and cytogenetic analysis of human oocytes that remained unfertilized after *in vitro* fertilization. *Fertil Steril* 1991; **55**: 958–63.

Dor J, Shulman A, Levran D, Ben-Rafael Z, Rudak E, Mashiach S. The treatment of patients with polycystic ovarian syndrome by *in vitro* fertilization and embryo transfer: a comparison of results with those of patients with tubal infertility. *Hum Reprod* 1990; **5**: 816–8.

Dor J, Itzkowic DJ, Mashiach S, Lunenfeld B, Serr DM. Cumulative conception rates following gonadotrophin therapy. *Am J Obstet Gynecol* 1980; **136**: 102–5.

Dunphy BC, Li T-C, Macleod IC, Barratt CLR, Lenton EA, Cooke ID. The interaction of parameters of male and female fertility in couples with previously unexplained infertility. *Fertil Steril* 1990; **54**: 824–7.

Edwards RG, Morcos S, Macnamee M, Balmaceda JP, Walters DE, Asch R. High fecundity for amenorrhoeic women in embryo transfer programmes. *Lancet* 1991; **338**: 292–4.

Elenbogen A, Lipitz S, Mashiach S, Dor J, Levran D, Ben-Rafael Z. The effect of smoking on the outcome of *in vitro* fertilization – embryo transfer. *Hum Reprod* 1991; **6**: 241–4.

Erickson GF, Magoffin DA, Garzo VG, Cheung AP, Chang RJ. Granulosa cells of polycystic ovaries: are they normal or abnormal? *Hum Reprod* 1992; **7**: 293–9.

Federation CECOS, Schwartz D, Mayaux MJ. Female fecundity as a function of age. Results of artificial insemination in 2193 nulliporous women with azoospermic husbands. *New Engl J Med* 1982; **306**: 404–6.

FIVNAT. French national IVF registry: analysis of 1096 to 1990 data. *Fertil Steril* 1993; **59**: 587–95.

FIVNAT. Infecondites inexpliquées bilan FIVNAT 1986–1991. *Contracept Fertil Sex* 1992; **20**: 821–3.

Fox H. The pathology of premature ovarian failure. *J Path* 1992; **167**: 357–63.

Fox R, Corrigan E, Thomas PG, Hull MGR. Oestrogen and androgen states in oligo-amenorrhoeic women with polycystic ovaries. *Br J Obstet Gynaecol* 1991; **98**: 294–9.

Glasier AF. Clomiphene citrate. *Baillière's Clin Obstet Gynaecol* 1990, **4**: 491–501.

Glazener CMA, Kelly NJ, Weir MJA, David JSE, Cornes JS, Hull MGR. The diagnosis of male infertility-prospective time-specific study of conception rates to seminal analysis and post-coital sperm-mucus penetration and survival in otherwise unexplained infertility. *Hum Reprod* 1987; **2**: 665–71.

Hill GA, Freeman M, Bastias MC, Rogers BJ, Herbert III CM, Osteen KG, Wentz AC. The influence of oocyte maturity and embryo quality on pregnancy rate in a program for *in vitro* fertilization–embryo transfer. *Fertil Steril* 1989; **52**: 801–6.

Hoff JD, Quigley ME, Yen SSC. Hormonal dynamics at midcycle: A reevaluation. *Journal of Clin Endoc Metab* 1983; **57**: 792–6.

Homburg R. Levy T, Berkovitz D, Farchi J, Feldberg D, Ashkenazi J, Ben-Rafael Z. Gonadotrophin-releasing hormone agonist reduces the miscarriage rate for pregnancies achieved in women with polycystic ovarian syndrome. *Fertil Steril* 1993; **59**: 527–31.

Hughes EG, Fedorkow DM, Daya S, Sagle MA, Van de Koppel P, Collins J. The routine use of gonadatropin-releasing hormone agonists prior to *in vitro* fertilization and gamete intrafallopian transfer: a meta-analysis of randomized controlled trials. *Fertil Steril* 1992; **58**: 888–96.

Hughes EG, YoungLai EV, Ward SM. Cigarette smoking and outcomes of *in vitro* fertilization and embryo transfer: a prospective cohort study. *Hum Reprod* 1992; **7**: 358–61.

Hull MGR, Joyce DN, McLeod FN, Ray BP, McDermott A. Human *in vitro* fertilization, *in vivo* sperm penetration of cervical mucus, and unexplained infertility. Lancet 1984; **ii**: 245–6.

Hull MGR. Epidemiology of infertility and polycystic ovarian disease: endocrinological and demographic studies. *Gynecol Endocrinol* 1987; **1**: 235–45.

Hull MGR, Glazener CMA, Kelly NJ, Conway DI, Foster PA, Hinton RA, Coulson C, Lambert PA, Watt EM, Desai KM. Population study of causes, treatment and outcome of infertility. *Br Med J* 1985; **291**: 1693–7.

Hull MGR. Gonadotrophin therapy in anovulatory infertility. In: Howles CM (ed) *Gonadotrophins, Gonadotrophin-Releasing Hormone Analogues and Growth Factors in Infertility: Future Perspectives.* 1991, pp. 56–69, Hove, UK: Medi-Fax International.

Jacobs HS, Homburg R. The endocrinology of conception. *Ballière's Clin Endocr Metab* 1990; **4**: 195–205.

Johnson P, Pearce JM. Recurrent spontaneous abortion and polycystic ovarian disease: comparison of two regimens to induce ovulation. *Br Med J* 1990; **300**: 154–6.

Kagawa T, Yamano S, Nishida S, Murayama S, Aono T. Relationship among serum levels of luteinizing hormone, estradiol, and progesterone during follicle stimulation and results of *in vitro* fertilization and embryo transfer (IVF-ET). *J Assisted Reprod Genet* 1992, **9**: 106–12.

Legro RS, Ary BA, Paulson RJ, Stanczyk FZ, Sauer MV. Premature luteinization as detected by elevated serum progesterone is associated with a higher pregnancy rate in donor oocyte *in vitro* fertilization. *Hum Reprod* 1993; **8**: 1506–11.

Lenton EA, Cooke ID, Hooper M, King H, Kumar A, Monks N, Turner K, Verma S. *In vitro* fertilization in the natural cycle. *Baillière's Clin Obstet Gynaecol* 1992; **6**: 229–45.

Lenton EA, Sexton L, Lee S, Cooke ID. Progressive changes in LH and FSH and LH:FSH ratio in women throughout reproductive life. *Maturitas* 1988; **10**: 35–43.

Lipitz S, Ravinovici J, Ben-Shlomo I, Bider D, Ben-Rafael Z, Mashiach S, Dor J. Complete failure of fertilization in couples with unexplained infertility: implications for subsequent *in vitro* fertilization cycles. *Fertil Steril* 1993; **59**: 348–52.

Liu DY, Gordon Baker HW. Tests of human sperm function and fertilization *in vitro*. *Fertil Steril* 1992; **58**: 465–83.

Liu HC, Lai YM, Davis O, Berkeley AS, Graf M, Grifo J, Cohen J, Rosenwaks Z. Improved pregnancy outcome with gonadotropin releasing hormone agonist (GnRH-a) stimulation is due to the improvements in oocyte quantity rather than quality. *J Assisted Reprod Genet* 1992; **9**: 338–44.

Lunenfeld B, Blankstein J, Kotev-Emeth, Kokia E, Geier A. Drugs used in ovulation induction. Safety of patient and offspring. *Hum Reprod* 1986; **1**: 435–9.

MacDougall MJ, Tan SL, Balen A, Jacobs HS. A controlled study comparing patients with and without polycystic ovaries undergoing *in vitro* fertilization. *Hum Reprod* 1993; **8**: 233–7.

Mackenna AI, Zegers-Hochschild F, Fernandez EO, Fabres CV, Huidobro CA, Prado JA, Roblero LS, Altieri EL, Guadarrama, Lopez TH. Fertilization rate in couples with unexplained infertility. *Hum Reprod* 1992; **7**: 223–6.

McNatty KP, Smith DM, Makris A, Osathondh R, Ryan KJ. The microenvironment of the human antral follicle, interrelationships among the steroid levels in antral fluid, the population of granulosa cells and the status of the oocyte *in vivo* and *in vitro*. *J Clin Endocrinol Metab* 1979; **49**: 8511–60.

Mahmood TA, Arumugam K, Templeton AA. Oocyte and follicular fluid characteristics in women with mild endometriosis. *Br J Obstet Gynaecol* 1991; **98**: 573–7.

Mattison DR, Plowchalk DR, Meadows MJ, Miller MM, Malek, London S. The effect of smoking on oogenesis, fertilization and implantation. *Sem Reprod Endocrinol* 1989; **7**: 291–304.

Michael AE, Gregory L, Walker SM, Antoniw JW, Shaw RW, Edwards CRW, Cooke BA. Ovarian 11β-hydroxysteroid dehydrogenase: potential predictor of conception by *in vitro* fertilization and embryo transfer. *Lancet* 1993; **342**: 711–2.

Mills MS, Eddowes HA, Cahill DJ, Fahy UM, Abuzeid MIM, McDermott A, Hull MGR. A prospective controlled study of *in vitro* fertilization, gamete intra-Fallopian transfer and intrauterine insemination combined with superovulation. *Hum Reprod* 1992; **7**: 490–4.

Mio Y, Sekijima A, Iwabe T, Onohara Y, Harada T, Terakawa N. Subtle rise in serum progesterone during the follicular phase as a predictor of the outcome of *in vitro* fertilization. *Fertil Steril* 1992; **58**: 159–65.

Molloy D, Harrison K, Breen T, Hennessey J. The predictive value of idiopathic failure to fertilize on the first *in vitro* fertilization attempt. *Fertil Steril* 1991; **56**: 285–89.

Morgan PM, Boatman DE, Bavister BD. Relationships between follicular fluid steroid hormone concentrations, oocyte maturity, *in vitro* fertilization and embryonic development in the rhesus monkey. *Molec Reprod Devel* 1990; **27**: 145–51.

Pattinson HA, Taylor PJ, Pattinson MH. The effect of cigarette smoking on ovarian function and early pregnancy outcome of *in vitro* fertilization treatment. *Fertil Steril* 1991; **55**: 780–3.

Pettigrew LA, Cahill DJ, Wardle PG, Hull MGR. Follicular dysfunction in endometriosis. *Hum Reprod* 1993; **8**(suppl 1): 77–8.

Polan ML, Daniele A, Russell JB, DeCherney AH. Ovulation induction with human menopausal gonadotrophin compared to human urinary follicle-stimulating hormone results in a significant shift in follicular fluid androgen levels without discernible differences in granulosa–luteal cell function. *J Clin Endocr Metab* 1986; **63**: 1284–91.

Polson DW, Adams J, Wadsworth J, Franks S. Polycystic ovaries – a common finding in normal women. *Lancet* 1988; **i**: 870–2.

Porter R, Honour JW, Holownia P, Adams J, Craft I, Jacobs HS. The intrafollicular environment of the developing oocyte–gonadotrophic and ovarian determinants. *J Endocrinol* 1986; **108**: (Abstracts) S79.

Richardson AJ, Nelson JF. Follicular depletion during the menopausal transition. *Ann NY Acad Sci* 1990; **592**: 13–20.

Rosevear S, Holt DW, Lee TD, Ford WCL, Wardle PG, Hull MGR. Smoking and decreased fertilization rates *in vitro*. *Lancet* 1992; **340**: 1195–6.

Roulier R, Mouzon J, Bachelot A, Logerot H. Unexplained infertility. French national *in vitro* fertilization, *Contracept Fertil Sex* 1992; **20**: 821–3.

Rowlands DJ, McDermott A, Hull MGR. Prognosis for assisted conception treatment after unexpected failure of fertilisation *in vitro*: a comparative study. *Hum Reprod* 1994; **9**: 2287–90.

Rowlands DJ, McDermott A, Hull MGR. Smoking and decreased fertilization rates *in vitro*. *Lancet* 1992; **340**: 1409–10.

Sagle M, Bishop K, Ridley N, Alexander FM, Michel M, Bonney RC, Beard RW, Franks S. Recurrent early miscarriage and polycystic ovaries. *Br Med J* 1988; **297**: 1027–28.

Sauer MV, Paulson RJ, Lobo RA. Pregnancy after age 50: application of oocytes donation to women after natural menopause. *Lancet* 1993; **341**: 321–3.

Saunders DM, Lancaster PAL, Pedisch EL. Increased pregnancy failure rates after clomiphene following assisted reproductive technology. *Hum Reprod* 1992; **7**: 1154–8.

Schoolcraft W, Sinton E, Schlenker T, Huynh D, Hamilton F, Meldrum DR. Lower pregnancy rate with premature luteinization during pituitary suppression with leuprolide acetate. *Fertil Steril* 1991; **55**: 563–6.

Scialli AR. *A Clinical Guide to Reproductive and Developmental Toxicology.* Vol. 1, pp. 51–67, 1992; London: CRC Press.

Shalet SM. Effects of cancer chemotherapy of gonadal function of patients. *Cancer Treatment Rev* 1980; **7**: 141–52.

Sher G, Herbert C, Maassarani G, Jacobs MH. Assessment of the late proliferative phase endometrium by ultrasonography in patients undergoing *in vitro* fertilization and embryo transfer (IVF/ET). *Hum Reprod* 1991; **6**: 232–7.

Shoham Z, Jacobs HS, Insler V. Luteinizing hormone: its role, mechanism of actions and detrimental effects when hypersecreted during the follicular phase. *Fertil Steril* 1993; **59**: 1153–61.

Shoham Z, Homburg R, Jacobs HS. Pulsed GnRH. *Baillère's Clin Obstet Gynaecol* 1990; **4**: 589–608.

Silverberg KM, Burns WN, Olive DL, Riehl RM, Schenken RS. Serum progesterone levels predict success of *in vitro* fertilization/embryo transfer in patients stimulated with leuprolide acetate and human menopausal gonadotrophins. *J Clin Endocr Metab* 1991; **73**: 797–803.

Testart J, Lefevre B, Gougeon A. Effects of gonadotrophin-releasing hormone agonists (GnRHa) on follicle and oocyte quality. *Hum Reprod* 1993; **8**: 511–18.

Thomas EJ, Edridge W, Weddell A, Mcgill A, McGarrigle HHG. The impact of cigarette smoking on the plasma concentrations of gonadotrophins, ovarian steroids and androgens and upon the metabolism of oestrogens in the human female. *Hum Reprod* 1993; **8**: 1187–93.

Tolis G, Bringer J, Chrousos GP. Eds. Intra-ovarian regulators and polycystic ovarian syndrome. *Ann NY Acad Sci* 1993; **687**: (310pp).

Toner JP, Philput CB, Jones GS, Muasher SJ. Basal follicle-stimulating hormone level is a better predictor of *in vitro* fertilization performance than age. *Fertil Steril* 1991; **55**: 784–91.

Trapp M, Kemeter P, Feichtinger W. Smoking and *in vitro* fertilization. *Hum Reprod* 1986; **1**: 357–8.

Turner K, Goldstein DJ, Rogers AW. Variation in the dry mass of mouse embryos throughout the preimplantation period. *Hum Reprod* 1992; **7**: 112–16.

Urman B, Fluker MR, Yuen BH, Fleige-Zahradka BG, Zouves CG, Moon YS. The outcome of *in vitro* fertilization and embryo transfer in women with polycystic ovary syndrome failing to conceive after ovulation induction with exogenous gonadotrophins. *Fertil Steril* 1992; **57**: 1269–73.

Van Steirteghem AC, Nagy Z, Joris H, Liu J, Staessen C, Smitz J, Wisanto A, Devroey P. High fertilization and implantation rates after intracytoplasmic sperm injection. *Hum Reprod* 1993; **8**: 1061–6.

Vanluchene E, Hinting A, Dhont M, De Sutter P, Van Maele G, Vandekerchove D.

Follicular fluid steroid lvels in relation to oocyte maturity and *in vitro* fertilization. *J Steroid Biochem Molec Biol* 1991; **38**: 83–7.

Walters De. Biometrical evaluation in fertility studies. *Hum Reprod* 1993; **8**: 2–7.

Wardle PG, McLaughlin EA, McDermott A, Mitchell JD, Ray BD, Hull MGR. Endometriosis and ovulatory disorder reduced fertilization *in vitro* compared with tubal and unexplained infertility. *Lancet* 1985; **ii**: 236–9.

Watson H, Kiddy DS, Hamilton-Fairley D, Scanlon MJ, Barnard C, Collins WP, Bonney RC, Franks S. Hypersecretion of luteinizing hormone and ovarian steroids in women with recurrent early miscarriage. *Hum Reprod* 1993; **8**: 829–33.

Witkin SS, Viti D, David SS, Stangel J, Rosenwaks Z. Relation between antisperm antibodies and the rate of fertilization of human oocytes *in vitro*. *J Assisted Reprod Genet* 1992; **9**: 9–13.

Wood JW. Fecundity and natural fertility in humans. *Oxf Rev Reprod Biol* 1989; **11**: 61–109.

Zheng CJ, Byers B. Oocyte selection: a new model for the maternal-age dependence of Down syndrome. *Hum Genet* 1992; **90**: 1–6.

13

Ovarian stimulation for assisted conception

J. L. YOVICH

Introduction

Ovarian stimulation was initially introduced as a medical therapy for women who were clearly anovulatory evidenced by amenorrhoea or severe oligo-menorrhoea. However, the role of ovarian stimulation currently has emerged as an integral treatment mode in different assisted conception procedures for a wide spectrum of infertility problems.

The spectrum of infertility

Involuntary infertility is a worldwide problem which causes a sense of personal failure as well as carrying a social stigma in many cultures. Infertile couples describe a sense of anguish, and often despair, when their desire to reproduce remains unfulfilled. Without contraception, 75% of couples would achieve pregnancy within 12 months, mostly within the first 4 months (Wilcox *et al.*, 1988). Thereafter the proportion conceiving is relatively low, and overall up to 15% of couples within the reproductive age range present for medical assessment, usually by 2 years of failed effort.

The aetiological factors underlying infertility are numerous and the predominant causes vary with geographical location, socio-economic factors and the changing face of health problems within different areas in given periods of time. For example, tuberculous disease of the genital tract is suspected to be the most prominent underlying condition in one recent study from Iran (Bahadori, 1986), whereas ovulatory dysfunction heads the list in an Australian report (Cox, 1975).

The broad categories of infertility recognized in industrialized societies are ovulatory dysfunction (25–45%), spermatozoal disorders (mostly unexplained; 20–35%), tubal disease (15–30%), pelvic endometriosis (10–15% as the attributed cause; up to 45% as an identified factor), poor sperm/mucus interaction (5–15%), antispermatozoal antibodies (ASABs; 5–15%), and completely unexplained (5–10%). With comprehensive investigations conducted on both partners, most cases will reveal a multifactorial basis although often a single condition will appear to have predominant relevance over other identified factors.

Uncommon causes of infertility include genital tract anomalies such as congenital absence of a vital structure (e.g. Rokitansky–Küster–Haüser syndrome androgen insensitivity syndromes, congenital absence of vasa deferentia) as well as those caused by diethylstilboestrol exposure *in utero,* and intrauterine synechiae causing Asherman's syndrome. Sexual dysfunctions and ejaculatory disorders are occasional causes of infertility owing to failure of sperm deposition in the vagina.

Therapeutic prognosis

Prior to 1960, it appears that less than 20% of couples who presented with infertility subsequently conceived – in fact, those conceptions which did occur were considered to be mostly unrelated to treatment (Jeffcoate, 1975). Subsequently the prognosis improved with the introduction of clomiphene citrate (CC) and gonadotrophins (from human menopausal urine; hMG and human pituitary glands; hPG) for ovulation induction. This was associated with inspired discoveries and developments in understanding the hypothalamic–pituitary–ovarian axis leading to the current improved level of knowledge regarding events concerning folliculogenesis, oocyte release and luteal function in the ovarian cycle. hPG was subsequently withdrawn from clinical use because of the aetiological relationship with Creutzfeld–Jacob disease which subsequently developed in some treated women (see later).

Further significant advances during the 1960s and 1970s included the introduction of laparoscopy as a primary diagnostic tool; the development of sensitive, specific and eventually, rapid hormone assay systems; the appreciation of the role of non-gonococcal anaerobic organisms such as *Bacteroides fragilis,* and later others such as *Chlamydia trachomatis,* in the causation of pelvic inflammatory disease; the recognition of hyperprolactinaemia and its successful treatment with bromocryptine; the establishment of donor semen banks using frozen straws; the development of microsurgery (initially on the female and subsequently on the male genital tract), advances in endoscopic operative procedures, and the detection of antibodies against gametes. Such advances improved the prognosis considerably and the understanding of human infertility sufficiently, to enable the introduction of techniques to assist human reproduction.

The integration of assisted reproductive methods with these developments in the comprehensive management of infertility has improved the potential prognosis to beyond 75% of couples who can now be successfully treated to achieve at least one livebirth. The main limiting factors to the successful treatment of infertility are no longer technical but relate to expense, ethical considerations and certain social aspects. These latter concerns have led to certain public anxieties in many countries and a perceived need to introduce legislative constraints in both service and research aspects of assisted reproduction.

Assisted conception procedures

Historical aspects

Although successful embryo transfers were described in the rabbit a century ago, the process of *in vitro* fertilization (IVF) has a much shorter history with the first mammalian success producing live offspring being reported in 1959, again achieved in rabbits (Chang, 1959). Interestingly, the rabbit model was not ideal with respect to spermatozoal capacitation *in vitro*, but this posed less problem with several other mammalian laboratory species where IVF was subsequently achieved. IVF has now been reported for a wide range of mammals, including non-human primates and domestic animals. Human IVF has proven to be relatively simple and current practice is based on the mouse model (Whittingham, 1968).

Crude attempts to achieve human IVF had been undertaken during the 1940s and 1950s but it is unlikely that normal cleaving embryos were generated prior to the combined efforts of Robert Edwards (physiologist and embryologist) and the late Patrick Steptoe (gynaecologist) with contributions by Barry Bavister and the late Jean Purdy (Evans, Mukherjee & Schulman, 1980). Edwards had earlier studied IVF in oocytes derived from surgical specimens of ovary and subsequently matured *in vitro*. The morphological quality of embryos was superior when pre-ovulatory oocytes were aspirated from mature follicles at laparoscopy following stimulation with human menopausal gonadotrophine (hMG) and fertilized *in vitro* in a modified Tyrode's solution. They reported the first human IVF pregnancy in 1976 (Steptoe & Edwards, 1976), but it proved to be an ectopic in the proximal segment of a distally occluded Fallopian tube. The team subsequently abandoned stimulated cycles as an onging pregnancy proved elusive, and it was considered that such cycles were unfavourable for implantation.

The first successful pregnancies were achieved in a series of 32 cycles which reached the stage of embryo transfer (ET) after monitoring natural, unstimulated follicle development with a sensitive immuno-bioassay for LH performed on urine (Edwards, Steptoe & Purdy, 1980). There were four pregnancies in that series and Louise Brown, a healthy female born in July 1978, became the first IVF infant (Steptoe & Edwards, 1978). A healthy male was also delivered a few months later but two other pregnancies miscarried, one in the first trimester shown to have triploidy, and another in the second trimester shown to have an inherited chromosomal anomaly (Steptoe, Edwards & Purdy, 1989). The next team to report success was from Australia where IVF had been studied for almost a decade and again this was achieved from a monitored natural cycle. However, natural cycle pregnancies proved to be relatively elusive and subsequent successes were derived from stimulated cycles. By 1983, IVF clinics were commenced in many countries but most were reporting sporadic successes only, amounting to the birth of around 50 infants. In the next 5 years clinics reported consistent pregnancy rates of 12–25%. However, worldwide reports from independent authorities published on data to 1987, showed the livebirth rate per IVF treatment cycle for those patients who reached the stage of oocyte recovery averaged only 9–10% (Yovich *et al.*, 1989).

During 1987–1992 improvements in methodology, increasing expertise and new knowledge in many aspects of reproductive medicine have led to higher rates of couples successfully completing their treatment cycles (>80%) and overall livebirth rates of 20–25% per cycle reaching the embryo transfer stage are becoming more common (Cohen, de Mouzon & Lancaster, 1993). By the end of 1992 it was estimated that there were in excess of 100 000 infants born as a result of IVF-related procedures worldwide. This achievement is the tangible consequence of advances in the science of human reproduction over the past 20 years. The new knowledge has also been applied effectively in a range of non-IVF treatments for infertility as well as opening the door to major advances in the management of genetic-based diseases, improved contraceptive methods and perhaps assisting the peoples of industrialized countries to sustain their population in a socio-economic climate causing reduced fecundity.

Physiological considerations

The ovarian stimulation protocols used in the various techniques of assisted conception are based on a clear understanding of existing knowledge in human reproduction, having evolved from major advances in knowledge of areas such as the hypothalamic–pituitary–ovarian axis and its relationship with apocrine events in the gonads and endometrium.

As advances in knowledge accrue, protocols can be adjusted accordingly. Reproductive medicine is advancing rapidly partly because of the establishment of dedicated clinics, with commitments to both service and research aspects. Such clinics are able to undertake fundamental research and develop new techniques.

Table 1. *Specific facilities required for the comprehensive management of infertility, preferably within a single unit functioning every day*

Consultation	–	● both partners
Counselling	–	● information
		● emotional support
Co-ordination	–	● senior nurse
		● tests/instructions/results
Laboratories	–	● andrology
		● embryology
		● cryopreservation
		● hormone assays
Ultrasound	–	● radiology
Results	–	● group meeting each afternoon
		● computer and hard-copy data registers
		● regular data analysis and evaluation
Treatment	–	● areas and facilities
Semen	–	● collection rooms
Theatre	–	● oocyte recovery/transfers
		● endoscopy facilities
		● ultrasound facility
		● operating microscope

Range of techniques

Modern treatments to assist conception can be categorized as specific, general or substitutive. Ideally, these modes are all carried out in a single unit structured to provide a comprehensive approach to infertility management (Table 1).

Specific treatments

Specific treatments include reconstructive pelvic and tubal microsurgery; the management of endocrine disorders including hyperprolactinaemia, hyper- and hypo-thyroidism, Cushing's disease and hypopituitarism; ovulation induction for discrete anovulatory disorders; and both medical and surgical treatments for pelvic endometriosis. These treatments are invariably followed by successful conception and pregnancy outcomes. The likelihood of success is dependent upon the relevance of the diagnosed disorder to the couple's infertility, the association

Table 2. *Optimal assessment prior to commencing infertility treatments*

1. Clinical examination	–	both partners
2. Routine tests	–	ECS and Pap smear
		Semen analysis
		ASABs–serum both partners
		–semen, cervical mucus
		Hep B and C, HIV screen both
3. Ovarian cycle	–	FSH, LH, Prolactin in early phase
	–	Androgen status in early phase
	–	Ultrasound in early phase
	–	E_2, P_4, LH in periovulatory phase
	–	Ultrasound in periovulatory phase
	–	Mucus score in preovulatory phase
	–	E_2, P_4 in mid-luteal phase
4. Post-coital test	–	8–12 h post coitus
		Immediate preovulatory phase
5. Laparoscopy	–	Pelvic assessment
	–	Tubal dye pertubation
6. Hysteroscopy	–	$\pm$ Hysterosalpingogram
7. Counselling	–	Early introduction

Further specific investigations and management required following the detection of abnormal results in any of the above areas.

of additional factors, and the effectiveness of the specific treatment to correct the disorder and reverse any underlying damage to reproductive mechanisms. These comments highlight the need for the comprehensive assessment of both partners and the sperm/cervical mucus interface prior to, or in association with, any proposed treatment mode (Table 2).

General treatments

General treatments provide solutions to multifactorial and poorly explained infertility problems as well as those resistant to or unsuitable for specific treatments. They include *ovarian stimulation* of women who appear to be ovulatory and the use of a range of procedures involving *gamete manipulation* in order to enhance the chance of fertilization or bypass the fallopian tubes for embryo placement. Whilst there may be a dominant single condition indicating the need for such assistance, in many cases more than one factor can be identified and

Table 3. *Infertility treatments involving gamete manipulation*

Insemination
DI	donor insemination
AIH	artificial insemination (husband)
IUI	intrauterine insemination

IVF-related
GIFT	gamete intrafallopian transfer
PROST	pronuclear stage tubal transfer*
IVF-ET	*in vitro* fertilization and embryo transfer
TEST	tubal embryo stage transfer*

Others
DIPI	direct intraperitoneal insemination
POST	peritoneal ovum and sperm transfer
FREDI	Fallopian replacement of eggs and delayed insemination
ICSI	intracytoplasmic sperm injection

* same as zygote intrafallopian transfer (ZIFT).

sometimes a range of factors appear to be relevant to the case. Indeed, the success of such treatments for poorly explained cases of infertility implies that other factors are operating even when diagnostic investigations reveal discrete abnormalities. A range of gamete manipulation procedures have now been described (Table 3) and these are often or usually combined with ovarian stimulation to achieve optimal results.

Substitution treatments

Substitution treatments provide the only methods currently possible for couples to achieve their own pregnancies when vital reproductive structures or suitable gametes are absent. These include *ovum donation, sperm donation, embryo donation and IVF surrogacy*. In the latter case, embryos generated from the gametes of an infertile couple are transferred to a surrogate who carries the pregnancy on behalf of the infertile couple.

Ovarian stimulation

Ovarian stimulation therapy with CC (Fig. 1) and gonadotrophins was introduced into clinical practice in the late 1960s for women with anovulation, usually presenting with amenorrhoea or marked oligomenorrhoea. Normogonadotrophic

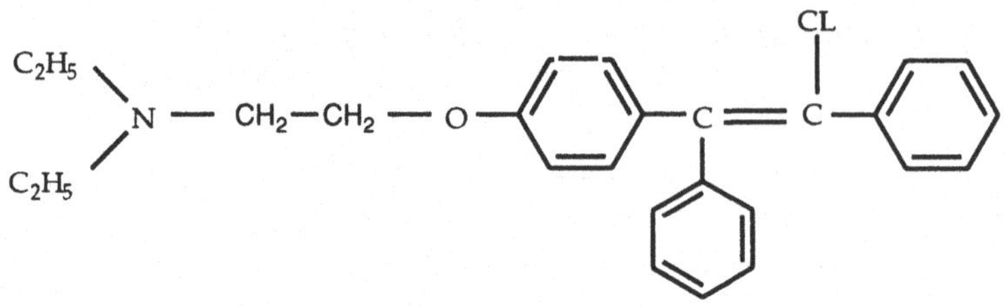

Fig. 1. Chemical structure of clomiphene citrate which has *cis-* and *trans-*isomeric forms, the former having greater biological activity. The molecule is structurally related to diethylstilboestrol.

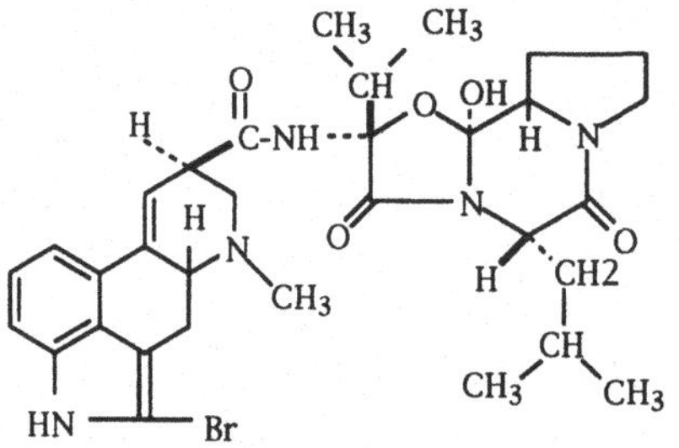

Fig. 2. Chemical structure of bromocryptine mesylate (2-bromo-α-ergocryptine), a peptide ergot alkaloid.

women are usually responsive to CC tablets (50 mg to 200 mg per day for 5 days) revealing signs of ovulation, but pregnancy occurs in only half of responding cases probably due to adverse actions such as cervical mucus inhibition, retention of oocytes within follicles and endometrial receptivity inhibition. Hypergonadotrophic women were found to be unresponsive to any form of stimulation due to ovarian failure and hypo-gonadotrophic cases with hypo-oestrogenism usually required gonadotrophins. These cases have an excellent prognosis with high rates of both ovulation and pregnancy (around 90%). Hyperprolactinaemic amenorrhoea is another anovulatory group with an excellent prognosis, responding well to oral bromocryptine (Fig. 2), usually in dose schedules of 2.5 mg to 10 mg per day. Hyperprolactinaemia requires careful assessment to determine any underlying aetiology such as abnormal thyroid function with thyroid stimulating hormone elevation and consideration of drug-related elevations.

Effective ovulation induction, particularly by bromocryptine and gonadotrophin therapy, generates high rates of pregnancy if other fertility factors for the couple are normal. However, the treatments are not without hazards.

Generally, ovarian stimulation has not been recommended for women who show evidence of ovulation. However, in clinical practice it is apparent that

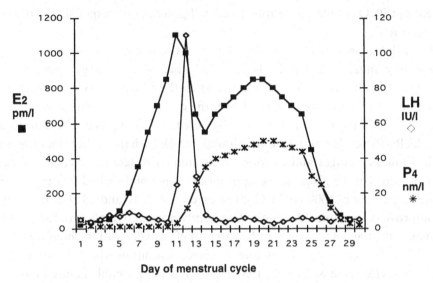

Fig. 3. Hormonal changes during a normal 'conception' ovulatory cycle showing serum oestradiol (E₂), luteinizing hormone (LH), progesterone (P₄) and, if pregnant, the pattern of detectable human chorionic gonadotrophin (βhCG) elevation.

conception can be enhanced by stimulation schedules applied empirically (Yovich *et al.,* 1987) and which probably correct minor disorders of ovulation; as an adjunct to insemination procedures if conception fails to ensue over 4–6 treatment cycles; and as a routine for IVF-related procedures to provide a number of oocytes for fertilization and the subsequent selection of optimal embryos for transfer.

Stimulation for disordered ovarian cycles and empiric stimulation

Women with unexplained infertility who are most likely to respond to ovarian stimulation are those who demonstrate some disorder when their cycles are closely monitored and compared to a normal 'conception' cycle (Fig. 3). Such normal cycles display oestradiol-17β (E$_2$) rises >620 pm/l prior to LH surge and the pre-surge LH levels throughout the follicular phase should be no greater than 1 standard deviation above the mean for conceiving women (Stanger & Yovich, 1985) (usually <10 i.u./l). The LH surge should be followed by an appropriate rise in progesterone (P$_4$) and the mid-luteal levels of E$_2$ and P$_4$ should be >500 pm/l and 30 nm/l, respectively. Ovarian ultrasound evaluation should exclude polycystic ovaries (PCO) (Adams, Polson & Franks, 1986) and demonstrate a dominant follicle ≥1.5 cm at the time of LH surge. Cycle length may also be relevant; in particular the luteal phase dated from LH surge should probably be >11 days. Women with clinical, ultrasound, androgen, or LH evidence of PCO should be identified and will generally be responsive to ovarian stimulation.

The author's preferred stimulation regimen is sequential as follows:

First, any underlying disorder is corrected where possible (e.g. weight control aiming for BMI between 20 and 25). Thereafter, the response to CC is monitored, beginning with 50 mg/day on days 2–6 of the cycle. The dose can be raised to a maximum of 200 mg/day but it is generally unrewarding to proceed beyond 50 mg b.d. Ideally the cycle should be monitored by BBT changes, hormonal assays, cervical mucus changes and ovarian ultrasound. A triggering injection of hCG 5000 IU can then be given at the appropriate stage of follicle development and booster injections of 1000 i.u. hCG given on days 4, 7, 10 and 13 after the trigger will improve corpus luteal function. Apparently normal ovulation occurs in 70% of cases but pregnancy ensues in less than half, usually within three treatment cycles. The discrepancy is partly due to mucus inhibition which occurs in 22% of CC cycles (Matson & Yovich, 1987), as well as the probable failure of follicles to disperse and release their oocytes properly (Stanger & Yovich, 1984).

If the response to CC has been ineffective, hMG should be added to the regimen. Depending upon the woman's age and weight, this is commenced with 75 to 150 i.u. i.m.i. alternate daily from day 3 of the cycle (i.e. the day after CC begins) increasing by 1 to 2 ampoules after 3 days if the response has been inadequate judged by the daily monitoring of E_2 levels from day 8 or 9 of the cycle. The aim is to generate a steady rise of E_2 over 6 days when the hCG trigger is given, followed by the luteal boosts as described above. One aims for peak E_2 levels between 1000 and 3000 pm/l which matches 1–3 mature follicles. Greater levels and follicle numbers signal a real danger of high-order multiple pregnancy and in such instances the couple should be counselled to consider the alternative options of avoiding intercourse in that cycle or converting to GIFT treatment where the oocyte numbers available for pregnancy can be controlled. The CC/hMG regimen (Fig. 4) is the most effective for empirical stimulation but some cases demonstrate continuing inhibition of cervical mucus (11%), raised LH or raised androgens which appear to be a consequence of the CC. Future cycles should be treated with hMG alone as described in combination with CC. In such cases the luteal hCG boosts are essential to avoid a markedly shortened luteal phase around 9 days.

The standard regimen therefore involves the progression from CC to CC/hMG to hMG alone. Bromocryptine may be used in conjunction to control hyperprolactinaemia and spironolactone to inhibit high androgen effects. However, certain groups of women may still fail to respond adequately to the regimen and are usually identified as those of advanced age, some cases of PCO disease in a partial or impending state of ovarian failure with mildly elevated

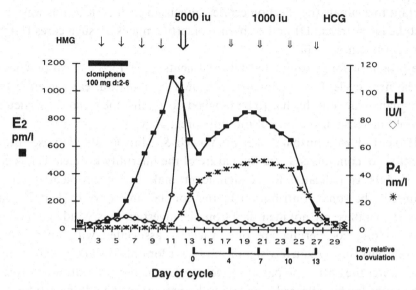

Fig. 4. Ovarian stimulation with clomiphene citrate combined with human meno-pausal gonadotrophin (CC/hMG) and including human chorionic gonadotrophin (hCG) for ovulation trigger and luteal support.

serum FSH, and others who simply demonstrate ovarian resistance even when 750 IU or more of hMG are given per day. Purified FSH (e.g. Metrodin, Serono) has been evaluated in several trials and may have conferred some benefit for those women with raised basal LH levels. Some cases may benefit from gonadotrophin suppression for 2–3 months using one of the higher strength oral contraceptive preparations. However, a more useful approach has followed the introduction of GnRH analogues which will be described in conjunction with IVF-related treatments.

Ovarian stimulation for insemination treatments

Donor insemination is generally applied as substitution therapy for severe male factor infertility, usually non-correctible azoospermia. The female partner usually has normal fertility or, at least, may not have had the opportunity to test her fertility. Furthermore donor insemination treatment relies on spermatozoal interaction with cervical mucus and the natural processes of sperm migration through the upper genital tract. Therefore ovarian stimulation is best avoided. However, if conception fails to ensue within four to six treatment cycles, ovarian stimulation will improve the chances if investigations of the female fail to detect any abnormalities other than minor disorders of ovulation. In such cases it is important to evaluate the effect on cervical mucus in each cycle as it is wasteful to undertake intracervical DI in the absence of fertile mucus. In such cases IUI with donor sperm can be applied.

The prognosis for unstimulated DI treatments is 10–15% clinical pregnancies per treatment cycle. IUI treatments with hMG stimulation can generate twice the pregnancy rate but this has to be weighed up against the hazards, particularly a five-fold increase in the rate of multiple pregnancy.

AIH (i.e. IUI with husband sperm) (Yovich & Matson, 1988*b*) poses quite a different set of conditions. First, the nature of the infertility problem is less clear. Even if AIH is indicated for a significant male factor problem, there will undoubtedly be some contribution to the couple's infertility by female-related factors, even if these are not identified from the investigations. Mild and moderate degrees of oligozoospermia are only variably associated with infertility and therefore constitute a relatively significant factor for only certain infertile couples. Furthermore, the sperm preparation technique and the procedure involved for AIH requires freshly released oocyte/s to be present in the fallopian tube at the time of insemination, and there is minimal reliance on the natural process of sperm transport in the female genital tract. For these reasons, ovarian stimulation, or at least ovarian cycle monitoring and usually an hCG trigger, are an integral part of the treatment in order to maximize the chance of viable sperm making contact with the oocyte.

The author's current programme involves the following:
(i) alternate day hMG injections; (ii) hMG dose according to age and previous response injection; (iii) hCG trigger when E_2 and ultrasound observations are optimal; (iv) single IUI at 42 h under ultrasound control; (v) husband's ejaculate collected 90 min prior for preparation.

The above regimen provides clinical pregnancy rates around 20–25% per cycle over three cycles if $\geqslant 5$ million motile sperm are available for insemination and the female genital tract is normal. The sperm may require enhancement accordingly to motility characteristics and acrosome reactivity (Yovich, 1993).

Ovarian stimulation for IVF-related procedures

The pioneer workers in human IVF used hMG stimulation in order to generate several ovarian follicles for oocyte recovery when techniques were relatively crude and to counter the problems of limited fertilization and limited developmental potential of oocytes. However, they recognized that the luteal phase was shortened to a degree which was directly related to the output of urinary oestrogens measured during the follicular phase (Edwards *et al.,* 1980). Subsequently, when a rapid immuno-bioassay (Hi-Gonavis; Mochida Pharmaceutical Co, Japan) became available for LH/βhCG detection, natural ovulatory cycles were monitored and the single oocyte was recovered where possible. The first IVF pregnancies were achieved from natural cycles but the method was seen to have major limitations. These included the expense and inconvenience of prolonged hospitalization for 8-hrly monitoring to detect the commencement of LH surge, the frustration of prolonged monitoring of disordered cycles, the difficulty of laparoscopic aspiration if the follicle was inconveniently located and inaccessible due to underlying pelvic pathology, and the need to access theatres outside a routine daytime schedule. Therefore stimulated cycles were seen to be a requirement if the IVF procedure was to be adopted into clinical service.

The first clinic to report success with stimulated cycles (Trounson, Leeton & Wood, 1981) utilized CC alone for stimulation and hCG 5000 IU for the ovulation trigger. Oocytes were recovered 33–35 h later and no luteal support was provided. Subsequently, others, particularly in the United States, reported success using hMG alone for stimulation (Jones *et al.*, 1982), triggering ovulation with hCG 10 000 IU and giving luteal support routinely in the form of progesterone i.m.i. 25–50 mg/day. The latter was continued throughout the first trimester if pregnancy ensued. By 1986, when many IVF clinics were established worldwide, one of the most popular stimulation regimens in use combined CC with hMG. Generally 50 mg CC was given b.d. days 2–6 or 5–9 and hMG 75 IU ampoules (1–3) were given beginning a day or two after the CC was commenced. Cancellation rates due to poor or inappropriate responses and premature LH surges were around 20%. Clinics varied in their opinion regarding a 'coasting' phase for hMG prior to the hCG trigger and also regarding the need or value of luteal phase support (see later).

Marked improvements in IVF results have recently ensued from the diminishing use of CC and the increasing use of GnRH analogues such as Buserelin (Suprefact, Hoechst Laboratories) and Leuprolide acetate (Lucrin, Abbott Laboratories). These agents can be used in various regimens combined with hMG. Optimum results appear with a *pituitary down-regulation schedule* (Tan *et al.*, 1992*a,b*). A successful regimen is shown in Fig. 5 and involves commencing Lucrin 1 mg s.c. daily in the mid-luteal phase of the preceding cycle. Pituitary down-regulation is usually achieved by day 3–5 of the ensuing cycle and is demonstrated by serum FSH and LH levels < 5 IU/l and E_2 < 200 pmol/l. Thereafter 0.5 mg Lucrin daily will maintain suppression and hMG injections are given daily with appropriate increases after 3 days of any given dosage in order to increase E_2 by approximately 50% per day and the hCG trigger is given on the 7th day of sustained E_2 rise. Spontaneous LH surges rarely occur with this regimen. Ultrasound monitoring can provide additional useful information and may occasionally lead to delaying the LH trigger until a cohort of follicles have reached 1.6 cms diameter or greater.

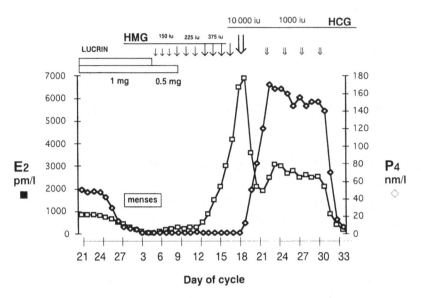

Fig. 5. Ovarian stimulation for *in vitro* fertilization (IVF) using leuprolide acetate (Lucrin) for pituitary down-regulation prior to hMG stimulation and hCG trigger and luteal support. The strength of hMG may be adjusted every 3 days to maintain a rising E_2 level over 7 days.

One aims for E_2 levels around 6000 pmol/l which indicates the likely recovery of 6–8 oocytes. If E_2 levels rise above 10 000 pmol/l there is a significant risk of ovarian hyperstimulation syndrome (OHSS).

The use of GnRH analogues has been shown to have significant benefits in patients of advanced age, with underlying PCO, with raised androgens, with raised basal LH or with previous premature LH surges (Cummins *et al.*, 1990). Those who have previously demonstrated poor ovarian responsiveness may often respond to the *'flare' technique* which involves commencing both the analogue and hMG together at the beginning of the cycle when the analogue will initiate pituitary release of gonadotrophins as a normal effect prior to down-regulation and so supplement the exogenous gonadotrophin. An *ultra-short 'flare' regimen* (Macnamee *et al.*, 1989) has also been described which is proving equally useful and has certain cost benefits although premature LH surges occur more frequently. However, the poor responder group remains a difficult group to treat effectively and cancellation rates due to an inadequate response are of the order of 10%. Current research indicates that the combined use of recombinant growth hormone (rGH) may improve the response or at least reduce the amount of hMG required to effect successful stimulation (Homburg *et al.*, 1990). However, the expense of such treatment is currently prohibitive for consideration in routine clinical service.

Other developments in ovarian stimulation for assisted reproduction include the use of recombinant FSH (Devroey *et al.,* 1993) and the use of GnRH antagonists (Hall, 1993). It remains to be seen if any advantages will be shown.

Timing the hCG trigger injection

Perhaps the main 'art' in assisted reproduction is deciding when to give the hCG trigger injection and upon what criteria to base the decision.

In normal unstimulated cycles, the LH surge occurs around day 12 when fertile mucus can be detected, ultrasound detects a follicle $\geqslant 15$ mm in diameter and he E_2 level is around 1000 pmol/L, usually on day 6 or 7 of the rise from the menstrual baseline (Yovich & Grudzinskas, 1990). In stimulated cycles, cervical mucus may become an unreliable guide as it may be inhibited, e.g. by CC, or enhanced over a prolonged phase, e.g. by hMG so that the chance of pregnancy bears no relationship to cervical mucus score at the time of trigger (Matson & Yovich, 1987). In stimulated cycles clinicians may choose to trigger on the basis of ultrasound findings e.g. leading follicle $\geqslant 18$ mm for IUI or leading follicle $\geqslant 18$ mm and at least 2 other follicles > 14 mm for IVF. They may enhance the decision by E_2 assays, aiming for a ratio of around 1000 pm E_2/L for each preovulatory oocyte. The author's preference is to trigger on day 7 of E_2 rise in GnRH analogue suppressed cycles which is often 2 days later than the aforementioned regimens and which has been shown to lead to a significant improvement in implantation and pregnancy rates (Tan *et al.,* 1992*a,b*). The timing may be modulated further by adjusting the trigger awaiting endometrial thickness measured on ultrasound to be at least 8 mm (Gonen *et al.,* 1989).

Luteal phase support

It would appear that regimens incorporating CC usually have normal luteal phase lengths and sustain a satisfactory output of P_4 and E_2. However, this can be ensured and improved, by giving hCG boost injections (Yovich, 1988) (Fig. 4). Although debate continues concerning the role of luteal support therapy, GIFT patients showed significant benefits from luteal support measured by implantation rate, pregnancy rate and livebirth rate, the latter showing the most marked benefit (Yovich, Edirisinghe & Cummins, 1991). Data modelling techniques implied that luteal support was of most value when the embryo quality factor was poorer. Although the author favours the hCG regimen, it was shown that daily progesterone injections i.m. (Proluton 50 mg; Schering UK) were equally effective. However, it appears that continuation of the Proluton injections is required throughout the first 10 to 12 weeks of the pregnancy as the corpus luteum may become suppressed and fail to respond to hCG secreted from the implanting embryo. The data also showed an apparent further benefit for a combined regimen of hCG and Proluton and early pregnancy support is usually not required. This combined regimen should be considered for cases with repeated failed implantations or poor hormonal profiles. As previously mentioned, cases undergoing hMG stimulation alone including those having either GnRH agonist down regulation or flare methods, have a high rate of luteal phase inadequacy with a very short luteal phase (usually around 9 days) unless luteal support is given. Each of the aforementioned three regimens has been found to be effective.

Hazards of ovarian stimulation

The various drugs used to stimulate folliculogenesis have proven to be relatively free from significant direct side effects, the major problems resulting from the secondary effects of excessive follicle stimulation – namely multiple pregnancies, ectopic and heterotopic pregnancies, OHSS and complications arising in enlarged ovaries.

Indirect hazards

Ovarian hyperstimulation syndrome

OHSS is the main serious and life-threatening complication of ovarian stimulation and is an iatrogenic disorder. A useful classification put forward by the WHO Scientific Group (Lunenfeld, 1976) describes three grades of severity. In its severe form there is massive ovarian enlargement, ascites, pleural effusions, haemoconcentration, oliguria, electrolyte imbalance and hypercoagulability. These changes can potentially lead to severe respiratory embarrassment, renal failure and disseminated intravascular coagulation, all life-threatening conditions. To date, the pathophysiological mechanisms have not been elucidated and studies have concentrated on plasma renin activity, changes in aldosterone and the renin–angiotensin cascade (Golan *et al.,* 1989).

OHSS requiring hospital admission is rare after CC alone but occurs in 1.5%–3% of cycles where HMG is used. Younger women with PCO and highly responsive ovaries are most prone (MacDougall, Tan & Jacobs, 1992). Conversely, those women requiring very high doses of HMG are least prone. Furthermore, the rates may be a little higher in GnRH analogue cycles. Implantation rates and pregnancy rates are significantly higher in cases complicated by OHSS, being around 50% per embryo and >80% per cycle respectively, and the multiple pregnancy rate may also be higher than in comparable stimulation groups. The incidence of OHSS appears to be lower in women undergoing ovarian stimulation for IVF than for GIFT and this may possibly relate to a beneficial effect of follicle aspiration (Draper & Yovich, 1988).

Treatment includes intravenous hydration, management of any electrolyte imbalance, careful attention to fluid balance and paracentesis with continuous drainage of the ascitic fluid. Such patients should not receive hCG injections during the luteal phase but may continue with progesterone support if luteal therapy is favoured. Abdominal drainage is continued over three to five days and 7 to 12 litres of straw coloured fluid may drain which can be proteinaceous towards the end. Intravenous human serum albumin infusions may also be beneficial. If the patient is not pregnant, the condition resolves spontaneously prior to the menstrual period, otherwise it recedes slowly by the eighth week of pregnancy.

A preventative approach to management involves continuation of the GnRH analogue throughout the luteal phase after oocyte recovery in cases suspected to be of high risk. Embryos are cryopreserved and transferred in the subsequent cycle which may be natural or controlled by a hormone replacement schedule similar to that used for ovum donation. The protocol appears to minimize any tendency to OHSS and the need for paracentesis is uncommon.

Multiple pregnancies

Ovarian stimulation increases the chance of pregnancy significantly for each of the assisted reproduction procedures, but the price is a rise in the rate and numeracy of multiple pregnancies. This is shown by data modelling using the binomial expansion in an IVF programme (Fig. 6). If the individual chance of implantation of a transferred oocyte (in GIFT) or embryo (in IVF) is 15% (a common rate among younger patients in efficient clinics), the pregnancy rate rises to 48% when four oocytes or embryos are transferred, but the multiple pregnancy rate will be 22% and include 1 quadruplet every 1000 pregnancies. The pregnancy rate can be further 'improved' to 56% by transferring five embryos but the multiple pregnancy rate will be 28% and include four quadruplets and possibly one quintuplet every 1000 pregnancies! For this reason, both voluntary and legislative controls place a maximum of three oocytes or embryos transferred, reduced to two in younger women with a favourable prognosis.

Subfertile women have a higher risk of preterm delivery even if a singleton pregnancy is achieved (14% as opposed to 7% in the general obstetric community). The rates are markedly increased for twin and triplet pregnancies with a consequential major rise in the risk of perinatal death or cerebral palsy in the survivors being 7-fold for a twin and 45-fold for a triplet infant when compared with background rates of term infants in the general population (Petterson *et*

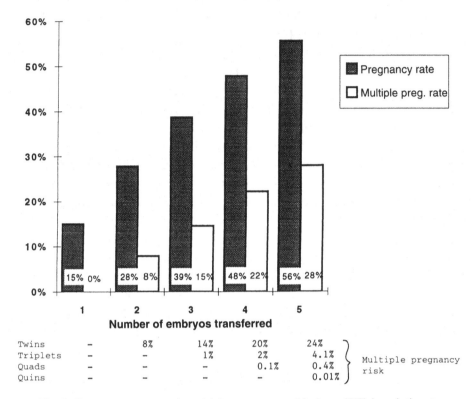

Fig. 6. Pregnancy rates and multiple pregnancy risk from IVF in relation to
number of embryos transferred. Data is modelled from binomial expansion, i.e.
Rate $= U(^n_r)E^r(1-E)^{n-r}$ using embryo implantation factor (E) of 0.15 and assumes
uterine receptivity factor (U) to be 1.0 in conceiving patients.

al., 1993). Again the need for care, control and monitoring of ovarian stimulation
is highlighted.

Ectopic and heterotopic pregnancies

Ectopic pregnancies arise in approximately 5% of women treated by assisted
reproduction (Yovich & Matson, 1988*a*) and the rate is mainly dependent upon
the degree of abnormality of the Fallopian tubes. The rate of ectopic pregnancy
in a fertile population is around 1% and this is the rate found in DI treatments
where the main basis for the infertility is a well-defined male factor. In GIFT
treatments performed in the presence of known tubal disorder, the rate may
approach 20%! (AIHW National Perinatal Statistic Unit, 1992) By confining
all cases with known tubal disorder to IVF-ET, and transferring the embryos
carefully to the mid-uterine cavity in a low fluid volume (Yovich, Turner &

Murphy, 1985), the ectopic rate can be reduced to 2%. However, some cases will still occur for unexplained reasons and occasionally the ectopic will occur in combination with an intra-uterine pregnancy, i.e. heterotopic (Yovich *et al.*, 1984, 1985; Molloy *et al.*, 1990; Svare *et al.*, 1993). The natural incidence of heterotopic pregnancies was calculated as 1 per 30 000 pregnancies but the incidence is now reported as high as 1 per 300 in assisted reproduction.

Complications to enlarged ovaries

These include ovarian torsion, ruptured luteal cysts and pelvic pressure symptoms. Serious sequelae appear to be infrequent.

The question of malignancies

Breast cancer and ovarian cancer have recently been suggested as potential hazards from repetitive ovarian stimulation treatments.

Breast cancer

This is a common malignancy, destined to affect 2% of women by 50 years rising markedly to 10% by 80 years of age. It is therefore inevitable that some women who had ovarian stimulation in the reproductive age will subsequently have breast cancer diagnosed. The risk may actually be higher in subfertile women (Folsom, Sellers & Kaye, 1993) in particular those women with polycystic ovaries who have high unopposed oestrogen levels (Toniolo & Whittemore, 1992), a sizeable group in any infertility clinic, but there appears not to be a direct causal effect from ovarian stimulation therapy. However, long-term prospective matched studies have yet to be reported.

Ovarian cancer

Two separate reports have attracted attention to the possible role of ovarian stimulation drugs – the first detailing epithelial ovarian cancers from an epidemiological study which included women who had a past history of ovarian stimulation (Whittemore, Harris & Itnyre, 1992); the second describing 12 cases of granulosa-cell ovarian cancers in women who had past treatment with CC (Willemsen *et al.*, 1993). However, in both reports the relationship between the treatments and the disease is unclear. Pregnancy and ovulation suppressing contraception both confer a protective effect for ovarian tumours (and also breast and endometrial cancers). Subfertile women may be more prone to ovarian cancer from incessant ovulation, possibly enhanced by repetitive ovarian stimulation, particularly if pregnancy is not achieved. However, the question of a causal relationship between fertility drugs and ovarian cancer can only be answered by appropriately designed prospective studies (Balasch & Barri, 1993).

Creutzfeld–Jacob disease (CJD)

Human pituitary hormones derived directly from human cadavers (usually young, ostensibly healthy, road accident victims at the time of autopsy) provided a major source of growth hormone and gonadotrophins from the mid-1960s to 1985. Worldwide, the programmes ceased when reports from the United States showed a clustering of CJD, a rare and fatal central nervous system disease which normally occurs in the general population at a rate of one case per million. To the end of June 1993, 45 CJD cases have been documented from 30 000 people treated with either human growth hormone (hGH) or hPG. In Australia, 4 women have died from CJD from only around 1500 treated.

The pituitary gland extracts were prepared in a way which precluded the survival of any known infective agent, either bacterial or viral. However, CJD is thought to be transmitted by a prion, an infectious protein particle which can behave like a virus influencing DNA activity within neural cells and inducing cerebral amyloidoses with spongiform encephalopathy (Brown *et al.*, 1993). The incubation period from presumed inoculation to clinical disease has been around 15 years and, as yet, there is no test to detect who is carrying the infection. hPG programmes were ceased in 1985 and recipients of hPG have been asked not to donate tissues or organs although there is no proof that CJD can be transmitted through blood transfusion.

Direct side effects of ovulation drugs

CC side effects are not prominent and are dose related. Vasomotor symptoms such as hot flushes caused by the anti-oestrogen action and visual symptoms described as scintillating scotomata, disappear on cessation of the drug. However, the author is aware of one case with some permanent partial visual loss. Whether this was a direct effect of CC or a secondary effect of raised E_2 is uncertain. Other oral stimulants include cyclofenil and tamoxifen and there may be some differences among them with respect to cervical mucus inhibition and effects on endometrial morphology (Suginami *et al.*, 1993; Asaad *et al.*, 1993; Thompson *et al.*, 1993).

Bromocryptine commonly causes nausea, dizziness and headaches during initiation of therapy and, less frequently, nasal congestion, a sense of fatigue and postural hypotension. These symptoms are usually not severe, and recede if the drug is introduced gradually and tolerance allowed to occur. Occasional serious side effects include seizures and depression.

Menopausal gonadotrophins, hCG and rGH appear to have no significant direct side effects although overdosage of the latter may cause disturbed glucose metabolism and, in long term overdosage, symptoms of acromegaly. GnRH agonists and antagonists also appear to have no significant direct side effects but a range of adverse reactions may arise from their known physiological function e.g. calcium depletion from bones in long-term use associated with prolonged hypo-oestrogenism.

Oocyte recovery techniques

Historically oocyte recovery developed as a laparoscopic procedure but has increasingly become replaced by ultrasound-directed techniques, particularly the trans-vaginal approach. The optimization of oocyte recovery has been shown to depend upon three main aspects (Yovich, Matson & Yovich, 1989):
1. Timing the recovery following LH surge or hCG induction and inducing the surge at the appropriate stage of follicle maturation;
2. The instrumentation and techniques applied for aspiration of the oocytes from follicles;
3. Accessibility of the ovaries for aspiration.

With respect to timing, the LH surge or hCG trigger should occur on day 6 or 7 of CC/HMG cycles and the optimal trigger is day 7 of cycles down-regulated with GnRH analogues (see earlier discussion). Thereafter, follicles are aspirated at 36 ± 2 h after initiation of the LH surge or hCG trigger. Oocytes aspirated earlier than 34 h may benefit by compensatory *in vitro* culture prior to insemination but embryo quality is poor and pregnancy rates are low if oocytes are recovered 4 or more h earlier than optimal. Oocytes collected up to 4 h after the optimal time remain equally suitable but the risk of spontaneous oocyte release increases. However this risk appears to be <10% up to 42 h in GnRH agonist cycles.

The matters of instrumentation and accessibility are considered separately for laparoscopic and ultrasound-directed recoveries.

Laparoscopic recovery

Laparoscopy requires general anaesthesia and endotracheal intubation. Access to follicles may be restricted by pelvic adhesions hence in the past preliminary pelvic adhesiolysis, ventrosuspension and plication of the ovarian ligaments have been recommended. Whilst this has significantly improved laparoscopic access, it may prejudice trans-vaginal access hence is no longer encouraged.

A wide range of single and double lumen needles are in common use but the latter are proving increasingly popular as they enable follicle flushing. Those which enable a fine spray-flush with a continuous flow-through system such as the PIVET-Cook laparoscopic/ultrasound double lumen ovum pickup needle provide optimal oocyte recovery rates, being around 90% of mature follicles. The technique involves needle puncture of the follicle under direct laparoscopic vision and aspiration of the contents into a 16 ml polystyrene test tube. Whilst the contents are being examined under stereomicroscopy by the embryologist in the adjacent IVF laboratory, the follicle is flushed with HEPES-buffered flushing medium (HTFM: human tubal fluid medium) up to 2 occasions (total 10 ml) prior to moving to the next follicle.

The post-operative recovery of women after laparoscopy is sometimes uncomfortable due to the anaesthetic drugs, the laparoscopic wounds and residual abdominal gas. Serious complications among IVF cases including deaths are usually anaesthetic related and occasionally due to the inadvertent puncture of bowel, bladder or vascular structures.

Ultrasound-directed recovery

The first reports using ultrasound guidance for follicle aspirations were reported from Scandinavia (Lenz, Lauritsen & Kjellow, 1981) and described a transcutaneous transvesical method. Subsequently a transurethral method was explored briefly and finally the transvaginal method has found popular acceptance (Wikland *et al.*, 1989). The optimization of transvaginal ultrasound-directed aspiration requires the following (Yovich & Grudzinskas, 1990):

1. Minimal anaesthesia, e.g. i.v. sedation with medazolam and fentanyl; propofol intravenous anaesthetic; or premedication combined with local anaesthesia.
2. Apply pressure band to lower abdomen to stabilize the ovaries and prevent them slipping away during attempts at needle penetration.
3. Use of very sharp, disposable needles with echo-enhanced tips and which enable an efficient follicle flushing technique. The PIVET–Cook needles were designed specifically for the purpose and are ideal.
4. Follicle aspiration and flushing is performed as previously described for laparoscopic access. It is ideal to have the theatre and IVF laboratory combined or adjacent. During follicle flushing, the follicle is only partially refilled so that flush and aspiration procedures proceed simultaneously. This requires a high-pressure fine jet to avoid 'short-circuiting' the follicle and again the PIVET–Cook needles are suitably designed.

5. The control of flow through the aspiration needles is governed by Poiseuille's Law hence aspiration pressures require adjustment depending upon needle length (factor of × 8 e.g. 35 cm 16 FG needle requires 180 mm Hg whilst 25 cm needle requires 100 mm Hg) and needle diameter (inversely related to fourth power of the radius).

6. High resolution ultrasound image required, e.g. General Electric electronic phased array sector scanner with 5.0 MHz vaginal probe and needle guide is widely and effectively used.

7. Ideally the vaginal probe is not covered although a non-toxic condom or clear plastic wrap can be used. The coupling medium is 10 ml culture medium placed in the vagina at the beginning of the procedure after saline washout. Sterilizing fluids are avoided hence it is imperative to exclude the presence of vaginal pathogens just before the treatment cycle. The probe can be sterilized in glutaraldehyde but must be washed thoroughly with sterile water and aired prior to use. Small traces of glutaraldehyde on the probe or within the theatre atmosphere are highly embryotoxic.

Using the above system, the overall oocyte recovery rate is 88% of follicles entered (Hussein, Balen & Tan, 1992). Of interest the vast majority of oocytes were recovered from the follicular aspirate of the first 2–3 ml flush and it was these which were most likely to generate pregnancies.

Outcome of assisted reproduction pregnancies

Early pregnancy wastage after IVF-related treatments appears to be increased above the normal expected rate, but is probably not increased above a matched group of subfertile patients who conceive spontaneously (Yovich & Matson, 1988a). As discussed previously, the ectopic pregnancy rate is high, around 5%, and the rate is influenced by both operator and patient factors. Heterotopic pregnancies are also increased. Blighted ovum pregnancies are more common following AIH and where GIFT has been applied for male-factor cases (Yovich, 1993). Preclinical pregnancies may be diagnosed in up to 10% but this rate may not be higher than found in normally fertile women monitored through the menstrual cycle into pregnancy (Wilcox *et al.*, 1988). Late pregnancy outcomes of IVF-related pregnancies reveal a high morbidity and mortality due to an increased risk of preterm delivery, mostly as a consequence of multiple pregnancies (Lancaster *et al.*, 1985). However, even singletons deliver preterm twice as commonly as women of normal fertility and this finding appears to be similar for subfertile women conceiving without assisted reproduction. The overall rate of major congenital abnormalities (IVF: 2.2%; GIFT: 3.1%) does not appear to be increased and the collaborative Australian and New Zealand data which earlier showed higher than expected observations of infants with spina bifida and transposition of the great arteries following IVF and of infants with major urinary tract malformations following GIFT is no longer sustained (AIHW National Perinatal Statistics Unit, 1992).

Ethical and legal status

IVF and related areas of assisted reproduction have generated unprecedented public interest in a medical area. Certainly, there are broader social, ethical, legal, religious and sometimes political issues which arise apart from the complexity of technical issues (Knoppers & Le Bris, 1993). There are four broad areas of concern:

  (i) standards of laboratory and clinical practice;
  (ii) accountability to the general community;
  (iii) protecting the welfare of children born following assisted reproduction; and
  (iv) ownership of stored gametes and embryos.

Guidelines and regulations should assist to limit the complications (e.g. high-order multiple pregnancies, ovarian hyperstimulation syndrome and anaesthetic mortalities) and ensure clinics are providing the best possible service to infertile couples, within the current limitations of knowledge. In this latter context, the need for continuing research into all aspects, including fundamental physiology as well as clinical applications, must be acknowledged and pursued. Public accountability can be incorporated within a self-regulatory mechanism by ensuring an accurate and current data reporting system which is accessible. The welfare of children, and potential children, means careful control over the disposal of gametes, avoiding mixed embryo transfers which might confuse the genetic identity of children, respecting confidentiality of donors but enabling those children who become aware of a donor background to have access to non-identifying information. Current topical debates concern access to identifying information and the question of respective responsibilities with regard to IVF surrogacy infants. Other concerns relate to ownership of stored embryos in the event of a couple's separation or death and ensuing disputation arising over the use of these embryos. Such matters can only be resolved by specific legislation.

Conclusions

Procedures in assisted reproduction have made a major impact in the area of infertility over the past decade, and have been based upon wide-ranging advances in knowledge concerning reproductive physiology. This has occurred at an appropriate time as the fecundity of many industrialized communities has decreased markedly in recent years. In their turn, the procedures themselves have created the opportunity to consider providing services for the fertile population, e.g. in controlling genetic disease, in gamete and embryo storage for the preservation of fecundity and in new considerations for contraception. The field has excited considerable public interest and has implications for other areas of medicine such as the team approach to the management of individual cases, control by Institutional Ethics Committees and other regulatory bodies, both voluntary and statutory. The main danger is the snowballing effect of a perceived need to introduce legislative controls, particularly in the area of embryo research, which may create an inhibitory or oppressive climate for further research (Braude & Johnson, 1989). Such legislation may effectively seal the current technology in its relatively inefficient state.

References

Adams J, Polson D, Franks S. Prevalence of polycystic ovaries in women with anovulation and idiopathic hirsutism. *Br Med J* 1986; **293**: 355–9.

Asaad M, Abdulla U, Hipkin L, Diver M. The effect of clomiphene citrate treatment on cervical mucus and plasma estradiol and progesterone levels. *Fertil Steril* 1993; **59**: 539–43.

AIHW National Perinatal Statistics Unit. *Assisted Conception Australia and New Zealand 1990.* Sydney: AIHW National Perinatal Statistics Unit and Fertility Society of Australia, 1992. 64.

Bahadori R. Tuberculosis and infertility in Azerbaijan, Iran. In: Ludwig H, Thomsen K, ed. *Gynecology and Obstetrics: Proceedings of the 11th World Congress of Gynecology and Obstetrics. Berlin 1985.* Berlin: Springer-Verlag, 1986: 675–6.

Balasch J, Barri PN. Follicular stimulation and ovarian cancer. *Hum Reprod* 1993; **8**: 990–6.

Braude P, Johnson M. Embryo research: yes or no? *Br Med J* 1989; **299**: 1349–51.

Brown P, Kaur P, Sulima MP, Goldfarb LG, Gibbs CJ, Gajdusek DC. Real and imagined clinicopathological limits of prion dementia. *Lancet* 1993; **341**: 127–9.

Chang MC. Fertilization of rabbit ova *in vitro. Nature London,* 1959; **184**: 466–77.

Cohen J, de Mouzon J, Lancaster P. *VIIIth World Congress on In Vitro Fertilization and Alternate Assisted Reproduction: Kyoto, September 12–15, 1993: World Collaborative Report: 1991.* International Working Group for Registers on Assisted Reproduction, 1993: 38.

Cox LW. Infertility, a comprehensive programme. *Br J Obstet Gynaecol* 1975; **82**: 2–6.

Cummins JM, Yovich JM, Edirisinghe WR, Yovich JL. Pituitary down-regulation using Leuprolide for the intensive ovulation management of poor prognosis patients having IVF-related treatments. *J In Vitro Fert Embryo Transfer* 1990; **6**: 345–52.

Devroey P, Mannaerts B, Smitz J, Bennink HC, van Steirteghem A. First established pregnancy and birth after ovarian stimulation with recombinant human follicle stimulating hormone (ORG-32489) – Case Report. *Hum Reprod* 1993; **8**: 863–5.

Draper RR, Yovich JL. Ovarian hyperstimulation syndrome. In: *Seventh Scientific Meeting of The Fertility Society of Australia.* Newcastle, Australia: Fertility Society of Australia (Inc), 1988: 26.

Edwards RG, Steptoe PC, Purdy JM. Establishing full-term human pregnancies using cleaving embryos grown *in vitro. Br J Obstet Gynaecol* 1980; **87**: 737–56.

Evans IE, Mukherjee AB, Schulman JD. Human *in vitro* fertilization. *Obstet Gynecol Survey* 1980; **35**: 71–81.

Folsom AR, Sellers TA, Kaye SA. Infertility linked to breast cancer. *Br Med J* 1993; **306**: 1065.

Golan A, Ron-El R, Herman A. Soffer Y, Weinraub Z, Caspi E. Ovarian hyperstimulation syndrome: an update review. *Obst Gynecol Survey* 1989; **44**: 430–40.

Gonen Y, Casper R, Jacobson W, Blankier J. Endometrial thickness and growth during ovarian stimulation: a possible predictor of implantation in *in vitro* fertilization. *Fertil Steril* 1989; **52**: 446–50.

Hussein EL, Balen AH, Tan SL. A prospective study comparing outcome of oocytes retrieved in the aspirate with those retrieved in the flush during transvaginal ultrasound directed oocyte recovery for *in vitro* fertilization. *Br J Obstet Gynaecol* 1992; **9958**: 841–4.

Hall JE. Gonadotropin-releasing hormone antagonists – effects on the ovarian follicle and corpus luteum. *Clin Obstet Gynecol* 1993; **36**: 744–52.

Homburg R, West C, Torresani T, Jacobs HS. Cotreatment with human growth hormone and gonadotropins for induction of ovulation: a controlled clinical trial. *Fertil Steril* 1990; **53**: 254–60.

Jeffcoate N. Sterility and subfertility. In: *Principles of Gynaecology*. London: Butterworths, 1975: 583–607.

Jones HW, Jones GS, Andrews MC *et al.* The program for *in vitro* fertillization at Norfolk. *Fertil Steril* 1982; **38**: 14–21.

Knoppers BM, Le Bris S. Ethical and legal concerns; reproductive technologies 1990–1993. *Curr Opin Obstet Gynecol* 1993; **5**: 630–5.

Lancaster PAL, Johnston WIH, Wood C *et al.* High incidence of preterm births and early pregnancy losses after *in-vitro* fertilization. *Br Med J* 1985; **291**: 1160–3.

Lenz S, Lauritsen JG, Kjellow M. Collection of human oocytes for *in vitro* fertilization by ultrasonically guided follicular puncture. *Lancet* 1981; **i**: 1163–4.

Lunenfeld B ed. *WHO Consultation on the Diagnosis and Treatment of Endocrine Forms of Infertility*. Geneva: World Health Organization, 1976.

MacDougall MJ, Tan SL, Jacobs HS. *In-vitro* fertilization and the ovarian hyperstimulation syndrome. *Hum Reprod* 1992; **7**: 597–600.

Macnamee MC, Taylor PJ, Howles CM, Elder KT, Edwards RG. Short-term luteinizing hormone-releasing hormone agonist treatment: prospective trial of a novel ovarian stimulation regimen for *in vitro* fertilization. *Fertil Steril* 1989; **52**: 264–9.

Matson PL, Yovich JL. Changes in cervical mucus following ovarian stimulation for *in vitro* fertilization. *Infertility* 1987; **10**: 267–77.

Molloy D, Deambrosis W, Keeping D, Hynes J, Harrison K, Hennessey J. Multiple-sited (heterotopic) pregnancy after *in vitro* fertilization and gamete intrafallopian transfer. *Fertil Steril* 1990; **53**: 1068–71.

Petterson B, Nelson KB, Watson L, Stanley F. Twins, triplets and cerebral palsy in births in Western Australia in the 1980s. *Br Med J* 1993; (in press).

Stanger JD, Yovich JL. Failure of human oocyte release at ovulation. *Fertil Steril* 1984; **41**: 827–32.

Stanger JD, Yovich JL. Reduced *in-vitro* fertilization of human oocytes from patients with raised basal luteinizing hormone levels during the follicular phase. *Br J Obstet Gynaecol* 1985; **92**: 385–93.

Steptoe PC, Edwards RG. Reimplantation of a human embryos with subsequent tubal pregnancy. *Lancet* 1976; **ii**: 1265.

Steptoe PC, Edwards RG. Birth after the reimplantation of a human embryo. *Lancet* 1978; **ii**: 366.

Steptoe PC, Edwards RG, Purdy JM. Clinical aspects of pregnancies established with cleaving embryos grown *in vitro*. *Br J Obstet Gyn* 1989; **87**: 757–68.

Suginami H, Kitagawa H, Nakahashi N, Yano K, Matsubara K. A clomiphene citrate and tamoxifen citrate combination therapy – a novel therapy for ovulation induction. *Fertil Steril* 1993; **59**: 976–9.

Svare J, Norup P, Thomsen SG *et al.* Heterotopic pregnancies after *in-vitro* fertilization and embryo transfer – a Danish survey. *Hum Reprod* 1993; **8**: 116–18.

Tan SL, Balen A, El Hussein E *et al.* A prospective randomized study of the optimum timing of human chorionic gonadotropin administration after pituitary dessensitization in *in vitro* fertilization. *Fertil Steril* 1992a; **57**: 1259–64.

Tan SL, Kingsland C, Campbell S *et al.* The long protocol of administration of gonadotropin-releasing hormone agonist is superior to the short protocol for ovarian stimulation for *in vitro* fertilization. *Fertil Steril* 1992b; **57**: 810–14.

Thompson LA, Barratt CLR, Thornton SJ, Bolton AE, Cooke ID. The effects of clomiphene citrate and cyclofenil on cervical mucus volume and receptivity over the periovulatory period. *Fertil Steril* 1993; **59**: 125–9.

Toniolo P, Whittemore AS, Polycystic ovaries and the risk of breast cancer. *Am J Epidemiol* 1992; **136**: 372–73.

Trounson AO, Leeton JF, Wood C. Successful human pregnancies by *in vitro* fertilization and embryo transfer in the controlled ovulatory cycle. *Science* 1981; **212**: 681–2.

Whittemore AS, Harris R, Itnyre J. Characteristics relating to ovarian cancer risk – collaborative analysis of 12 United States case-control studies .2. Invasive epithelial ovarian cancers in white women. *Am J Epidemiol* 1992; **136**: 1184–203.

Whittingham DG. Fertilization of mouse eggs *in vitro*. *Nature London,* 1968; **220**: 592–3.

Wikland M, Hamberger L, Enk L, Nilsson L. Technical clinical aspects of ultra-sound guided oocyte recovery. *Hum Reprod* 1989; **4**: 79–82.

Wilcox AJ, Weinberg CR, O'Connor JF *et al.* Incidence of early loss of pregnancy. *N Eng J Medicine* 1988; **319**: 189–94.

Willemsen W, Kruitwagen R, Bastiaans B, Hanselaar T, Rolland R. Ovarian stimulation and granulosa-cell tumour. *Lancet* 1993; **341**: 986–8.

Yovich JL, Stanger JD, Tuvik A, Hahnel R. Combined pregnancies following gonadotrophin therapy. *Am J Obstet Gynecol* 1984; **63**: 855–8.

Yovich JL, McColm SC, Turner SR, Matson PL. Heterotopic pregnancy from *in vitro* fertilization. *J In Vitro Fert Embryo Transf* 1985; **2**: 146–50.

Yovich JL, Turner SR, Murphy AJ. Embryo transfer technique as a cause of ectopic pregnancies in *in vitro* fertilization. *Fertil Steril* 1985; **44**: 318–21.

Yovich JL, Tuvik AI, Matson PL, Willcox DL. Ovarian stimulation for disordered ovulatory cycles. *Asia-Oceania J Obstet Gynaecol* 1987; **13**: 457–63.

Yovich JL. Treatments to enhance implantation. In: Chapman M, Grudzinskas G, Chard T, ed. *Implantation: Biological and Clinical Aspects.* London: Springer-Verlag, 1988. 237–54.

Yovich JL, Matson PL. Early pregnancy wastage after gamete manipulation. *Br J Obstet Gyn* 1988a; **95**: 1120–7.

Yovich JL, Matson PL. The treatment of infertility by the high intrauterine insemination of husband's washed spermatozoa. *Hum Reprod* 1988b; **3**: 939–43.

Yovich JL, Matson PL, Yovich JM. The optimization of laparoscopic oocyte recovery. *Int J Fertil* 1989; **34**: 390–400.

Yovich JL, Turner S, Yovich JM *et al. In Vitro* Fertilization today. *Lancet* 1989; **ii**: 688–9.

Yovich JL, Grudzinskas G. *The Management of Infertility: A Manual of Gamete Handling Procedures.* Oxford: Heinemann Medical, 1990: 276 p.

Yovich JL. Pentoxifylline: actions and applications in assisted reproduction. *Hum Reprod* 1993; **8**: 1786–91.

Yovich JL, Edirisinghe WR, Cummins JM. Evaluation of luteal support therapy in a randomized controlled study within a GIFT program. *Fertil Steril* 1991; **55**: 131–9.

Yovich JL. Transabdominal GIFT. In: Chapman M, Grudzinskas JG, Chard T, Djahanbakhch O eds. *The Fallopian Tube: Biological and Clinical Aspects.* London: Springer-Verlag, 1994: 213-27.

14

The zona pellucida

M. PATERSON AND R. J. AITKEN

Introduction

The zona pellucida is a translucent, extracellular, glycoprotein matrix that surrounds the oocytes of all Eutherian mammals (see Fig.1). This oocyte-specific structure is secreted during folliculogenesis and persists throughout the pre-implantation stage of pregnancy. Within its relatively short life span the zona pellucida plays key roles in ensuring that both fertilization of the oocyte and implantation of the resulting embryo are successfully accomplished. During fertilization the zona pellucida is the site at which sperm–egg recognition occurs and where the spermatozoa become activated, undergoing the acrosome reaction and generating a plasma membrane domain that is capable of recognizing and fusing with the vitelline membrane of the oocyte. Following sperm–oocyte fusion, the zona pellucida plays a major role in the prevention of polyspermy and the physical protection of developing embryo during its passage to the uterine cavity.

An understanding of the biochemical composition of the zona pellucida and the molecular mechanisms by which it fulfils its biological functions is of clinical importance in the context of both infertility and the development of new approaches to contraception. In terms of infertility, bioassays of sperm–zona interaction suggest that a significant proportion of such patients exhibit a pathology associated with a failure to bind to, or penetrate, the zona pellucida (Oehninger, 1992). In the field of contraception, advances in our knowledge of zona biochemistry are facilitating the development of contraceptive vaccines that target the fertilization process (Aitken, Paterson & Koothan, 1993).

Sperm–zona interaction

Before spermatozoa can physically penetrate the zona pellucida they must first be able to recognize and bind this structure. The act of sperm–zona recognition

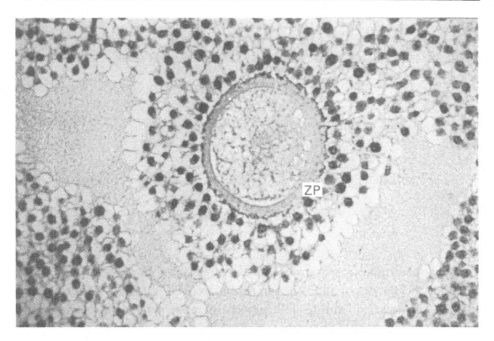

Fig. 1. Section through a marmoset ovary illustrating the structure of the zona pellucida (ZP). Antibodies raised against the zona pellucida, inhibit sperm–zona interaction by masking the binding sites for spermatozoa.

is a key event that sets in motion a cascade of events which ultimately results in fertilization. The specificity of this interaction is due to receptors on the surface of spermatozoa which recognize one of the major glycoprotein components of the zona pellucida, namely ZP3. This glycoprotein is highly conserved in evolutionary terms exhibiting a homology of around 60% between amino acid sequences of species as diverse as the mouse and human. In spite of this homology, the process of sperm–egg recognition mediated by ZP3 possesses great species specificity which is thought to depend on the carbohydrate side chains of this glycoprotein, and in particular, a class of O-linked oligosaccharides (Florman & Wassarman, 1985).

ZP3 also plays a secondary role in activating the spermatozoa. In the mouse, an interaction between the sperm plasma membrane and the O-linked oligosaccharides of ZP3 initiates, via a cross-linking mechanism that requires the presence of the polypeptide backbone, a secretory event known as the acrosome reaction (Wassarman, 1991). During this exocytotic event, the sperm plasma membrane fuses with the outer acrosomal membrane resulting in the activation and release of proteolytic enzymes and exposure of the inner acrosomal membrane.

These acrosome-reacted spermatozoa remain tightly bound to the zona pellucida via secondary sperm receptors located in another zona glycoprotein, ZP2 (Bleil, Greve & Wassarman, 1988a). Aided by acrosomal enzymes such as acrosin, the fertilizing spermatozoon then penetrates through the zona matrix in a narrowly defined path and ultimately engages the vitelline membrane of the oocyte.

Once the spermatozoon has fused with the vitelline membrane, the zona pellucida plays a key role in the mechanisms by which the oocyte prevents polyspermic fertilization. The block to polyspermy proceeds in two stages: to begin with the spermatozoa in the perivitelline space are prevented from fusing with the oolemma by a rapid depolarization of this membrane (Sato, 1979). Subsequently cortical granules containing proteases and glycosidases fuse with the plasma membrane of the fertilized egg and release their contents into the perivitelline space. Interaction between the constituents of the cortical granules and the zona pellucida, effects a secondary phase in the block to polyspermy known as the zona reaction. This event is characterized by a hardening of the zona pellucida and a loss of sperm receptor activity as a consequence of which this structure can no longer bind, or be pentrated by, spermatozoa. It is proteolytic cleavage of ZP2 which is though to account for the hardening of the zona pellucida (Moller & Wassarman, 1989), while modification of the oligosaccharide side chains of ZP3 by glycosidases in the cortical granules, results in a loss of both sperm receptor activity and the ability of ZP3 to induce the acrosome reaction (Wassarman, 1991).

Biochemistry of the zona pellucida

The mammalian zona pellucida comprises three or four major glycoprotein species (ZP 1–4) named in order of decreasing molecular weight. In the mouse, the zona is composed of interconnecting filaments of heterodimers of ZP2 ($Mr = 120\,000$) and ZP3 ($Mr = 83\,000$) which are held together by dimers of ZP1 ($Mr = 200\,000$) to give an open, porous, matrix (Greve & Wassarman, 1985; Wassarman, 1988). These proteins are heavily glycosylated and possess both N-linked and O-linked oligosaccharide side chains which are linked to the polypeptide backbone by asparagine and serine/threonine residues respectively.

ZP3, which contains the sperm receptor, has been extensively studied and shows considerably homology between species. In general, this protein is approximately 424 amino acids long and is particularly rich in serine and threonine residues, the potential sites of O-linked glycosylation. There is also a proline rich region in the centre of ZP3 which may explain why the molecule possesses very few α-helices. An additional conserved feature is the number and location of cysteine residues; the human, marmoset, mouse and hamster ZP3 sequences all possessing 15 cysteine residues at identical sites (Koothan, van Duin & Aitken, 1993). This would suggest that intra-molecular disulphide bonds place important architectural constraints on the molecule, which may be essential to its biological activities. Despite the similarity in the amino acid sequences, there are considerable differences in relative molecular mass within this family of ZP3 glycoproteins (human ZP3 $Mr = 57$–$73\,000$, mouse $Mr = 83\,000$, hamster $Mr = 56\,000$) presumably due to differences in glycosylation. Recent evidence, based on immunological and molecular cloning techniques, have suggested that there may be two isoforms of human ZP3 (van Duin *et al.*, 1992; Shabanowitz, 1990).

In the murine system, species specificity is determined by a specific class of O-linked oligosaccharides linked to ZP3 via serine and threonine residues (Florman & Wassarman, 1985). If these active structures are removed and purified they retain the properties of a sperm receptor and, at nanomolar concentration, are able to block sperm-zona interaction in competition assays (Wassarman, 1990). However, the purified oligosaccharides lose their ability to induce the acrosome reaction, emphasizing the importance of the polypeptide backbone in mediating this effect through the cross-linking of zona binding sites on the sperm surface (Leyton & Saling, 1989*b*; Wassarman, 1991). The composition and structural configuration of these carbohydrate side-chains have yet to be elucidated; however, the significance of certain sugar residues has been determined. In particular, a galactose residue, located at the non-reducing terminus has been shown to be essential for sperm binding (Bleil & Wassarman, 1988*b*). Removal of the galactose by digestion with α-galactosidase or oxidation of its C-6 hydroxyl to an aldehyde group can lead to a complete loss of sperm receptor activity. An alternative model involving a sperm surface β-1,4-galactosyl transferase, that behaves like a lectin by binding to a specific glycoside substrate of ZP3, has also been reported (Miller, Macek & Shur, 1992).

Zona adhesion proteins

Our understanding of the nature of the complementary receptor on sperm plasma membrane that binds to ZP3 is not so well advanced, although several candidate antigens have been proposed. Bleil & Wassarman (1990) have identified a $Mr = 56\,000$ protein, SP-56, on the surface of mouse spermatozoa that recognizes and binds to ZP3. Using purified, ZP3, that had been modified by covalently attaching to it a hetero-bifunctional cross-linking reagent, they were able to isolate the complementary sperm protein which binds to ZP3. SP-56 is also capable of binding to galactose affinity columns in keeping with the data suggesting that a galactose residue at the terminus of the carbohydrate side chains of ZP3 is essential for sperm binding (Bleil & Wassarman, 1988*b*). This protein is located on the sperm head of acrosome intact spermatozoa only and is not present on acrosome-reacted spermatozoa, a feature consistent with a zona adhesion protein.

Recently it has been suggested that the enzyme β-1,4-galactosyltransferase (gal-transferase), present on the sperm surface and the oligosaccharides of ZP3 are complementary adhesion proteins that mediate sperm–zona interaction in the mouse (Miller *et al.,* 1992). This interaction is specific for ZP3 as gal-transferase shows no affinity for other glycoproteins. If the gal-transferase binding sites on purified ZP3 are either blocked or removed, its ability to inhibit sperm-zona interaction in a competition assay is reduced. It has been suggested that sperm gal-transferase binds to terminal N-acetylglucosamine residues of ZP3 oligo-saccharides. Since each oligosaccharide side chain is able to bind 2-3 gal-transferase molecules, it is possible to visualize how the latter become aggregated by ZP3, inducing a state of receptor oligomerization that results in the activation of the spermatozoa and the induction of the acrosome reaction. Following the acrosome reaction, gal-transferase is thought to relocate to a new membrane domain where it is no longer able to bind to ZP3.

Another pathway by which sperm–zona interaction may result in the activation of spermatozoa is through the stimulation of tyrosine kinase activity. In 1989, Leyton & Saling (1989*a,b*) postulated that acrosomal exocytosis could be triggered by receptor aggregation, an activation mechanism which is a characteristic feature of the tyrosine kinase class of receptor. They identified a $Mr = 95\,000$ protein in the plasma membrane of mouse spermatozoa overlying the acrosomal region that could be aggregated by ZP3. The aggregation of these receptors is then thought to result in the stimulation of tyrosine kinase activity that leads, in turn, to acrosomal exocytosis (Leyton & Saling, 1989*b*; Leyton *et al.,* 1992). Intriguingly, a similar $Mr = 95\,000$ phosphotyrosine protein has also been identified in the plasma membrane of human spermatozoa (Naz, Ahmad & Humar, 1991).

Binding of guinea pig spermatozoa to the zona pellucida is thought to be mediated by receptors on the inner acrosomal membrane. This recognition event can be blocked by using fucoidan, a fucose-rich, sulphated polysaccharide (Huang &Yanagimachi, 1984). Using radiolabelled [125]-I fucoidan as a probe, Jones & Williams (1990) demonstrated that several guinea-pig sperm proteins could be recognized on SDS–PAGE. Several of the bands observed with $Mr = 48\,000$, $34\,000$ and $30\,000$ could also be identified by [125-I]zona glycoproteins and are thought to represent proacrosin and acrosin(s), respectively. These proteins are located within the acrosomal vesicle and there is evidence to suggest that acrosome-reacted spermatozoa retain some proacrosin/acrosin bound to the inner acrosomal membrane. This supports the hypothesis that secondary tight binding of acrosome-reacted spermatozoa to ZP2 may be mediated by a carbohydrate binding domain located at the N-terminus of acrosin (Töpfer-Peterson & Henschen, 1987; Mortillo & Wassarman, 1991; Jones & Williams, 1990; Calvete, Sanz & Töpfer-Peterson, 1992) except that in the guinea pig, this mechanism has assumed importance as the primary mechanism by which sperm–zona interaction is achieved.

From this brief view of the molecules thought to be involved in the mediation of sperm-zona interaction, it is clear that no single dominant entity is involved. Instead, a number of ZP binding proteins have been identified in spermatozoa the precise function of which may depend on the species under consideration and the stage of sperm–egg interaction being examined. In common with other cell recognition events, it is likely that gamete interaction during fertilization involves multiple components many of which may be acting in parallel.

Development of the zona pellucida

During oogenesis, when zona pellucida formation occurs, levels of ZP3 mRNA increase from undetectable levels in non-growing mouse oocytes to maximum levels in growing oocytes in concert with the increase in cell size (Roller *et al.*, 1989; Kinloch & Wassarman, 1989). A steady state level of ZP3 mRNA is then maintained until ovulation, when levels of ZP3 mRNA rapidly decline and become virtually undetectable in fertilized eggs (Roller *et al.*, 1989).

The site of synthesis of the components of the zona pellucida has been a controversial issue over many years. Numerous morphological, immunohisto-chemical and biochemical studies have debated over whether the site of zona glycoprotein synthesis is the oocyte (Guraya, 1974), the follicle cells that surround the growing oocyte (Greve *et al.*, 1982), or both (Wolgermuth *et al.*, 1984; Dunbar, Maresh & Washenisk, 1989*a*). There is now a considerable body of evidence in the literature to suggest that in the mouse, at least, oocytes and not follicular cells synthesize and secrete the glycoproteins of the zona pellucida (Haddad & Nagai, 1977; Shimizu, Tsuji & Dean, 1983; Ringuette *et al.*, 1986; Philpott, Ringuette & Dean, 1987). Using probes for ZP3 mRNA, *in situ* and gel hybridization studies have suggested that ZP3 is expressed exclusively in growing oocytes during oogenesis in both the mouse (Philpott *et al.*, 1987; Roller *et al.*, 1989) and marmoset (Koothan *et al.*, 1993). However, these results are in contrast to a recent study by Lee & Dunbar (1993), who have demonstrated in rabbit ovaries that both the oocyte and granulosa cells express zona glycoproteins. Expression of the $Mr = 55\,000$ glycoprotein predominantly occurred in the early stages of follicular development after the granulosa cells had differentiated from squamous to cuboidal cells (Lee & Dunbar, 1993). Whether these variations in the synthesis of zona glycoproteins may reflect a difference in the source and formation of the zona pellucida between species, has still to be resolved.

Clinical aspects

The current high incidence of male factor infertility ($\sim 30\%$ of infertile couples) has led to the development of a variety of *in vitro* diagnostic tests to evaluate the fertilizing potential of human spermatozoa. Successful fertilization is the culmination of a cascade of interactions initiated by the act of sperm–zona recognition. Key steps in this sequence of events constitute the basis of bioassays that aim to provide information on the functional competence of human spermatozoa for diagnostic purposes. There are three categories of *in vitro* diagnostic tests which investigate the early events in fertilization including: 1) sperm–zona recognition and binding, 2) sperm–zona penetration, 3) sperm–oolema fusion.

Sperm–zona recognition assays

The act of sperm–zona recognition is of crucial importance because a spermatozoon may make contact with hundreds, or even thousands, of other cells on its journey through the female reproductive tract and yet must instantly recognize when it has located the surface of the ovum. This initial recognition event is mediated via receptors on the sperm plasma membrane for the zona glycoprotein, ZP3. The spermatozoon is then induced to undergo the acrosome reaction and bind tenaciously to the zona glycoprotein ZP2, possibly through a fucose binding domain contained within the acrosin molecule (Töpfer-Peterson & Henschen, 1987; Calvete *et al.*, 1992). These crucial steps of recognition and tight binding of the spermatozoa to the zona pellucida can be clinically evaluated through the use of salt-stored human zonae pelludicae (Kruger *et al.*, 1991) in *in vitro* bioassays employing the whole zona pellucida or part of this structure, as in the case of the hemi-zona assay (HZA; Franken *et al.*, 1989, 1993).

The first *in vitro* assay to investigate sperm–zona interaction was performed by Overstreet and Hembree (1976) using oocytes from human ovaries recovered from cadavers. Although initially developed as a sperm penetration assay, it has evolved into a method to evaluate the tight binding of spermatozoa to the zona. In the HZA oocytes are bisected into two equal halves by a micromanipulator. These matching hemi-zona surfaces provide an internal control with which to compare the zona binding capacity of spermatozoa from an infertile patient and a fertile donor. Each hemi-zona is introduced into a 100 μl droplet of spermatozoa (at 500 000 ml), under oil and after 4 h co-incubation the hemi-zona are washed free of loosely adherent spermatozoa and the remaining tightly bound spermatozoa are counted. The hemi-zona index (HZI) can then be calculated as follows:

$$\frac{\text{number of spermatozoa from the infertile patient bound to the zona}}{\text{number of spermatozoa from the fertile donor bound to the zona}} \times 100$$

The value of the HZI is held to be predictive of the fertilizing capacity of the spermatozoa *in vitro*. Thus, initial experiments by Oehninger *et al.* (1989) showed that semen samples which had given poor results in IVF by failing to fertilize, or had a poor fertilization rate ($<65\%$), had a significantly lower HZI value than normal semen samples. They also found that tight binding correlated significantly with sperm motility, morphology, and concentration. Menkveld *et al.* (1991) have suggested that the human zona pellucida is capable of positively selecting for morphologically normal spermatozoa under HZA conditions. Whether morphologically abnormal spermatozoa are unable to bind to the zona pellucida, or whether the lack of binding is a secondary phenomenon reflecting a primary loss of motility, is still unknown (Morales *et al.*, 1988). In contrast to many animal species, human spermatozoa exhibit extreme heterogeneity in their morphology. Although this pleomorphism is found in both fertile and infertile men, infertility is frequently associated with an abnormally high incidence of morphologically abnormal spermatozoa (Kruger *et al.*, 1986; Aitken *et al.*, 1982). The inherent inability of morphologically abnormal spermatozoa to bind to the human zona pellucida may be of particular significance in the context of predicting the suitability of male patients for *in vitro* fertilization therapy. On the basis of correlative studies, a HZI of 36 was found to represent a threshold value below which a high risk of failure in IVF could be predicted (Oehninger *et al.*, 1989).

The oocytes used in such bioassays can come from several sources. Oocytes may be recovered from post-mortem ovarian tissue, from surgically removed ovaries, or from IVF programmes where they have failed to fertilize. Franken *et al.* (1989, 1991*a*) have shown that no significant differences in sperm binding curves were obtained whether fresh, DMSO-frozen or salt-stored (1.5 M $MgCl_2$ supplemented with 0.1% dextran buffered with HEPES at 4°C) ova were used. Irrespective of the method of storage, inter-oocyte variability does occur and has been estimated to be $\sim 10\%$ for eggs at the same stage of maturation. This is taken into account in the HZA as each hemi-zona is of the same quality. However, to account for the poor quality of some zonae a lower cut off value of 20 (Franken *et al.*, 1991*b*) spermatozoa bound per hemi-zona using normal donor sperm has been suggested.

An alternative protocol for accounting for the differences between zonae in their capacity to bind spermatozoa, involves using fluorescent probes to differentially label the patient's and donor's sperm populations. The zona binding capacity of the patient's spermatozoa can then be compared with the fertile donor by using different fluorescence filters to determine the relative numbers of spermatozoa bound to each zona pellucida (Lui *et al.*, 1988, 1989).

Sperm–zona penetration tests

In order to penetrate the zona pellucida the spermatozoon must have first completed its acrosome reaction. Hyperactive motility and sperm enzymes such as acrosin assist the spermatozoon entering and penetrating the zona along a sharply defined path. The precise mechanism by which zona penetration occurs is not clearly understood; it may rely purely on the propulsive force of the penetrating spermatozoon or involve a bind-and-cut mechanism due to the capacity of acrosin to act as both a proteolytic enzyme and as a binding site for the zona glycoprotein, ZP2 (O'Rand, Welch & Fisher, 1986). The capacity of spermatozoa to penetrate the human zona pellucida was first evaluated in non-living oocytes from post-mortem tissue (Overstreet & Hembree, 1976). In this study, spermatozoa from 11 out of 16 infertile patients were able to penetrate the zona pellucida although the penetration rate was lower than that obtained with fertile donors (12.9% and 46.6%, respectively). When these oocytes were incubated with a mixed population containing equal numbers of patient and donor spermatozoa, identified by a fluorescent label, again a significant difference in penetration rate was observed (12.9% and 50%, respectively). However, no correlation could be found between the number of motile sperm with which the oocytes were incubated and the penetration rate. A positive result in this assay, where spermatozoa are observed to penetrate through to the perivitelline space, may be used to assist in the process of selecting patients for IVF treatment. However, whether such information significantly enhances the diagnostic information generated by the binding assay has not been systematically investigated.

Sperm–oocyte fusion test

The hamster oocyte, once denuded of its zona pellucida, is capable of fusing with all species of mammalian spermatozoa tested to date. The ability of the hamster oolemma to fuse with human spermatozoa is the basis of a prognostic test to assess male infertility *in vitro* (Yanagimachi, Yanagimachi & Rogers 1976; Aitken, 1986). This heterologous bioassay measures the ability of human spermatozoa to undergo a series of biological changes including capacitation, the acrosome reaction, fusion with the oolemma and nuclear decondensation in the ooplasm. Modifications of the initial assay have been introduced to improve its predictive value in IVF treatments (Aitken *et al.*, 1983). In particular, induction of the acrosome reaction with a calcium ionophore has been found to increase the sensitivity and specificity of the assay (Aitken, Irvine & Wu, 1991; WHO, 1987).

A homologous system for assessing the competence of human spermatozoa to fuse with the oocyte has also been developed using zona-free human eggs prepared from oocytes that failed to fertilize during *in vitro* fertilization therapy (Tesarik, 1989). Despite previous *in vitro* ageing, most of these human oocytes are still capable of being penetrated by multiple spermatozoa if re-inseminated and can go on to develop pronuclei. Although such a homologous system may generate useful information on the competence of both the male and female gametes to participate in sperm–oocyte fusion, there may be ethical restraints on its widespead use.

These bioassays of sperm–zona interaction and sperm–oocyte fusion constitute valuable tools in the assessment of sperm–egg interaction and elucidation of the possible causes of infertility in some couples. If these tests are used in concert it may be possible to develop a diagnostic scheme that will help direct the therapeutic management of any given couple in which male factor infertility is suspected. If a specific problem in sperm–zona interaction can be identified while the capacity for sperm–oocyte fusion is normal, micromanipulation techniques such as partial zona dissection (PZD) or sub-zonal insemination (SUZI) might be used to assist fertilization. If both sperm–zona interaction and sperm–oocyte interaction are defective, the only logical course of action would be to inject a spermatozoon directly into the cytoplasm of the oocyte (ICSI), a technique which is now being used to great effect in certain centres (Palermo *et al.*, 1993).

Contraceptive vaccines

The general concept of a contraceptive vaccine which would provide a safe and reliable means of regulating fertility, is an attractive one, given the inexorable upward trend in the rate of world population growth. The notion of an immunological approach to contraception involving the disruption of sperm-zona recognition, stems from experimental work dating back nearly two decades (Shivers *et al.*, 1972; Sacco & Shivers, 1973; Jivek & Pavlok, 1975; Aitken & Richardson, 1980). These early studies showed that an antiserum raised against an aqueous extract of hamster ovarian tissue could block fertilization of hamster ova *in vitro*. It was rapidly established that the antibodies responsible for this effect were directed against antigens on the zona pellucida. Since then our understanding of sperm–egg recognition at biochemical and molecular levels has increased enormously and the components on the surface of the zona pellucida responsible for this contraceptive effect have been identified and characterized.

The two most extensively studied systems are those of the mouse and pig. Porcine zona antigens, in particular, have received a great deal of attention because of their cross-reactivity with the human zona pellucida and the ability of anti-porcine zona antibodies to block human sperm–egg interaction *in vitro* (Paterson *et al.*, 1992). Anti-zona antibodies are thought to exert their contraceptive effect *in vitro* in one of two ways, either by direct interaction with the sperm receptor, or by binding to epitopes in close proximity to the receptors, and cross-linking to form an immunoprecipitate which masks the receptor by steric hindrance. In the heterologous system, where antibodies against the zona pellucida antigens expressed by one species are used to block sperm–zona interaction in another, the latter mechanism is though to predominate as it has been demonstrated that univalent antibodies (Fab), which cannot cross-link antigens, have no contraceptive effect (Aitken *et al.*, 1982).

Several active immunization programmes have been undertaken to investigate the contraceptive potential of anti-zona antibodies *in vivo*. These studies have demonstrated that in a variety of species, including dog (Mahi-Brown *et al.*, 1985), rabbit (Skinner *et al.*, 1984), primates (Sacco *et al.*, 1987; Gulyas, Gwatkin & Yvan, 1983; Paterson *et al.*, 1992) and horse (Kirkpatrick *et al.*, 1992), immunization with heterologous zona antigens will result in an antibody-mediated loss of fertility. Although these studies have been encouraging, with several authors reporting a long term reversible loss of fertility, there has been an increasing accumulation of data suggesting that anti-zona antibodies may also act at the level of the ovary by inducing an ovarian pathology. This pathology is characterized by a loss of secondary and tertiary follicles and a depletion of the primordial follicle pool resulting in a cessation of folliculogenesis. In addition, the appearance of follicular clusters containing actively growing granulosa cells but no oocytes are often observed (see Fig. 2).

Numerous research groups have tried to investigate the cause of this pathology however the results of these active immunization experiments with zona antigens have been conflicting. It was thought that the observed pathology may be attributed to the relatively impure antigen or mixture of zona antigens used in early studies (Skinner *et al.*, 1984; Mahi-Brown *et al.*, 1988; Gulyas *et al.*, 1983). However, studies using purified ZP3 as an immunogen have also found that the infertility observed may be due, in part, to a disruptive effect by anti-ZP3 antibodies on folliculogenesis as well as sperm–egg interaction (Paterson *et al.*, 1992). Studies by Sacco *et al.* (1987, 1991) have suggested that these disturbances in ovarian functions are reversible in primates and that the ovaries of immunized

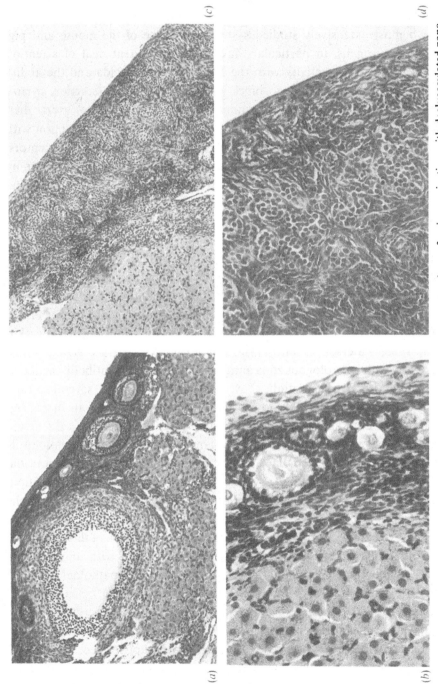

Fig. 2. Photomicrographs of sections through the ovary of marmoset monkeys after immunization with deglycosylated zona antigens or control immunization with adjuvant alone. (a) × 450 and (b) × 750, ovarian sections from control marmosets immunized with adjuvant alone, (c) × 450 and (d) × 750 ovarian sections from marmosets immunized with deglycosylated zona antigens. In those animals immunized with zona antigens, large numbers of follicular clusters and a complete absence of any primordial or developing follicles are observed in contrast to the control group where active folliculogenesis is ongoing.

animals show signs of recovery a year or more post-immunization. In contrast, Paterson *et al.* (1992) have shown that the induction of high titre antibodies against ZP3 resulted in a permanent depletion of the primordial follicle pool, from which fertility cannot be recovered. This side effect could not be alleviated by the use of deglycosylated zona antigens (Dunbar, Powell & Stevens, 1989*b*; Paterson *et al.*, 1992) despite the importance of the oligosaccharide side chains in enhancing the immunogenicity of ZP3 (Sacco, Yurewicz & Subramanian, 1986). These results are in contrast to Keenan *et al.* (1991) who suggested that active immunization of rabbits resulted in ovarian pathogenesis only when glycosylated antigens were used and that normal ovarian function was maintained when deglycosylated or partially glycosylated ZP3 antigens were used as immunogens. This discrepancy may reflect genuine differences between species in the mechanism responsible for the ovarian dysfunction. Alternatively, the presence of carbohydrate greatly enhances the immunogenicity of the zona polypeptides (Paterson & Aitken, 1990; Paterson *et al.*, 1992) and the resulting high tires obtained after immunization with glycosylated antigens may influence the onset of this pathology. The choice of adjuvant may also affect the outcome of these active immunization programmes but again the data in this area is not consistent (Upadhyay *et al.*, 1989; Sacco *et al.*, 1991; Paterson *et al.*, 1992).

The mechanism responsible for this loss of primordial follicles is currently under intense investigation and represents a key issue in the viability of a contraceptive vaccine based on antigens of the zona pellucida. It has recently been suggested that the cause of this ovarian dysfunction may be attributed to a cell-mediated immune response resulting from cytotoxic T-cell epitopes residing within the ZP3 sequence. Using monoclonal antibodies raised against mouse ZP3 Miller *et al.* (1989) were able to identify a seven amino acid peptide representing amino acid residues 336–342 with the potential to impair fertility without inducing the oophoritis responsible for the unacceptable depletion of the primordial follicle pool. Female Swiss mice were immunized with this peptide (coupled to a carrier protein) and produced anti-peptide antibodies which resulted in a long-lasting contraceptive effect and an absence of any ovarian pathology. Miller *et al.* (1989) have suggested that this may be due to the absence of a T-cell epitope within this sequence. Further studies by Rhim *et al.* (1992) have shown that it is possible to induce oophoritis in $B6AF_1$ mice by adoptive transfer by $CD4^+$ T-cells derived from affected animals, without any antibodies to ZP3 being detected in the recipients. If this is the case in primates, the future of a contraceptive vaccine clearly depends on the successful identification and segregation of epitopes responsible for the contraceptive and pathological effects.

Conclusions

The zona pellucida plays a central role in the sequence of events that leads to the fertilization of an ovum by a single spermatozoon. Over the past decade considerable advances have been made in our understanding of sperm–zona interaction and we are now beginning to identify the molecular mechanisms by which the zona pellucida fulfils its biological functions. Complementary adhesion proteins on the surface of the spermatozoon and ovum that may be involved in the early recognition steps, have recently been identified and characterized. In particular, the glycoprotein ZP3 is thought to play a dual role in both the mediation of this initial recognition step and the induction of the acrosome reaction. Once the acrosome has reacted, the spermatozoa remain tightly bound to the zona pellucida through secondary binding sites on ZP2 which appear to interact with sperm-bound acrosin in a bind-and-cut mechanism in order to achieve penetration of the zona matrix and thereby gain access to the perivitelline space. Following sperm–oocyte fusion, the zona pellucida is again involved in mediating the secondary block to polyspermy as well as the protection the pre-implantation embryo.

An understanding of the biological function of the zona pellucida has been of clinical importance in the context of infertility, through the development of bioassays in which the ability of spermatozoa to bind to or penetrate the zona pellucida can be evaluated. The zona antigens are also clinically important in the development of new contraceptives. The biochemical composition of the major glycoprotein ZP3, has been fully characterized and the epitopes with contraceptive potential mapped and identified. One major problem with this approach has been the observed loss of primordial follicles following active immunization. However, recent studies have suggested that it may be possible to identify contraceptive epitopes which avoid the T-cell responses thought to be responsible for the appearance of this ovarian pathology. If this is so, it will lead the way to developing contraceptive vaccines which provide a safe and effective means of controlling fertility.

References

Aitken RJ. The zona-free hamster oocyte penetration test and the diagnosis of male fertility. World Health Organisation Symposium. *Int J Androl* 1986; supplement 6.

Aitken RJ, Richardson DW. Immunisation against zona pellucida antigens. In: Hearn J, ed. *Immunological Aspects of Reproduction and Fertility Control.* Lancaster: MTP Press, 1980: 173–201.

Aitken RJ, Best FSM, Richardson DW, Djahanbakhch O, Mortimer D, Templeton AA, Lees MM. An analysis of sperm function in cases of unexplained infertility:

conventional criteria, movement characteristics and fertilising capacity. *Fertil Steril* 1982; **38**: 212–21.

Aitken RJ, Irvine DS, Wu FC. Prospective analysis of sperm–oocyte fusion and reactive oxygen species generation as criteria for the diagnosis of infertility. *Am J Obst Gyn* 1991; **164**: 542–51.

Aitken RJ, Wang YF, Lui J, Best F, Richardson DW. The influence of medium composition, osmolarity and albumin content on the acrosome reaction and fertilising capacity of human spermatoza: development of an improved zona-free hamster egg penetration test. *Int J Androl* 1983; **6**: 180–3.

Aitken RJ, Holmes E, Richardson DW, Hulme MJ. Properties of intact and univalent (Fab) antibodies raised against isolated solubilized mouse zonae. *J Reprod Fertil* 1982; **66**: 327–34.

Aitken RJ, Paterson M, Thillai Koothan P. Contraceptive vaccines. *Br Med Bull* 1993; **49**: 88–99.

Bleil JD, Greve JM, Wassarman PM. Identification of a secondary sperm receptor in the mouse egg zona pellucida: role in maintenance and binding of acrosome reacted sperm. *Devel Biol* 1988*a*; **128**: 376–85.

Bleil JD, Wassarman PM. Galactose at the non-reducing terminus of O-linked oligosaccharides of mouse egg zona pellucida glycoprotein ZP3 is essential for the glycoprotein's receptor activity. *Pro Nat Acad* 1988*b*; **85**: 6778–82.

Bleil JD, Wassarman PM. Identification of a ZP3-binding protein on acrosome intact mouse sperm by photoaffinity cross-linking. *Proc Nat Acad Sci* 1990; **87**: 5563–7.

Calvete JJ, Sanz L, Töpfer-Peterson E. Carbohydrate-binding domains involved in gamete interaction in the pig. In: Nieschlag E, Habenicht UF, ed. *Spermatogenesis–Fertilisation–Conception*. Berlin: Springer-Verlag, 1992: 395–418.

Dunbar BS, Maresh GA, Washenick K. Ovarian development and the formation of the mammalian zona pellucida. In: Dietl J, ed. *The Mammalian Egg Coat. Structure and Function*. Berlin: Springer-Verlag, 1989*a*: 38–48.

Dunbar BS, Lo C, Powell J, Stevens VC. Use of a synthetic peptide adjuvant for the immunization of baboons with denatured and deglycosylated pig zona pellucida. *Fertil Steril* 1989*b*; **52**: 311–18.

Florman HM, Wassarman PM. O-linked oligosaccharides of mouse egg ZP3 account for its sperm receptor activity. *Cell* 1985; **41**: 313–24.

Franken DR, Burkman LJ, Oehninger SC, Veeck LL, Kruger TF, Coddington CC, Hodgen GD. Hemi-zona assay using salt stored-human oocytes: evaluation of zona pellucida capacity for binding human spermatoza. *Gamete Res* 1989; **22**: 15–26.

Franken DR, Coddington CC, Burkman LJ, Oosthuizen WT, Oehninger S, Kruger TF, Hodgen GD. Defining the valid hemizona assay: accounting for binding variability within zonae pellucidae and within semen samples from fertile males. *Fertil Steril* 1991*a*; **56**: 1156–61.

Franken RD, Oosthuizen T, Coope S, Kruger TF, Burkman LJ, Coddington CC, Hodgen GD. Electron microscope evidence on the acrosomal status of bound sperm and their penetration into human hemi zonae pellucidae after storage in a buffered salt solution. *Andrologia* 1991*b*; **23**: 205–8.

Franken DR, Acosta AA, Kruger TF, Lombard CJ, Oehninger S, Hodgen GD. The hemi-zona assay: its role in identifying male factor infertility in assisted reproduction. *Fertil Steril* 1993; **59**: 1075–80.

Greve JM, Salzmann GS, Roller RJ, Wassarman PM. Biosynthesis of the major zona pellucida glycoprotein secreted by oocytes during mammalian oogenesis. *Cell* 1982; **31**: 749–59.

Greve JM, Wassarman PM. Mouse egg extracellular coat is a matrix of interconnected filaments possessing a structural repeat. *J of Mol Bio* 1985; **181**: 253–64.

Gulyas BJ, Gwatkin RBL, Yvan LC. Active immunization of Cynomolgus Monkeys (*Macaca fascicularis*) with porcine zonae pellucidae. *Gamete Res* 1983; **4**: 299–307.

Guraya SS. Morphology, histochemistry and biochemistry of human oogenesis and ovulation. *Int Rev Cyto* 1974; **37**: 121–52.

Haddad A, Nagain MET. Radio autographic study of glycoprotein biosynthesis and renewal in the ovarian follicles of mice and the origin of the zona pellucida. *Cell Tiss Res* 1977; **177**: 347–69.

Henderson CJ, Braude P, Aitken RJ. Polyclonal antibodies to a 32 kDa deglycosylated polypeptide from porcine zonae pellucidae will prevent human gamete interactions *in vitro*. *Gamete Res* 1987; **18**: 251–65.

Huang TTF Jr., Yanagimachi R. Fucoidan inhibits attachments of guinea pig spermatozoa to the zona pellucida through binding to the inner acrosomal membrane and equatorial domains. *Exp Cell Res* 1984; **153**: 363–73.

Jivek F. Pavlok A. Antibodies against mouse ovaries and their effect on fertilization *in vitro* and *in vivo* in the mouse. *J Reprod Fertil* 1975; **42**: 377–80.

Jones R, Williams RM. Identification of a zona- and fucoidin-binding protein in guinea pig spermatozoa and mechanism of recognition. *Development* 1990; **109**: 41–50.

Keenan JA, Sacco AG, Subramanian MG, Kruger M, Yurewicz EC, Moghissi KS. Endocrine response in rabbits immunized with native verses deglycosylated porcine zona pellucida antigens. *Biol Reprod* 1991; **44**: 150–6.

Kinloch RA, Wassarman PM. Profile of a mammalian sperm receptor gene. *New Biol* 1989; **1**: 232–8.

Kirkpatrick JF, Lui IMK, Turner JW Jr., Naugle R, Keiper R. Long-term effects of porcine zonae pellucidae immunocontraception on ovarian function in feral horses (*Equus caballus*). *Fertil Steril* 1992; **94**: 437–44.

Koothan TP, van Duin M, Aitken RJ. Cloning, sequencing and oocyte-specific expression of the marmoset sperm receptor protein, ZP3. *Zygote* 1993; **1**: 93–101.

Kruger TF, Menkveld R, Stander FSH, Lombard LT, Van der Merive JP, van Zyl JA, Smith K. Sperm morphologic features are a prognostic factor in *in vitro* fertilization. *Fertil Steril* 1986; **46**: 1118–23.

Kruger TF, Oehninger S, Franken DA, Hodgen CD. Hemi-zona assay: use of fresh versus salt-stored human oocytes to evaluate sperm binding potential to the zona pellucida. *In Vitro Fertilization Embryo Transfer* 1991; **8**: 154–6.

Lee VH, Dunbar BS. Developmental expression of the rabbit 55-kDa zona pellucida protein and messenger RNA in ovarian follicles. *Dev Bio* 1993; **155**: 371–82.

Leyton L, Saling PM. Evidence that aggregation of mouse sperm receptors by ZP3 triggers the acrosome reaction. *Cell Biol* 1989a; **108**: 2163–8.

Leyton L, Saling PM. 95kD sperm proteins bind ZP3 and serve as tyrosine kinase substrates in response to zona binding. *Cell* 1989b; **57**: 1123–30.

Leyton L, LeGuen P, Bunch D, Saling PM. Regulation of mouse gamete interaction by a sperm tyrosine kinase. *Proc Nat Acad Sci* 1992; **89**: 11692–5.

Lui DY, Clarke GN, Lopata A, Johnston WIH, Baker GHW. A sperm–zona pellucida binding test and *in vitro* fertilization, *Fertil Steril* 1989; **52**: 281–7.

Lui DY, Lopata A, Leung A, Johnston WIH, Baker GHW. A human zona pellucida binding test using oocytes that failed to fertilise *in vitro. Fertil Steril* 1988; **50**: 782–8.

Mahi- Brown CA, Yanagimachi R, Hoffman JD, Huang TTF. Fertility control in the bitch by active immunication with porcine zonae pellucidae: use of difference adjuvants and patterns of estradiol and progesterone levels in oestrus cycles. *Biol Reprod* 1985; **32**: 761–72.

Mahi-Brown CA, Yanagimachi R, Nelson ML, Yanagimachi H, Palumbo N. Ovarian histopathology of bitches immunized with porcine zonae pellucidae. *Am J Reprod Immunol* 1988; **18**: 94–103.

Menkveld R, Franken DR, Kruger TF, Oehinger S, Hodgen GD. Sperm selection capacity of the human zona pellucida. *Mol Reprod Dev* 1991; **30**: 346–352.

Miller DJ, Macek MB, Shur BD. Complementarity between sperm surface β-1,4-galactosyl-transferase and egg-coat ZP3 mediates sperm binding. *Nature* 1992; **357**: 589–93.

Miller SE, Chamow SM, Baur AW, Oliver C, Robey F, Dean J. Vaccination with a synthetic zona pellucida peptide produces long term contraception in female mice. *Science* 1989; **246**: 935–8.

Moller CC, Wassarman PM. Characterization of a proteinase that cleaves zona pellucida glycoprotein ZP2 following activation of mouse eggs. *Dev Biol* 1989; **132**: 103–12.

Morales P, Katz DF, Overstreet W, Samules SJ, Chang RD. The relationship between the motility and morphology of spermatozoa in human semen. *J Androl* 1988; **9**: 241–7.

Mortillo S, Wassarman PM. Differential binding of gold-labelled zona pellucida glycoprotein in mZP2 and mZP3 to mouse sperm membrane compartments. *Development* 1991; **112**: 141–9.

Naz RK, Ahhad K, Kumar R. Role of membrane phosphotyrosine proteins in human spermatozoal function. *J Cell Sci* 1991; **99**: 157–65.

Oehninger S. Diagnostic significance of sperm-zona pellucida interaction. *Reprod Med Rev* 1992; **1**: 57–81.

Oehninger S, Coddington CC, Scott, R, Franken DR, Burkman LJ, Acosta AA, Hodgen GD. The hemi-zona assay: assessment of sperm dysfunction and prediction of IVF outcome. *Fertil Steril* 1989; **51**: 665–70.

Overstreet JW, Hembree WC. Penetration of zona pellucida from non-living human oocytes by human sperm *in vitro. Fertil Steril* 1976; **27**: 815–31.

Palermo G, Joris H, Derde M-P, Camus M, Deurosy P, van Steirteghem A. Sperm characteristics and outcome of human assisted fertilization by sub-zonal insemination and intracytoplasmic sperm injection. *Fertil Steril* 1993; **59**: 826–35.

Paterson M, Atiken RJ. Development of contraceptive vaccines targeting the zona pellucida. *Cur Opin Immunol* 1990; **2**: 743–7.

Paterson M, Thillai Koothan P, Morris KD, O'Byrne KT, Braude P, William A, Aitken RJ. Analysis of the contraceptive potential of antibodies against native and deglycosylated porcine ZP3 *in vivo* and *in vitro. Biol Reprod* 1992; **46**: 523–34.

Philpott CC, Ringuette MJ, Dean J. Oocyte-specific expression and developmental regulation of ZP3, the sperm receptor of the mouse zona pellucida. *Dev Biol* 1987; **121**: 568–75.

O'Rand MG, Welch JE, Fisher SJ. Sperm membrane and zona pellucida interactions during fertilization. In Dhinsay DS., Bahl OP, ed *Molecular and Cellular Aspects of Reproduction.* New York: Plenum Press, 1986: 131–44.

Rhim SH, Millar SE, Robey F, Luo AM, Lou YH, Yule T, Allen P, Dean J, Tung KSK.

Autoimmune disease of the ovary induced by a ZP3 peptide from the mouse zona pellucida. *Clin Inves* 1992; **89**: 28–35.

Ringuette MJ, Sobieski DA, Chamow SM, Dean J. Oocyte-specific gene expression: molecular characterization of a cDNA coding region for ZP3, the sperm receptor of the mouse zona pellucida. *Proc Nat Acad Sci* 1986; **83**: 4341–4.

Roller RJ, Kinloch RA, Hiraoka BY, Li SS-L, Wassarman PM. Gene expression during mammalian oogenesis and ealy embryogenesis: quantification of three messenger RNAs abundant in fully grown mouse oocytes. *Development* 1989; **106**: 251–61.

Sacco AG, Shivers CA. Localisation of tissue-specific antigens in the rabbit oviduct and uterus by the fluorescent antibody technique. *J Reprod Fertil* 1973; **32**: 415–20.

Sacco AG. Antigenic cross-reactivity between human and pig zona pellucida. *Biol Reprod* 1977; **16**: 164–73.

Sacco AG, Yurewicz EC, Subramanian MG. Carbohydrate influences the immunogenic and antigenic characteristics of the ZP3 macromolecule ($Mr = 55\,000$) of the pig zona pellucida. *J Reprod Fertil* 1986; **76**: 575–86.

Sacco AG, Pierce DL, Subramanian MG, Yurewicz EC, Dukelow WR. Ovaries remain functional in Squirrel Monkeys (*Saimiri sciureus*) *Biol Reprod* 1987; **36**: 481–90.

Sacco AG, Yurewicz EC, Subramanian MG, Lian YE, Dukelow WR. Immunological response and ovarian histology of squirrel monkeys (*Saimiri sciureus*) immunized with porcine zona pellucida ZP3 ($Mr = 55\,000$) macromolecule. *Am J Primatol* 1991; **24**: 15–28.

Sato K. Polyspermy-preventing mechanisms in mouse eggs fertilized *in vitro*. *J Exp Zool* 1979; **210**: 353–9.

Shabanowitz RB. Mouse antibodies to human zona pellucida: evidence that human ZP3 is strongly immunogenic and contains two distinct isomer chains. *Biol Reprod* 1990; **43**: 260–70.

Shimizu S, Tsuji M, Dean J. *In vitro* biosynthesis of three sulphated glycoproteins of murine zonae pellucidae by oocytes grown in culture. *J Biol Chem* 1983; **258**: 5858–63.

Shivers CA, Dudkiewicz AB, Franklin LE, Fussel EN, Inhibition of sperm–egg interaction by specific antibody. *Science* 1972; **178**: 1211–13.

Skinner SM, Mills T, Kirchick HJ, Dunbar BS. Immunization with zona pellucida proteins results in abnormal ovarian follicular differentiation and inhibition of gonadotrophin induced steroid secretion. *Endocrinology* 1984; **115**: 2418–32.

Tesarik J. The potential use of human zona-free eggs prepared from oocytes that failed to fertilise *in vitro*. *Fertil Steril* 1989; **52**: 821–4.

Töpfer-Peterson E, Henschen A. Acrosin shows zona and fucose binding, novel properties for a swine proteinase. *Fed Eur Biochem Soc Lett* 1987; **226**: 38–42.

Tsunoda Y, Change MC. Effect of antisera against eggs and zonae pellucidae on fertilization and development of mouse eggs *in vivo* and in culture. *J Reprod Fertil* 1978; **54**: 233–7.

Upadhyay SN, Thillaikoothan P, Bamezai A, Jayaraman S, Talwar GP. Role of adjuvants in inhibitory influence of immunization with porcine zona pellucida antigen (ZP3) on ovarian folliculogenesis in bonnet monkeys: a morphological study. *Biol Reprod* 1989; **41**: 665–73.

van Duin M, Polman J, Verkoelen C, Bunschoten H, Heyerink J, Olijvie W, Aitken RJ. Cloning and characterisation of the human sperm receptor ligan ZP3: evidence for a second polymorphic allele with a different frequency in the Caucasian and Japanese population. *Genomics* 1992; **14**: 1064–70.

Wassarman PM. Zona pellucida glycoprotein. *Ann Rev Biochem* 1988; **57**: 415–22.

Wassarman PM. Role of carbohydrate in receptor-mediated fertilization in mammals. In: Bock G., Harnett S, ed. *Carbohydrate Recognition in Cellular Function*. London: Ciba Foundation Symposium, vol. 145, 1989: 135–55.

Wassarman PM. Profile of a mammalian sperm receptor. *Development* 1990; **108**: 1–17.

Wassarman PM. Cellular and molecular elements of mammalian fertilization. In: Dale B, ed. *Mechanisms of Fertilization*. Berlin: Springer-Verlag, 1991: 305–14.

Wolgemuth DJ, Celenza J, Bundam DS, Dunbar BS. Formation of the rabbit zona pellucida and its relationship to ovarian follicular development. *Dev Biol* 1984; **106**: 1–14.

World Health Organisation. *WHO Laboratory Manual for the Examination of Human Semen and Semen–Cervical Mucus Penetration*. 2nd ed. Cambridge: The Press Syndicate of the University of Cambridge, 1987: 55–58.

Yanagimachi R, Yanagimachi H, Rogers BJ. The use of zona-free animal ova as a test system for the assessment of the fertilizing capacity of human spermatozoa. *Biol Reprod* 1976; **15**: 471–6.

15

Oocyte storage

S. AL-HASANI AND K. DIEDRICH

Introduction

After the birth of Louise Brown 1978, *in vitro* fertilization (IVF) heralded a new era in the understanding and management of human infertility. It brought a major breakthrough into the field of human reproduction and provided hope for infertile couples. IVF is now an integral and important part of gynaecology and is widely practised in industrialized countries. Since transfer of more than one embryo increases the likelihood of achieving pregnancy, it is necessary to obtain a large number of oocytes to generate embryos for replacement. Unfortunately, such procedures lead to the problem of excess oocytes and consequently a high number of embryos which, if all replaced, would increase the risk of high order multiple pregnancy. To minimize this risk, most centres have adopted the approach of replacing three or fewer embryos. In Germany as in other countries the law requires that not more than three fertilized oocytes or embryos are transferred. Such a policy obviously creates the issue of excess oocytes and embryos. The surplus embryos thus created raise complex ethical, social, legal, moral and religious issues concerning their future use or disposal. A practical solution for this dilemma is to consider cryopreservation of the embryos. Unfortunately this may serve only to postpone confrontation of these problems. Many religious groups are opposed to embryo cryopreservation because of their belief that the embryo is the beginning of human life. An alternative approach to the problem of spare or excess embryos is to inseminate only the required number of oocytes and to store the surplus oocytes by cryopreservation for later use. With the current controversy surrounding embryo cryopreservation, there is clearly a need to investigate the possibility of freezing human oocytes as an alternative. Of equal importance is the need for research into cryopreservation of the human oocyte. Little is known about the effects of deep freezing on the oocyte, its survival after thawing and its subsequent performance and development following exposure to sperm in the *in vitro* system. The potential significance and practical application of this research is clearly far-reaching.

History of oocyte cryopreservation

Attempts have been made in the past to preserve mammalian oocytes at very low temperatures. Early work in the 1950s provides evidence of this research although with little success. Sherman and Lin (1958 a,b, 1959) using unfertilized ovulated mouse oocytes and glycerol as cryoprotectant, obtained survival among oocytes when cooled to -10 °C. None of them, however survived at temperatures below -20 °C. The most significant demonstration in the 1950s on the survival of oocytes after freezing and thawing was provided by Parkes (1958) in experiments where slices of rat ovaries were tested for viability by subcutaneous grafting after freezing-thawing procedure. Although all the oocytes within Graafian follicles appeared to be degenerating, numerous primordial follicles survived freezing.

A temporary lull ensued until the 1970s when interest was revived. Leibo (1977), in a study of mouse ova and embryos, obtained a higher proportion of ova surviving after deep freezing to -196 °C. Survival was found to bear an inverse relationship to cooling rates and the formation of intracellular ice. These observations were fundamental to an understanding of cryobiological processes involving cells held at very low temperatures. In another important study, Whittingham (1977), using dimethyl sulphoxide (DMSO) as cryoprotectant, succeeded not only in cooling unfertilized ovulated mouse oocytes to a temperature of -196 °C, permitting storage from between 24 hours to 3 months, but also in obtaining 70% survival among those oocytes, thus clearly demonstrating the feasibility of oocyte cryopreservation. Fertilization *in vitro* of the frozen–thawed oocytes was significantly lower than those of freshly collected control oocytes. However, living, healthy, normal fetuses were obtained after transfer of the oocytes into the oviducts of recipient females when mated with fertile males. Successful oocyte cryopreservation was achieved by Kasai, Iritani & Chang (1979) in the rat. The oocytes were frozen at -196 °C using DMSO, with 60% surviving after thawing and 47% showing fertilization *in vitro*.

Parkening and Chang (1977) stored hamster oocytes at -75 °C, whilst Quinn, Barros & Whittingham (1982) obtained an 80% survival rate of these oocytes after slow cooling to -80 °C prior to storage at -196 °C. In rabbit, most of the cryopreservation experiments were done either with fertilized or cleaved oocytes. The first of these experiments was done by Smith (1952). She used fertilized rabbit ova and glycerol as a cryoprotectant. One year later, (1953) Chang observed that fertilized rabbit oocytes are easier to cryopreserve than the unfertilized ones. Until 1977 there was no interest in regarding cryopreservation of rabbit oocytes.

In this year Ogawa and Tomada claimed to be able to fertilize successfully rabbit oocytes after freezing them, but their method could not be reproduced. The first report of successful cryopreservation of rabbit oocytes leading to the production of living, healthy, normal offspring was published by our group (Al-Hasani *et al.*, 1989).

In a recent study by De Mayo *et al.* (1985), an attempt was made to freeze monkey oocytes as a forerunner to similar procedures to that of human oocytes. The monkey oocytes were collected by laparoscopy after appropriate ovarian hyperstimulation, and then frozen in DMSO before storage at −196 °C. Ova were stored for 1 to 12 weeks in liquid nitrogen. The stored ova were thawed either slowly or rapidly and then subjected to xenogenous fertilization in the rabbit oviduct. Survival after freezing–thawing procedure varied between 20% and 40%, with xenogenous fertilization rates of about 30%. Whilst animal studies clearly showed that the mammalian oocyte could be frozen and stored successfully, there was little evidence to indicate that this was possible in humans. Indeed, some IVF researchers thought cryopreservation of human oocytes to be extremely difficult or even technically impossible because of the potential instability of the oocyte chromosome spindle when subjected to freezing and thawing. In one study, however, ten human ova were exposed to 35% glycerol and then frozen in liquid nitrogen (Burks *et al.*, 1965). Nine retained their morphological integrity after thawing. In another study, Trounson (1984) obtained more than 80 oocytes from ovarian wedge samples and cultured them for 48 hours *in vitro* prior to freezing. Only four oocytes survived both freezing and subsequent thawing. In a preliminary experiment done in our centre (Tolksdorf *et al.*, 1985), five human oocytes were cryopreserved to −196 °C and DMSO was used as cryoprotectant, two oocytes did survive after thawing. After *in vitro* fertilization, one of those two oocytes showed two visible pronuclei 24 hours after insemination. In the same year, Bernard *et al.* (1985), using glycerol as cryoprotectant, found that none of their oocytes were fertilizable after cryopreservation–thawing procedure. In this study they also used 1,2 propanediol instead of glycerol and both fertilization and cleavage to the eight-cell stage occurred in one ova before termination of the experiment. Later more publications appeared concerning the cryopreservation of human oocytes with successful results.

Advantages of cryopreservation of human oocytes and the practical application

In case of serious risk of developing hyperstimulation syndrome by women undergoing IVF it is advantageous to freeze the supernumerary oocytes to attempt conception at a later date. This has also the advantages of reducing the risk of multiple pregnancies as well as the number of operative interventions. It also offers a greater chance of success from embryo transfer in a natural ovulatory cycle and a significant reduction in costs to the patient.

Oocyte cryopreservation is also expected to increase the results of IVF by increasing the number of pregnancies from several eggs obtained in a single IVF treatment cycle. It may provide an alternative to embryo freezing especially in countries in which freezing of embryos is not acceptable due to ethical, moral and legal reasons. It also creates possibilities for patients with cancer to become pregnant after chemo- and radiotherapy which has rendered them sterile. Another possibility is the establishment of oocyte banking. Thus patients who suffer from diseases that endanger the function of the ovaries (such as cancer, endometriosis, recurrent cysts and infections) may wish to store oocytes for future use. Should their ovaries require removal to cure their disease, they could still become pregnant through IVF, using their stored oocytes.

Oocyte cryopreservation may provide a means for family planning. Thus women who defer child bearing because of the pursuit of a career, the unavailability of a marriage partner or illness may at a young age opt to have their oocytes stored for later use. The storage of the oocytes at the time of sterilization may also be of importance for those women who later regret the operation and desire a family, especially if a reversal operation is not possible. Stored oocytes may find their use in oocyte donation programmes to provide embryos for women with congenital or surgical absence of the ovaries, the presence of hypoplastic ovaries, the failure to produce ovulation from stimulation regiments, premature menopause, genetic diseases and ovaries which are inaccessible to both laparoscopic and ultrasonic collection of oocytes.

Consideration should also be given to disadvantages that can arise through oocyte cryopreservation. These include technical problems of prolonged storage of the oocytes, as well as patient related matters such as difficulties with fees for the storage, or failing marital partnerships.

The human oocyte

Oocyte maturation and its meiosis

During the embryological development, oocytes enter the prophase of the first meiotic division and then become arrested in the dictyate stage. This stage extends through infancy until just prior to the onset of puberty and ends with the menopause (Chandly, 1971; Baker, 1976; Ohno, Klinger & Atkin, 1962; Zamboni, 1970). With the onset of reproductive life, the meiotic process is resumed and the first meiotic division is then completed. The second meiotic division occurs and the oocyte is ovulated at the metaphase II stage, with the first polar body extruded and the chromosomes arranged on spindle at the second meiotic metaphase. Meiotic division then arrests again at the second phase. During this stage the oocyte may be regarded as relatively unstable. It is characteristic of ovulated oocytes that if fertilization does not occur, the spindle subsequently breaks down, the chromosomes forming micronuclei. It is the view of cryobiologists that the oocyte should best be cryopreserved at the ovulated phase (Polge, 1977; Al-Hasani *et al.*, 1986*b*). Following fertilization, resumption of meiotic maturation occurs and the second polar body is extruded, and shortly after that the third polar body appears for a short while.

Feature of the human oocyte

According to the cryobiologists, the most important feature of mammalian egg for cryopreservation is its size. The oocyte at the time of ovulation is generally the largest cell found in most mammals, being a sphere varying in diameter from about 70–80 μm in the mouse, rat and hamster to about 130 μm in the rabbit bovine and human. The oocyte is surrounded by a transparent non-cellular membrane, the zona pellucida, and a layer of follicular cells, the corona radiata and cumulus cells. The ovum is therefore just visible to the naked eye as a tiny white speck. In freezing most investigators tried to reduce the size of oocyte–cumulus complex by removing the cumulus complex either mechanically or chemically to increase the success of survival after freezing and thawing. Polge (1977) found that the size can adversely affect the survival rate after freezing. In mouse the size of the oocyte is about half of the size of human egg, therefore the success is twice as high as in human and rabbit (Whittingham 1977; Al-Hasani 1986*a*, 1988). The time exposure of the oocyte to the cryoprotectant can also affect the survival and the further development as it was observed in mouse (Damien *et al.*, 1990). The larger the size of the oocyte the longer the exposure to cryoprotectants is necessary. Therefore the solute exchange has to be quicker to reduce the time of exposure and in case of oocyte, another phenomenon which affects the survival rate after freezing is that the solute exchange of unfertilized oocytes takes a longer time than that of the fertilized ones.

Cryobiology of oocyte freezing

Action of cryoprotectants

Before starting any work on oocyte and embryo cryopreservation, a general understanding of cryobiological concepts in cell freezing is essential. Successful cryopreservation is due to the application of theoretical considerations and empirical observations derived from studies in different species and cellular system. There are two factors of utmost important in cryopreservation work: the presence of molar concentration of a protective solute or cryoprotectant and appropriate rates of cooling and thawing. Cryoprotective agents which are of low molecular weight are thought to prevent the potentially deleterious exposure of cells to elevated concentrations of electrolytes by their colligative action in reducing the quantity of ice formed intracellularly at any sub-zero temperature. Also precise control of the cooling and warming rate determines the ultimate fate of water that is present intracellularly during the cryopreservation process. If the cooling rate during freezing is sufficiently slow, cytoplasmic water will flow out of the cell and will freeze extracellularly, resulting in a gradual dehydration of the cell. However, damage to the cell at slow rates of cooling may be caused by solution effects which again can be reduced by the use of cryoprotectant media. On the other hand, if cooling is too rapid, the cytoplasm will not have sufficient time for dehydration so it will supercool and freeze eventually. The formation of intracellular ice is a lethal factor and leads to cell-damage and death. Generally for different cells there is an optimal cooling rate that varies accordingly to the cell-size and type (Chen, 1990).

Cellular events during cryopreservation

If a cell suspended in physiological medium-like saline solution is cooled progressively to temperatures slightly below 0 °C, ice forms first in the extracellular solution. Consequently, the dissolved solutes become more concentrated as water is removed in the form of ice. As the temperature of the cell suspension is lowered further, more ice forms, resulting progressively in a more concentrated extracellular solution. The higher the concentration, the lower the chemical potential of water. The cell responds osmotically to equalize the chemical potentials of water across its membranes hence, during freezing, it loses water extracellularly. If the cell is cooled sufficiently slowly, it will progressively lose more water as the temperature is lowered so as to maintain an osmotic equilibrium and as the temperature falls the cell content will become increasingly supercooled, until suddenly the cell water freezes within the cell itself, resulting in cell death. Seeding or the induction of ice formation in the medium overcomes this problem of supercooling and the deleterious effect of thermal changes following the release of the latent heat fusion.

As cooling proceeds further and the temperature reaches −40 °C, 74% of the solution becomes crystallized and the solute concentration in the remaining liquid increases to 47% weight (Rall, Reid & Polge, 1984). Many small ice crystals form and surround the cell, thereby obscuring it from view on cryomicroscopy.

The next phase is a critical one when cell death can happen. As the temperature falls further, the intracellular contents freeze and the cell suddenly reappears. This is cause by the diffraction of the light by the ice crystals formed intracellularly – a phenomenon termed 'blackening out' or 'flashing'. If the cell is now cooled rapidly by plunging it into liquid nitrogen at −196 °C, there is no additional crystallization, that is, a 'glass' forms and the residual liquid 'vitrifies'. Cooling to −196 °C results in an arrest biological time for the cell that can then be stored virtually indefinitely. During thawing the physical events depend on whether warming is slow or rapid. Slow warming is accompanied by a complex series of changes: a 'flashing' of the cytoplasm at −90 °C 'first flash', the gradual growth of a dark crystalline material extracellularly between −90 °C and −70 °C, gradual disappearance of the dark material between −70 °C and −42 °C, and 'second flash' at −55 °C. With rapid warming, that is rates in excess of 100 °C/minute, the extracellular ice merely melts when the temperature increases above −40 °C. There is insufficient time for the formation of ice nuclei or 'detrification' and the glassy solid therefore 'liquefies'. The final step is a critical one of diluting out the cryoprotectant and a return to physiological conditions. The most cryodamage occurs to the biological material at this final step.

These cryobiological concepts described are clearly of great importance. The role of the cryoprotectant is protection of the cell during freezing; in addition the avoidance of supercooling by seeding, careful control of the cooling-rate, the prevention of significant intracellular ice formation, the establishment of osmotic and thermal equilibrium during freezing and the control of warming-rates are of importance. Both the understanding of these concepts and meticulous attention and control of these factors during freezing and thawing are influential in a successful outcome of the cryopreservation process (Chen, 1990).

Factors influencing successful cryopreservation

Various factors are thought to affect the successful outcome of rabbit and human oocytes freezing and thawing. They include oocyte selection, its size, time exposure to cryoprotectant, seeding and assessment of survival.

Oocyte selection

We faced a problem in selecting mature oocytes for cryopreservation in our IVF centre because most of the oocytes of good quality were taken for the conventional *in vitro* fertilization procedure, while the surplus oocytes were either of intermediate or immature quality. To compensate for this problem the oocytes were first cultured for about 24 hours and then cryopreserved. A very small number of mature oocytes could be obtained for freezing. It is important to mention that only oocytes that appeared morphologically normal under the dissecting microscope were considered to be suitable for cryopreservation.

Size

The oocyte volume in the freezing process plays an important role. The larger the size of the oocyte, the lower is the survival rate after freezing and thawing. According to Polge (1977) the cell size could adversely affect freezing because the time of equilibration is longer than in the case of a small sized cell. A good example of this is the freezing of semen. The survival rate in this case is much higher than oocyte freezing, presumably because the size of sperm is about 1/180 of the size of the oocyte in both the human and rabbit. Another example for the importance of size is in the case of mouse oocyte that is half as large as the human and rabbit oocyte, mouse oocytes having a better survival rate than the other two species (Whittingham 1977; Al-Hasani 1987, 1986*b*; Al-Hasani *et al.,* 1989). Fuller and Bernard (1984) used the microscope to observe the time required by mouse eggs to reach their appropriate volume after the addition of glycerol. They concluded that the unfertilized mouse oocytes would need at least one hour to allow sufficient glycerol to permeate the cells.

Time exposure to cryoprotectant

The duration of exposure to cryoprotectant is again of importance and the shorter the time of exposure to the cryoprotectant the better is the survival rate after freezing and thawing. If the time of exposure is too long it can alter the intracellular pH as well as the developmental potential as seen in mouse zygotes by Damien *et al.* (1990). Recently Pickering, Braude & Johnson (1991) found that inappropriate exposure of human oocytes to DMSO reduces the fertilization rate. In our freezing procedure the time of exposure to propanediol was 20 min which may be long for human oocytes. We believe that shortening this time to half might improve the survival rate.

Seeding

Controlling the seeding process by naked eye is an important procedure especially in the case of automatic seeding because in such cases some of the materials will not be seeded and super cooling may occur in these straws, a lethal process for the oocytes. Seeding can be induced at $-7\,°C$. A period of 15 min for equilibration till the crystals form in the whole straw is seen to be a favourable interval before starting with further cooling.

Assessment of survival

Survival assessment after cryopreservation is also of importance, the oocytes being observed immediately after dilution of the cryoprotectant and again shortly before the insemination *in vitro*. In case of cryopreservation of rabbit oocytes five assays are used to identify the surviving oocytes after thawing (see above) whereas with human oocytes only one assessment is undertaken namely the morphological examination under the dissecting microscope. This examination is found to be enough for assessing the surviving from the non-surviving oocytes. The intact oocyte appears shiny without discolouration of the ooplasm, cell disruption or pyknosis. The cytoplasm adheres to the zona pellucida without any zona fracture whereas the damaged oocyte has a dark ooplasm and the cytoplasm is contracted and pyknotic. Sometimes the zona is fractured also. The best test of survival in cryopreservation is the subsequent performance of the intact oocyte namely fertilization and cleavage of the embryo.

Possible cryodamage

The spindle apparatus

The mature oocyte shortly before, and at, ovulation is in the metaphase II of the second meiotic division. At this stage the chromosomes are arranged on a spindle which is an unstable phase. The microtubuli of this stage can be affected by changing the temperature (Sathanathan, Trounson & Freeman, 1987). This change in temperature or the addition of cryoprotectant will cause the chromosomes not to arrange themselves and they will be scattered in the cytoplasm. Scattering of chromosomes leads to their dislocation and aberration. Therefore the rate of abnormality or malformation will be higher after oocyte cryopreservation.

Magistrini & Szellosi (1980), Pickering & Johnson (1987) observed that the depolymerization of the microtubuli of mouse eggs was reversible. Vincent *et al.* (1988) found that the addition of cryoprotectant is responsible for the depolymerization of the microtubuli. These changes are reversible after the removal of the cryoprotectant and a short period of culture. Recently Aigner *et al.* (1991) observed, that a higher number of frozen–thawed mouse oocytes showed normal spindle apparatus using either slow freezing or ultrarapid freezing.

The cortical granules

The oocytes surviving after thawing show a high percentage of polyploidy in *in vitro* fertilization. This phenomenon is observed in mouse (Wood, 1986; Glenister

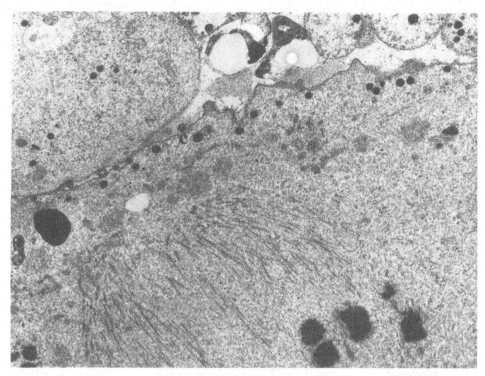

Fig. 1. Surface of a mature unfertilized rabbit oocyte collected 13 h after HCG injection. C, cortical granules under the cytoplasmic membrane. × 5300.

et al., 1987) and in human (Al-Hasani *et al.,* 1989, Mandelbaum *et al.,* 1986). Normally the cortical granules are diffused under the oolemma in mature oocytes. The zona reaction in human oocyte occurs after the movement of these granules to the periphery of the cytoplasm and this reaction is responsible for hindering the penetration of more than one spermatozoa (polyspermy block). An electron microscopic examination is done on the frozen–thawed and on the freshly collected oocytes from rabbit and human. In rabbit the number of the cortical granules is seen to be reduced and the margin not sharp, some showing signs of disappearance or lysis (Figs. 1, 2). This observation may explain the high incidence of polyploidy in frozen–thawed and *in vitro* fertilized oocytes. Conversely, these findings may explain that the freezing process can damage and reduce the number of cortical granules thus leading to a high frequency of polyploidy. Similar findings are observed in humans (Figs. 3, 4). Johnson, Pickering & George (1988) found that the fertilization rate was reduced in mouse oocytes after thawing, suggesting that the rapid cooling to 4 °C may promote release of cortical granules and a premature zona reaction.

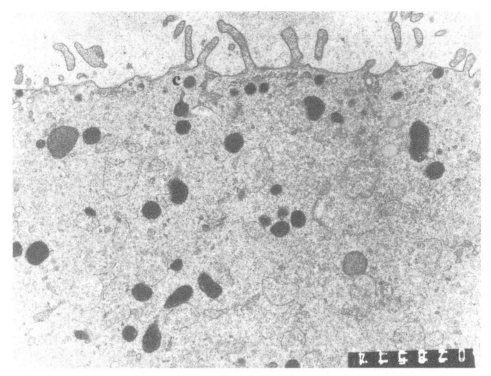

Fig. 2. Surface of mature unfertilized rabbit oocyte frozen–thawed from propanediol.
C, cortical granules reduced in number and not well distinct. × 5000.

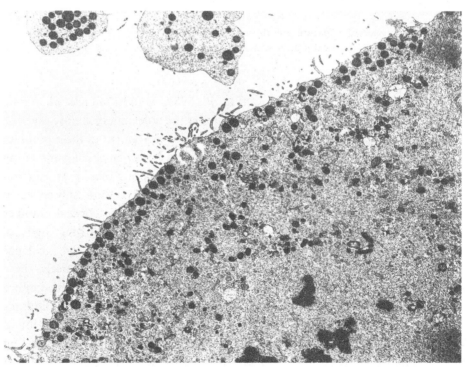

Fig. 3. Surface of a mature unfertilized human oocyte. C, cortical granules are
aggregated under the cytoplasmic membrane and high in number. × 5000.

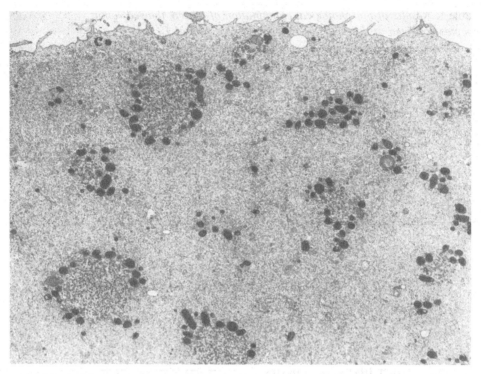

Fig. 4. Surface of a mature unfertilized human oocyte frozen–thawed with propanediol. C, cortical granules reduced in number and not well distinct. × 5000.

Freezing of rabbit oocytes

We have used a rabbit model to develop the techniques of freezing and thawing
in humans (Al-Hasani *et al.*, 1984, 1986*a*).

Our microscopic observations of frozen–thawed oocytes after different times
of collection and culture in both DMSO and propanediol experiments are
summarized in Table 1. 22 of 405 frozen oocytes (5,4%) which were collected 6
hours after LH application were morphologically intact. 63 out of 315 oocytes
(20%) of the ova collected 9 hours after LH injection appeared to have survived.
The highest survival rates of 28.8% in case of DMSO and 32% in case of
propanediol were obtained in the group of ovulated oocytes 2–3 hours after
ovulation. A total of 52 oocytes that were considered viable after freezing and
thawing were incubated for 2 min in Ham's F-10 medium containing fluoroscein
diacetate (FDA) (Table 2). All examined oocytes were fluorescent. No oocytes
that was considered to be degenerated showed fluorescence. Table 3 summarizes
the results of the chromosomal analyses. In oocytes collected 6 hours after LH

Table 1. *Results of morphological examination of frozen–thawed rabbit oocytes collected at different times after the injection of LH*

Type of cryoprotectant	Time of collection after LH (h)	Period of culture after thawing (h)	Number of frozen/ thawed oocytes	Number and (%) of oocytes morphologically intact after culture	
DMSO	6	14	405	22	(5.4)
DMSO	9	7	315	63	(20)
DMSO	12	4	320	92	(28.8)
PROH	12	1/2	774	246	(32)

Table 2. *Results of FDA examination of morphologically intact oocytes after freezing/thawing*

Time of collection after LH (h)	Number of oocytes examined	FDA test	
		Positive	Negative
6	11	11	–
9	18	18	–
12	23	23	–

Table 3. *Results of chromosomal analyses of frozen–thawed oocytes collected at different times after injection of LH*

Time of collection after LH (h)	Period of culture after thawing (h)	Number of fixed oocytes	Number of oocytes with visible chromosomes	Stages of
6	14	14	2	2Xmetaph. II
9	7	46	19	9Xmetaph. II
				10Xmetaph. II
12	4	71	23	1Xtelophase
				22Xmetaph. II

Table 4. *Results of frozen/thawed oocytes fertilized* in vitro *and cultured for a further 6 h*

Type of cryoprotectant	Number of oocytes inseminated	Number (%) of oocytes fertilized in 2- to 4-cell stage		Number (%) of blastocysts	
DMSO	30	18	(60)	1	(5.5)
PROH	246	161	(61)	no	culture

injection, only 3 metaphase II stages were observed out of 14 fixed oocytes. 19 out of 46 oocytes collected 9 hours after LH application and cultured for 7 hours after thawing could be fixed successfully. 10 out of these 19 oocytes reached the metaphase II and none were still in metaphase I. 71 thawed eggs were fixed on slides after 4 hours of culture. The chromosomes were visible in 23 preparations. They were all in metaphase II. The success rates for fixing oocytes on slides were higher in the last groups than in the first.

Morphologically intact oocytes are capable of being fertilized *in vitro* (Table 4). 18 of 30 (60%) and 161 of 246 (61%) oocytes which were incubated with capacitated spermatozoa for 5 hours could be fertilized and cleaved to 2- and 4-cell stages 20 hours later than in case of DMSO and propanediol experiments, respectively.

The overall implantation rate and pregnancy outcome are summarized in Table 5, an overall implantation rate of 9.4% being seen.

Freezing of human oocytes

The two different freezing methods, developed using rabbits, have been used for freezing human oocytes.

Oocytes and oocyte retrieval

Oocytes were collected by either laparoscopy or by transvaginal puncture after ovarian stimulation with HMG/HCG or GnRH agonist/HMG/HCG.

The oocytes in excess of the 4–6 committed for IVF were used for cryopreservation. After retrieval excess oocytes were incubated for about 24 hours to let them reach maturity since many oocytes used for cryopreservation were immature or at intermediate stages of maturity at the time of recovery.

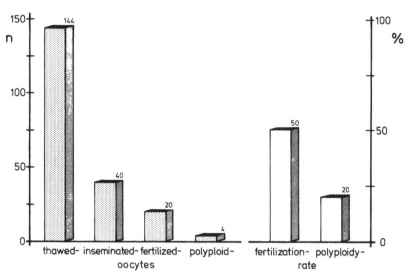

Fig. 5. *In vitro* fertilization results of frozen–thawed human oocytes (frozen with DMSO). Number of cycles = 39.

Furthermore, before cryopreservation of excess oocytes, it was useful to observe two pronuclei in the inseminated oocytes indicating that fertilization had occurred.

The freezing and thawing process similar to that used in rabbit has been described in detail elsewhere (Al-Hasani, 1986*a*).

Results

217 excess oocytes from 39 cycles were frozen slowly to −33 °C using 1.5M DMSO. Of 144 oocytes that have been thawed, 40 oocytes seemed to be morphologically intact (28%), only 20 oocytes could be fertilized *in vitro*, the polyploidy rate being 20%.

Fig. 6 summarizes observations on freezing human oocytes by the method described previously by Lassalle, Testort & Renard (1985). 66 excess oocytes from nine cycles were frozen. Twelve of 38 oocytes thawed were morphologically intact and nine could be fertilized *in vitro*, the polyploidy rate being 44%.

The importance of oocyte quality for the success of cryopreservation is shown in Table 6, the maturational stage of oocytes before freezing playing an important role in the success of cryopreservation and the subsequent IVF procedures. Oocyte maturation at the time of oocyte retrieval is also important. The embryos from the only two pregnancies which have been achieved originated from mature oocytes.

Table 5. *Transfer results of cryopreserved and in vitro fertilized rabbit oocytes cultured for 24–26 h using propanediol*

	Number of recipients	Number of embryos transferred	Implantations at day 15		Fetuses		Resorptions		Number of born
			Number	%	Number	%	Number	%	
a	2	17	3	18	2	12	1	6	2
b	2	18	–	–	–	–	–	–	–
c	2	18	2	11	2	11	–	–	2
Total	6	53	5	9.4	4	7.5	1	1.9	4

Recipients were given HCG 30, 24 and 18 h before embryo transfer

Table 6. *In vitro fertilization results of frozen–thawed human oocytes (in relation to the oocyte quality)*

Number of patients	Number of quality* of frozen oocyte			Thawed oocytes	Found after thawing	Number of oocytes inseminated (intact)			Number of fertilized oocytes (%)			Number of pregnancies
	+	++	+++			+	++	+++	+	++	+++	
48	141	101	29	182	159	10	28	16	3(30)	16(57)	19(69)	2
		283					54			30		

*Oocytes maturity was estimated morphologically at the time of oocyte retrieval.
+ = immature. + + = intermediate. + + + = mature.

Table 7. *Worldwide reported pregnancies resulting from freezing human oocytes*

Reference	Year	Pregnancies	
Chen	1986	Twins (M + F) delivered	
(Adelaide, Australia)	1987	Single	(F) delivered
van Uem *et al.*	1987	Single	(F) delivered
(Erlangen, Germany)			
Diedrich	1987	Miscarriages	(2)
(Bonn, Germany)			
Kolodziej *et al.*	1991	Single	(F) delivered
(Essen, Germany)	1991	Miscarriage	(1)

M, male; F, female

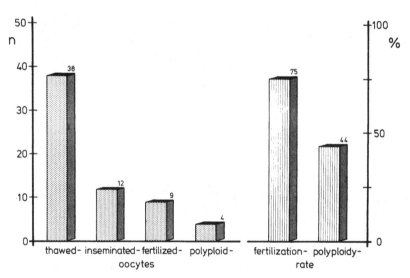

Fig. 6. *In vitro* fertilization results of frozen–thawed human oocytes (frozen with propanediol). Number of cycles = 9.

Results of pregnancies worldwide after human oocyte cryopreservation

To date, a total of seven pregnancies derived from frozen human oocytes have been reported (Table 7). All the pregnancies were achieved by using a slow-freeze and fast-thaw technique, with DMSO as cryoprotectant. Four of the pregnancies have delivered and all of the infants a male and four females are healthy and normal. The remaining three pregnancies resulted in first trimester miscarriages.

Perspective

The human preovulatory oocyte can be successfully frozen and stored. Mouse oocytes had already been successfully cryopreserved by Whittingham (1977) who reported that oocytes could survive deep freezing at $-196\,^{\circ}C$ with a survival rate of about 70%. These thawed mouse oocytes were capable of fertilization *in vitro* although with lower rates than control unfrozen oocytes and on transfer to recipient females who produced normal live offspring. However, the technique may not be applicable to the human oocyte because of species differences, as there are structural differences between the chromosomes of mouse and man (Chen, 1990).

Parthenogenetic activation of frozen–thawed oocytes has not been seen in either rabbit or human oocytes. With human oocytes there is clear morphological evidence of the appearance of both male and female pronuclei with subsequent syngamy and cell cleavage. The only and most practical means of assessing the survival and subsequent performance of the fertilized frozen–thawed human oocyte is by its morphological appearance on light microscopy. Polyploidy rates are higher after cryopreservation of human oocytes regardless of which cryoprotectant is used. Reducing the number of inseminating spermatozoa may reduce the polyploidy rate. The risk of fetal malformation resulting from freezing–thawing of the human oocytes is not known as only five normal children have been born without malformation after cryopreservation of oocytes. Presumably only the most robust normal cells survive.

References

Aigner S, Siebzehnruebl E, van der Eilst J, Spitzer M, van Steirteghem AC, Lang L. Veränderungen des meiotischen Spindelapparetes von Mäuseeizellen nach verschiedenen Einfrierverfahren. *Freiländertagung Fertilität und Sterilität Goslar* 1991: 267–8.

Al-Hasani S, Hahn J, Dankowski K, Schneider U. *In vitro* fertilization and embryo transfer of rabbit oocytes collected at different times after P-LH injection. *Europ J Obstet Gynec Reprod Biol* 1984; **17**: 417–23.

Al-Hasani S, Tolksdorf A, Diedrich K, van der Ven H, Krebs D. Successful *in vitro* fertilization of frozen–thawed rabbit oocytes. *Hum Reprod* 1986a; **1**: 309–12.

Al-Hasani S, van der Ven H, Diedrich K and Krebs D. Successful *in vitro* fertilization of frozen–thawed human oocytes. In: *Workshop on Embryos and Oocytes Freezing (Reports). Collection Fondation Marcel Merieux* 1986b Annecy: 25–39.

Al-Hasani S, Diedrich K, van der Ven H, Reinecke A, Hartje M, Krebs D. Cryopreservation of human oocytes. *Hum Reprod* 1987; **2**: 695–700.

Al-Hasani S, Kirsch J, Diedrich K, Blanke S, van der Ven H, Krebs D. Successful embryo of cryopreserved and *in vitro* fertilized oocytes. *Hum Reprod* 1989; **4**: 77–9.

Baker TG. Oogenesis and ovulation. In: Austin CR, RV Short (Eds). *Fortpflanzungsbiologie der*

Säugetiere, Bd. 1, Keimzelle und Befruchtung, Parey-Verlag, Berlin und Hamburg 1976: 19–42.

Burks JL, Davies ME, Bakken AH, Tomasovic JJ. Morphologic evaluation of frozen rabbit and human ova. *Fertil Steril* 1965; **16**: 638–64.

Brackett BG, Williams WL. Fertilization of rabbit ova in a defined medium. *Fertil Steril* 1968; **19**: 144–55.

Bernard A, Imoedemhe DA, Shaw RW, Fuller B. Effects of cryoprotectants of human oocyte. *Lancet* 1985; **1**: 632–3.

Chandly AC. Culture of mammalian oocytes. *J Reprod Fertil Suppl* 1971; **14**: 1–6.

Chang MC. Storage of unfertilized rabbit ova: subsequent fertilization and the probability of normal development. *Nature, London* 1953; **172**: 353.

Chen C. Pregnancy after human oocyte cryopreservation. *Lancet* 1986; **1**: 884–6.

Chen C. Pregnancies after human oocyte cryopreservation. *Fifth World Congress on* In Vitro *Fertilization and and Embryo Transfer*. Norfolk, USA, Abstr. 1987; **51**: 19.

Chen C. Oocyte freezing. *Clinical* In Vitro *Fertilization,* Carl Wood and Alan Trounson (eds), Second edition, Springer-Verlag 1990: 113–26.

Damien M, Luciano AA, Peluso JJ. Propanediol alters intracellular pH and developmental potential of mouse zygotes independently of volume change. *Hum Reprod* 1990; **5**: 212–16.

De Mayo FJ, Rawlins RG, Dukelow WR. Xenogenous and *in vitro* fertilization of frozen–thawed primate oocytes and blastomere separation of embryos. *Fertil Steril* 1985; **43**: 295–300.

Diedrich K. Cryopreservation of rabbit and human oocytes *Abstracts of 5th World Congress on* In Vitro *Fertilization and Embryo Transfer. Norfolk, Virginia, 5–10 April* 1987.

Fraser LR, Dandekar PV, Vaidya RA. *In vitro* fertilization of tubal rabbit ova partially or totally denuded of follicular cells. *Biol Reprod* 1971; **4**: 229–33.

Glenister PH, Wood MJ, Kirby C, Whittingham DG. Incidence of chromosome anomalies in first cleavage mouse embryos obtained from frozen–thawed oocytes fertilized *in vitro*. *Gamete Res* 1987; **16**: 205–16.

Fuller BJ, Bernard A. Successful *in vitro* fertilization of mouse oocytes after cryopreservation using glycerol. *Cryo-Letters* 1984; **5**: 307–12.

Hahn J, Sulzer H, Schneider U. Ergebnisse von *in vitro* Befruchtungsversuchen mit Kanincheneizellen. A: Einflüsse der Samenzellkonzentrationen und der Kapazitationsdauer. *Zuchthygiene* 1974; **9**: 178–84.

Johnson MH, Pickering SJ, George MA. The influence of cooling on the properties of the zona pellucida of the mouse oocyte. *Hum Reprod* 1988; **3**: 383–7.

Kasai M, Iritani A, Chang MC. Fertilization *in vitro* of rat ovarian oocytes after freezing and thawing. *Biol Reprod* 1979; **21**: 839–44.

Lassalle B, Testort B, Renard JP. Human embryo features that influence the success of cryopreservation with the use of 1,2-propanediol. *Fertil Steril* 1985; **44**: 645–51.

Leibo SP. Fundamental cryobiology of mouse ova and embryos. In: Elliot K. Whelan J. (eds) *The Freezing of Mammalian Embryos*. Elsevier Excerpta Medica, Amsterdam 1977; 69–96. (Ciba Foundation 52 (new series)).

Magistrini M, Szollosi D. Effects of cold and isopropyl-N-phenylcarbamate on the second meiotic spindle of mouse oocytes. *Eur J Cell Biol* 1980; **22**: 699–707.

Mandelbaum J, Junca A, Plachot M, Alnot MO, Tibi C, Cohen C, Salat-Baroux J. Cryopreservation of human oocytes and embryos using 1–2 propanediol with or without sucrose as cryoprotective agents. *Workshop on Embryos and Oocytes Freezing* recovery and fertilization of frozen–thawed rodent eggs. *Biol Reprod* 1977; **17**: 527–31.

Parkes AS. Factors of the viability of frozen ovarian tissue. *J Endocrinol* 1958; **17**: 337–43.

Pickering SJ, Johnson MH. The influence of cooling on the organization of the meiotic spindle of the mouse oocyte. *Hum Reprod* 1987; **2**: 207–16.

Pickering SJ, Braude PR, Johnson MH. Cryopreservation of human oocytes: inappropriate exposure to DMSO reduces fertilization rates. *Hum Reprod* 1991; **6**: 142–3.

Polge C. The freezing of mammalian embryos: perspectives and possibilities. In: *Elliott K, Whelan J. (eds) The Freezing of Mammalian Embryos*. Elsevier Excerpta Medica. Amsterdam (Ciba Foundation 52 (new series)); 1977: 3–18.

Quinn P, Barros C, Whittingham DG. Preservation of hamster oocytes to assay the fertilizing capacity of human spermatozoa. *J Reprod Fertil* 1982; **66**: 161–8.

Sathanathan AH, Trounson A, Freeman L. Morphology and fertilization of frozen human oocytes. *Gamete Res* 1987; **16**: 343–54.

Sherman JK, Lin TP. Survival of unfertilized mouse eggs during freezing and thawing *Proc Soc Biol Med* 1958*a*; **98**: 902–5.

Sherman JK, Lin TP. Effect of glycerol and low temperature on survival of unfertilized mouse eggs. *Nature, London* 1958*b*; **181**: 785–6.

Sherman JK, Lin TP. Temperature shock and cold storage of unfertilized mouse egg. *Fertil Steril* 1959; **10**: pp 384–96.

Smith AU. Behaviour of fertilized rabbit eggs exposed to glycerol and to low temperatures. *Nature, London*, 1952; **170**: 374–5.

Tolksdorf A, Al-Hasani S, Diedrich K, van der Ven H, Krebs D: An attempt to freeze rabbit follicular oocytes. *Hum Reprod Bonn FRG* 1985 23–26 June 1985, abstract 93, 33.

Trounson A. *In vitro* fertilization and embryo preservation. In: Trounson A, and Wood C. (eds). In Vitro *fertilization and embryotransfer*. Churchill Livingstone, Edinburgh 1984: 111–30.

Vincent C, Heymann Y, Garnier V, Renard JP. Cryopreservation of ovulated rabbit oocytes: cryoprotectant effect in microfilament and microtuble organization. *In vivo* survival after freezing. *25th Annual Meeting of Cryobiology Society, Aachen-Germany*, 1988: abstr. 157.

Whittingham DG. Fertilization *in vitro* and development to term of unfertilized mouse oocytes previously stored at −196 °C. *J Reprod Fert* 1977; **49**: 89–94.

Wood MJ. An increased incidence of polyploidy in embryos derived from frozen oocytes. *In Workshop on Embryos and Oocytes Freezing (Reports). Collection Fondation Marcel Merieux, Annecy* 1986: 41–51.

Zamboni L. Ultrastructure of mammalian oocytes and ova *Biol Reprod Suppl.* 1970; **2**: 44–63.

16

Bioethics and the oocyte: reproductive choice

R. P. S. JANSEN

Oocytes kept: reproductive choice

Unless impregnation has been forced, a woman nowadays can more or less choose to whom her ovulating eggs will be bared. She can exercise choice over who her sexual partner will be and who shall father her offspring. Ordinarily she will be the genetic, gestational and social mother of the child or children who result. In the modern family, love, sex, procreation, and companionship are meant, ideally, to go together.

This chapter's purpose is to explore from biological and modern cultural perspectives the moral codes and ethical rules that society is developing to give couples, and especially women, responsibility for their reproduction through the exercise of choice. The position I take (as I have in a companion chapter on the ethics of spermatozoa in *The Spermatozoon*) is that the wisdom of ethical principles should be able to be tested and that what is an ethical, moral or wise course of action or inaction should be responsive to evidence; it should, in principle if with caution, be alterable.

Awareness of reproductive destiny and exercise of reproductive choice are the two sides, at once sociological and biological, to responsible, determined reproductive behaviour. Reproductive destiny is the theme of the chapter in Volume 3; reproductive choice is this chapter's theme. The differentiation of the two chapters is contrived. I encourage readers again to excuse inadvertent, nonbiological distinctions of gender, and to make their own philosophical integrations of matters that for convenience are presented separately.

Choosing a mate, having sex and having children

A successful marriage needs wisdom, foresight and luck. Compared with historical times, marriage can now last an unprecedentedly long time. While it lasts, just one of its purposes is procreation, and nowadays that too is optional. But if the option is exercised, procreative or reproductive choice includes the ancient process of anticipating one's mate's reproductive fitness.

Mate choice

In the animal kingdom, competition between males for reproductive rights to females occurs through the defeat of competitors or, with monogamous or near-monogamous species, through an individual's talent in attracting females. In both cases, in evolutionary and sociobiological terms, it is the female's reproductive needs and receptiveness that has determined and governed male sexual strategy (Short, 1984). It is only among humans, now for long periods in history and probably prehistory, that the female's primacy in matters of sex has been lost and that female choice in reproduction has been suppressed.

In nature, at least among the more monogamous species, both males and females can, and usually do, exercise reproductive choice. Behind that choice there is a premium placed on correctly anticipating mutual duties – one's own and, especially, those of one's partner. The premium is not so much in anticipating one's own conjugal *rights* as it is in anticipating one's partner's reproductive *duties*. Let me digress on this distinction.

When does one person's duty become another person's right? There can be no moral rights without moral duties; they are correlatives. It is said, for example, that citizens of a democracy have the *right* to vote in elections; but if you stay at home on election day and no one has the *duty* to bring you a ballot paper then your right to vote is meaningless. So, duties and rights are reciprocal. The rights of wives can be seen as the duties of husbands; the rights of husbands are the duties of wives; and the rights of single mothers need to be the duties or obligations of third parties (or they will find they have none). The rights of children are really the correlative duties and obligations of parents and others in society. Animals have rights when humans acknowledge a duty to them. Mutual conjugal rights are really mutual conjugal duties – and they can become a pleasure if they are matters of choice.

Sexual and reproductive choice is particularly important for women, after all they receive the sperm and they carry the baby. A woman's potential for expressing fecundity is thus more constrained than a man's, being limited by ability to gestate, and to bear and to nurse the young to independence. For this she expends so much energy that, until the most modern of times, health and wellbeing for women has meant division of labour between the sexes, with a home-based strategy for women and a roving role for men. The unprecedented modern possibility of exceptions to this rule is biologically luxurious – but it is also culturally exciting.

In a number of species, female reproductive choice is a trait of behaviour that has now been shown to have a heritable basis (Majerus, O'Donald & Weir, 1982; Watt, Carter & Donohue, 1986). The preference shown is often for males who are or who appear nurturant (Clutton-Brock, 1991) as well as capable. There are several agencies by which such behaviour and genetic selection may come about. There may simply be an intuitive female preference for straightforward displays of male care: female stickleback fish, for example, are attracted to male sticklebacks that are already guarding the spawned eggs of another female – to the point where male sticklebacks will steal eggs from other nests in order to attract females (Gwynne, 1991). More complicatedly, genes that govern choice and reproductive display, for example the splendour of a peacock's tail, and which are in linkage disequilibrium with genes that affect fitness, will be co-inherited (Maynard Smith, 1989). Lastly, a gene that causes the female carrying that gene to be fussy in picking a mate, instead of having impregnation follow the first or the slightest temptation, will especially favour persistent, adept and fussy males, more likely perhaps to be endowed with genes for fitness; studies have shown that this advantageous effect is displayed more often in some species among older, more experienced and more discriminating females (Watt, Carter & Donohue, 1986).

Sex

The zoologist Desmond Morris almost 20 years ago summarized what was known of the pressures there probably were for monogamy among early man. His and others' conclusions on the evolutionary reasons for monogamous mating, breaking with the established primate pattern of sexual promiscuity (Small, 1993), are now hardly controversial (Short, 1984; Morris, 1986). The theory is a strong one.

At the time in prehistory that increasing brain-size demanded lengthening gestation times, and when increasing intelligence and education required lengthening times of infancy and pre-pubertal childhood (see below), paleontological studies tell us that the forests of the earth were giving way to grasslands and to less predictable supplies of food. Early men and women turned omnivorous, supplementing the gathering of primitive vegetables and fruits (we believe by women) with the hunting of game (we believe by men). An upright gait improved speed and freed the forelimbs for the use of tools, implements and weapons. It also enabled the pelvis to enlarge to accommodate the larger fetal head size at birth.

Monogamy and sexual fidelity for males meant, as it has repeatedly meant through evolution, surer paternity and an increase in certainty that offspring themselves will reach maturity and reproduce. For females there was the security of being materially provided for. If the rule of monogamy in human society is sometimes defined better in its breach than in its observance, there none the less is no mistaking the reciprocal importance of making a correct or best choice of mate.

The observer of animal mating systems is soon struck by the extraordinary reciprocity there is between the behaviour of males and females in diverse species and circumstances. Evolution has had no room for inefficient battles between the sexes (between the genders). Sex is virtually confined to female oestrus, when pregnancy is possible, and male sexual arousal at other times is uncommon; forced mating of unreceptive females is rare in the extreme (though young male orang-utans pressing their needs on older females appears to be an exception (Fleagle, 1988). M. Small has pointed out that sexuality, female and male, is well-developed among most primates (Small 1993). Thus it would cause little surprise if a shift in the role of having sex for apparently casual, if social, mutual pleasure among emerging humans towards a more calculated, if less frequent, conjugal activity (accompanied by the evolution of greater penile and vulval size) too was a reciprocal development.

The human female can and does enjoy sex at almost any time during the menstrual cycle, and throughout pregnancy and lactation – times when sex can have no reproductive and procreative purpose other than the fostering of monogamy through pleasure. It should be absurd that the Pope and the bishops of the Roman Catholic church can, in the name of the 'inseparability of the unitive-procreative dimensions of sexuality', as expressed in Pope John Paul II's *Humanae Vitae* and *Familiaris Consortio,* promote this principle for every act of sex, and on this basis condemn both contraception and assisted conception (McCormick, 1989), yet not condemn sex during pregnancy and lactation.

Spacing children

The arboreal environment in which the monkeys and apes evolved suited their generally vegetarian diet, their lack of nesting or fixed abode, their quadrupedal gait, and (though gibbons are one exception) their non-monogamous mating systems. In this environment they came to need longer times for gestation, to cope with the evolutionary pressure for bigger brains. The limits set by the anatomy of the pelvis to the size of the fetal head at birth meant a relative shift of cerebral development from prenatal to postnatal life. This, in turn, meant longer times devoted to dependent infancy and childhood. The time from birth to maturity increased considerably.

R.V. Short points out that female chimpanzees and gorillas in the wild start having menstrual cycles at the age of 8 to 9 years, and first become pregnant at 9 to 12 years. In primitive human societies, menarche is at about 16.5 years and first pregnancy is not until about 18 years (Short, 1984). Childhood is needed for cerebral development and education. Children are just too silly to be allowed to get pregnant while they are still children. Thus we have a reproductive strategy in which delaying sexual maturity turns out to be reproductively advantageous.

From amoebae to man, a successfully reproducing organism marshalls resources so that the genetic endowment it gets is on average outweighed by the genetic legacy it leaves its descendants; quantitatively or qualitatively, there should be a genetic gain from generation to generation. Population scientists talk of two general strategies by which this can be achieved. The first strategy, known as r-selection, shows rapid sexual maturity, superabundant egg production with relatively low survival rates of offspring, and a short life for the parent. r-Selection is typically favoured by or forced on smaller species, whose numbers wax and wane with changes in the environment. Many r-selected species see parents die soon after a single, explosive event of reproduction. The second strategy, known as K-selection, shows slow attainment of sexual maturity, limited egg production with relatively high survival rates of offspring, and a longer life for the parent, usually with several episodes of gestation, and invariably with a premium placed on parental care, so that the offspring can reach the sexual maturity they need for their parents' genetic potential to be realized. K-Selected species are generally animals that in one way or another smooth out the environment's cycles – perhaps because there aren't any (as in the tropics), perhaps because the animals accumulate spare capacity or bulk (K-selection typifies bigger animals), or in our own case because ingenuity and intelligence overcome the effects of the environment's fluctuations. The differences between r-selected and K-selected species can be overdone – big animals always need longer to grow than small animals – but it is none the less instructive to examine how the primates generally, and encultured H. sapiens in particular, have come to be quintessentially K-selected and have lengthened their birth intervals by spacing their pregnancies. This consideration is basic to understanding what we today call infertility.

Reproductive pressure for pregnancy spacing in nature is most obvious for the largest mammals, the young of which need the longest time physically to grow to a size where they can fend for themselves (Short, 1984). The African elephant, for example, has a 22-month gestation, and a typical birth interval of 3 to 4 years. Sperm whales have a 15.5-month gestational period and a birth interval of 4 to 5 years. As humans, we rival these long birth intervals, despite our much lower body mass, because the time our young need to become reasonably independent has for different reasons become the same.

Spacing of pregnancies among these different mammals is accomplished in several ways, such as gestational infertility, lactational infertility and seasonal breeding, which all operate by inhibiting ovulation.

Lactational amenorrhoea is the chief natural contraceptive of the great apes and humans. To be an effective physiological contraceptive, though, breast feeding must be exclusive, and not be complemented by exogenous foodstuff. The hunter–gatherer !Kung nomads of the Kalahari Desert in southern Africa feed their babies several times an hour for the first two or three years of life, and sleep with them at the breast; in consequence the average birth interval is 4.1 years despite apparently high intrinsic fertility (Short, 1984). There is no way of knowing, though, for what time in human history and prehistory such intensive suckling has been usual. Modern primitive societies such as the !Kung may have evolved considerably from our own anticedent tribes.

Seasonal breeding is apparent among the lesser apes, such as the lar gibbon of the Malayan rain forest (Kavanagh, 1983), but among humans, other than higher sperm concentrations being found in winter (Levine *et al.*, 1988), seasonal changes in fertility are not conspicuous. Not the least of the likely reasons for this is that men and women have, through clothing, shelter and sometimes migration, successfully adapted the environment to provide rough constancy among the seasons.

Environmental constraints on human fertility are seen, however, in the hypothalamic hypogonadotrophic amenorrhoea that occurs when a woman loses weight to below menarcheal levels (Frisch, 1987). Hypothalamic production of gonadotrophin releasing hormone is singularly sensitive to body mass. The physiological corollary of this sensitivity is that the improvement in human nutrition that has taken place in the last 100 years has produced an important lowering in the age at Menarche, from the age of 15 to 16 in the mid-nineteenth century to 12 to 13 years in Western societies today (Wyshak & Frisch, 1982). At the same time, the need for enculturation of our young is raising the age at which emotional maturity and educational maturity are reached. This counter-K selective secular trend in age at menarche has increased further the split between the ages of physical and mental maturity – a split that has already become a gulf with clear and deep social consequences.

Fertility, culture and contraception

One suspects that environmental and lactational anovulation has not been contraceptive enough over the last several hundred thousand years alone to accommodate the need for a longer and longer hominid childhood. Prehistoric biological pressures for hominids – and, in historical times, social conventions that have become part of human culture – doubtless have been important too. and in the last generation or so the invention of effective contraception has added a technical solution to the educational priorities and K-selection imperatives modern civilization demands.

Infertility's paradox

Necessity may seem to precede invention, but in evolution it is preadaptation that is invention's real mother. Species under significant strain are too hardpressed to adapt to change, whereas successful species fill voids and diversify before they need to. It is a species' success that affords its members the luxury of change for its own sake. The biological variations that result may not find application straight away, but the diversity that comes from it will sooner or later be rewarded by peculiar advantages when the environment changes, when competition tightens, or when new opportunities present. It is then that the luxury of diversity becomes both the necessary seed of survival and the mother of evolutionary invention. It is then, too, that what manifests as adaptation turns out to be the realisation of prior preadaptation.

When flowering opportunity of intelligence demanded a quickly lengthening childhood, what was it, then, that the evolving hominids turned to in order to lengthen the birth interval? How could the number of young raised safely to maturity be increased by reducing fecundity and thus improve reproductive fitness? One adaptive option that was by now closed was limiting sexual attractiveness and interest: sexuality – the realization of a primate preadaptation – had become the cement to the monogamy that ensured that female hominids had the paternal support they and their dependent offspring needed.

Clinical reproductive medicine tells us that human fertility is not only low by primate standards, but that several conditions associated with diminished fertility have a genetic basis. Any (and probably all) of these clinical conditions may have acted to limit hominid fecundity and in this way to have bettered ultimate reproductive success.

High *embryonic* mortality can serve a useful purpose in extremely *K*-selected species, according to Short (1984), who draws attention to the advantages brought by 'a sprinkling of genetically defective gametes [to produce] a measure of non-recurrent infertility through early embryonic death'. Evidence of high rates of early pregnancy failure among humans (Biggers, 1981) shows that no more than 25–50% of fertilizations will produce a normal, viable pregnancy – a lower proportion than among the other primates, and, in evolutionary terms, a shift that is apparently convergent with a similar evolutionary development among species highly *K*-selected because of the demands of huge adult size. Elephants too have high rates of embryonic death (Short, 1984).

Endometriosis is a condition of the female pelvic structures in which tissue with characteristics of endometrium develops in locations other than the mucosa of the uterus, changing the internal environment of the woman's reproductive organs and resulting in relative infertility. The prevalence of endometriosis increases with age during the reproductive years, as the modern woman, generally neither pregnant nor lactating, accumulates the legacy of an historically and prehistorically unprecedented number of ovulatory menstrual cycles.

Endometriosis is rarely severe enough to be an undoubted cause of sterility, but several lines of evidence show that fertility is reduced even in mild endometriosis (Tulandi & Mouchawar, 1991; Jansen, 1986; Hammond, Jordan & Sloan, 1986). Such information fits a model in which endometriosis reduces fertility in a dose-dependent way (Jansen, 1993).

Among 123 patients with clinically proven endometriosis studied by Simpson *et al.* (1980), 9 of 153 female siblings aged over 18, and 10 of 123 mothers, had also had a diagnosis of endometriosis confirmed by similar criteria, giving a prevalence of clinically important endometriosis among first-degree relations of 19/276, or 6.9%; on the other hand, endometriosis had been diagnosed in only one of 104 female siblings of patients' husbands and in only one of 107 husbands' mothers, giving a prevalence among non-genetic relations of 2/211, or 0.9%. This relative risk of 7.3, given a positive family history, is consistent with polygenic or multifactorial inheritance of endometriosis.

Endometriosis has also been found in the other menstruating mammals, namely the non-human primates (D'Hooghe *et al.*, 1991), occasionally causing severe debilitation (McClure, Ridley & Graham, 1971). We do not know whether the condition has evolved independently in hominids or if nature seized on a once innocuous primate histological concomitant of menstruation dating from more than 40 million years ago (which is when the old world monkeys diverged from the hominoid line). Either way, endometriosis is so common in women that, given its hereditary basis, it is plausible that nature – at the cruel expense of significant symptoms for many modern sufferers – developed it or preserved it for a purpose. That purpose may have been to improve reproductive fitness through diminishing fecundity.

The irregularity of ovulation that accompanies the polycystic ovary syndrome (PCOS) is another, often inherited, impediment to human female fertility (Jansen, 1994). Clinically there is evidence of increased male sex hormone activity, with both the anovulation and the masculinization accentuated if the woman gains weight to become obese. Conversely, fertility is enhanced in women with PCOS by a loss of weight to levels which, in ordinary women, would cause anovulation and infertility. Indeed, mild PCOS is so common (perhaps 20% of all women), that calling it abnormal might be questioned. Evolution may have given it a dual purpose: a brake on fertility during times of plenty; preservation of fertility of a population during times of famine (J Eden, personal communication; Jansen, 1994).

The inheritance of *oligospermia* has a similar effect in systematically diminishing fertility. It is well demonstrated that variability in sperm counts and the size of the testes in primates is determined genetically (Short, 1979; Moller, 1988). It also seems that inherited sperm production rates and motility fractions are related to the way mating practices have evolved in primate societies (with, for example, a low 7% motility among monogamous gibbons – see Volume 1). But it is also true that those apes who have low sperm counts are extremely fertile during the few months in which, as seasonal breeders, they copulate. Whatever limitation the male's low sperm count places on fecundity among gibbons, apparently happily monogamous, is made up by high female fertility. The American urologist Sherman Silber has drawn my attention to the advantages that genetically determined oligospermia may paradoxically have for monogamous human reproduction through limiting fecundity without limiting the expression of sexuality (personal communication, and Silber, 1990).

Oligospermia in the male and endometriosis of PCOS in the female are common clinical combinations among infertile couples (e.g. Mahmood & Templeton, 1989). One often suspects that if the conditions were isolated and mild there would be no serious difficulty with conception, and that it is their chance coexistence or their chance exaggeration to a more severe form that pushes the once desirable retardation they put on fecundity into the realm of reproductive disability through infertility (Jansen, 1993).

What is a reproductive disability in term of infertility in western society today, however, is not the same as it was during prehistory. Conversely, an involuntarily wait of 4 or 5 years for conception to take place is no longer considered to be the pinnacle of *K*-selected human reproductive achievement that, it seems, it once was.

High fertility disability

There was an old woman, who lived in a shoe; she had so many children, she knew not what to do. English nursery rhyme, approximately the sixteenth century.

In about 1500 in England, a boom began in the practice of wet-nursing. It put a stop to millenia of lactational contraception (Fildes, 1986; Stone, 1977). Restricted at first to the aristocracy and the gentry, by the early eighteenth century many more ordinary women were foregoing what was, and is, the most natural break on fecundity; at least while their resources allowed it, mothers were sending off their infants shortly after birth to nurses in the country in order to preserve their busts – and, inadvertently, to be pregnant again within a few months (Stone, 1977). Well-to-do English women of that time had anywhere from a dozen to 20 babies, and 30 babies was not unusual (Kolata, 1987). Childhood mortality was high and parental concern about it generally low, but none the less, with still so many surviving children who required education or placement, family wealth was dissipated. The 'commodification of children' is a popular perjorative slogan heard today from some critics of modern reproductive technology. But, if ever children were a commodity, it was in England and societies like it in the early modern period. High fertility, at this unique crossroads in civilization, was a stark disability.

Among at least the aristocracy in Britain, the social response to the disability of high fertility, before the invention of effective contraception, was a quickly escalating age at marriage, seen between the sixteenth and nineteenth centuries (Stone, 1977), together with a social taboo that was placed on premarital conception. The social *K*-selection that came about by lengthening further the interval between sexual maturity and commencement of procreation was as important in limiting family size then as it is today in enabling adolescents to be adequately educated before adulthood and parenthood.

Low natural fecundity, perhaps for the last time, showed its human evolutionary advantages.

Contraception

The history of modern contraception is well known. These unparalleled devices for implementing human reproductive choice have been championed by women's liberationists since the last century. To discuss the profoundness of this development further is to risk numbing the reader to the comprehensively important place that effective contraceptive practice has in human social and ethical history.

In brief, contraception has removed the disability from the high part of nature's distribution of fertility in human societies. For those couples with average or above-average fecundity, reproducing or choosing not to is essentially no longer a problem.

Modern infertility and its treatment

We turn thus to the disability of infertility – the low end of fecundity's distribution among couples intent on reproducing. More than 50% of infertile women regard infertility to be the most upsetting experience of their lives, remembering it to be as stressful or more stressful than divorce or the death of a close friend or family member (Mazure & Greenfeld, 1989). Given that about 10% of married couples experience it, infertility's threat to reproductive choice is one of, if not the, major cause of psychological morbidity among women, and a lesser but still important one among men.

Infertility and sterility

To consider the laws, ethics and morality of treating infertility let us first be sure of its causes and the real options for treating it. The ordinary medical investigation of infertility as it is presented by a couple who seek a doctor's help leads generally to one of three conclusions.

First, there may be a cause found for *sterility* (or absolute infertility), namely: an absence of sperm production; an absence of oocyte production or ovulation (sometimes the result of premature depletion of eggs from the ovaries); or an anatomical obstruction in man or woman that prevents sperm from reaching an ovulated oocyte before, during or after sexual intercourse.

Secondly, a cause may be found for *relative infertility*, such as a low sperm count, irregular ovulation, a problem of anatomy or physiology that reduces the probability of sperm or oocyte arriving at the prospective site for fertilization, or some cause of embryopathy or gametopathy, like endometriosis or uterine fibroids. In these cases, medicine faces a task that in principle is difficult. Pushing a clinical circumstance that is a departure from normal *back* to normal (which, after all, is medicine's reason for being) is most likely to work when the departure from normal is major. Because any medical or surgical intervention risks introducing disturbances attributable to the intervention itself, the more minor the departure from normal the less likely it is that the intervention will, on balance, improve the circumstance instead of making it worse. The difficulty is multiplied when there is more than one abnormality present and separate but simultaneously effective manoeuvres need to be devised.

Thirdly, investigations may show *no* departure from presently known standards of anatomical and physiological normality, or *unexplained infertility*. The temptations here are (a) to invent new causes of infertility (but not one such cause has been characterised in the last 15 years, despite the unprecedented opportunity IVF technology has provided us to obtain new insights), or (b) to call the infertility psychosomatic. The objective evidence for this last possibility is threadbare, provided ovulation and sexual intercourse both continue to happen; the once-credited anecdotal accounts that conception commonly follows adoption have been refuted by no fewer than five of five prospective studies (Lamb & Leurgans, 1979).

We are left with the conclusion that unexplained infertility, as well as much not-well-explained infertility, is the inevitable product of the evolution of highly *K*-selective (and otherwise successful) reproductive strategies. Although a five-year or longer natural birth interval is a worry for modern couples, it did not become a disability in hominid evolution and human society until very, very recently.

What then is infertility? Like any symptom that causes a person or persons to consult a doctor, infertility is subjective: it is when the couple think that too much time has elapsed in trying to conceive, often made worse by a nowadays all-to-true fear that little time is left in which to trust that conceiving naturally will happen. The doctor's, and the couple's, three options, after investigations have been done, are (a) to do nothing, (b) to seek to correct the underlying abnormality, if one or more of these is obvious from the investigations, or (c) to address the disability directly via a programme of assisted conception, this being defined as one or other therapeutic manoeuvre that increases the chance of becoming pregnant during the month or the cycle in which the treatment is invoked (Jansen, 1987*a*).

Assisting conception

The medical indications for helping conception, then, are properly based on time: the time it has taken for conception demonstrably not to have happened (the duration of infertility); and the time available for more attempts at conceiving naturally to work. The actual diagnosis made is then a guide to choosing the form which assisted conception should take.

It is noteworthy that the extreme *K*-selective pressure that evolution has imposed on humans through biological mechanisms has now been advanced by the cultural effects of human civilisation and modern society. For several hundred years the demands of birth control and adolescent education have postponed pregnancy past the first third of a woman's potentially reproductive years. Many couples today, however, are choosing to delay reproduction further, well into the second half of the female partner's potentially fertile time (DeCherney & Berkowitz, 1982). Whereas in many cases this may not matter much (Bongaarts, 1982), the age of women seeking assistance with conception through reproductive technology is already high (in our programme in Australia the average age is now 37) (unpublished information from Sydney IVF, Sydney, Australia). Normal reproduction and assisted reproductive technology alike are being stretched to extraordinary lengths, mainly because of the social postponement that has occurred in deciding to have children. The IVF-related clinical activity that in 1993 is causing much social comment involves security pregnancies by young-oocyte donation for women who are much older than what, until 1990, was considered the age of reproductive competence, women in their 50s and 60s.

There is therefore no clear distinction between fertility and infertility. Fertility, like contraception, ought to be a matter of reproductive choice for the couple concerned, especially for the woman. The question of who should pay the money needed to enable such reproductive choice, given that assisted conception techniques are much more expensive than contraceptive techniques, is a matter for the plural voices of democratic societies to come to terms with. None the less the principle should be clear that no society will wish or will be able to pay for each possible manoeuvre that can be devised, for the number of times it might be necessary, for every couple wanting to push the limits of what is reproductively possible (Jansen, 1987b). The more extreme the case, especially with advancing age, ageing oocytes, and sparser and sparser spermatozoa, the more at the frontier is the technology, the more unproven are the methods, and the more remote may be the chance of success.

Reproductive medicine is an area where medical research has become medical practice with unmatched speed, causing less-clear-thinking critics of its technology to be confused over its aims (which are to improve reproductive choice) and its practice (which makes childless women pregnant). This is not 'social engineering' (ironically a popular feminist criticism of it), even if putting an end to infertility and enabling conception-on-demand turns out, as it no doubt will, to be a part of a change in the nature of society. IVF is not social engineering any more than the invention of contraception, the discovery of antibiotics, and the development of safe obstetric practice were, even though each of these developments changed the social nature of the family and increased the importance attached to individual human life. The legal development of divorce, just 150 years ago, was a singularly more important device for social change than the treatment of infertility and most other medical discoveries will ever be. Feminists' related criticisms that it is men that are forcing IVF technology on women (Klein, 1989) and that men are the dominant partner in reproductive decisions (Rowland, 1992) does not sit well with the history of IVF (especially in America, where the pioneers were Georgeanna Segar Jones and Lucinda Veeck - Jones, 1984; Veeck, 1991), nor with the empirical finding that, whereas 50% of infertile women regard infertility as the greatest stress of their lives, this is true of just 15% of men (Mazure & Greenfeld, 1989).

Feminists and others, including IVF doctors, may still question just whose reproductive choice is being exercised when programmes of assisted conception are taken to extremes. The vulnerabilities of desperate couples – usually personified as the female partner who undergoes the ovarian stimulations, the follicle aspirations, the gamete or embryo transfers, the physical and emotional lurching of an amplified luteal phase, and the disappointment and pain of menstruation – have been an object of an earlier essay (Jansen, 1987c). The pitfalls and opportunities there are for exploitation when novel medicine is played to the grandstands need to be anticipated and avoided. Ultimately, though, assisted conception is, and should be, a matter of informed choice for the childless woman. It is usually true that there is satisfaction to be found in just having tried IVF.

But for this to be the case it will need to have been made available carefully and compassionately.

Where more radical feminists put themselves on the least secure ground is when, for convenience, they ally themselves with those who are against reproductive technology for very different reasons, especially those who are against IVF on moral or religious grounds. R. Rowland, for example, self-servingly joins the most conservative of society's patriarchs in wanting to stop embryo research (Dwyer, 1992), while resting her harsh criticism of IVF (Rowland, 1992) on its still relatively low success rate, condemning it as a 'failed technology'. It is the embryo research that she wants to put an end to, after all, which is the very means of improving its effectiveness.

Research with oocytes and spermatozoa

It was once a virtue not to make an issue of a matter without good cause. Today, issues are kept alive for the sake of it – or at least to benefit academic careers which owe nothing to the detached or systematic enquiry that should distinguish the social scientist. Research involving the fertilization of human oocytes *in vitro* remains popularly contentious despite its repeated acceptance in surveys of public opinion and despite agreement to it, after exhaustive presentation of arguments, by better than two-thirds majorities of both houses of the British parliament. Research involving human eggs that are fertilized *in vitro* and which are then ruined by not being placed in someone's uterus has been called destructive or 'non-therapeutic' embryo research (Senate Select Committee on the Human Embryo Experimentation Bill 1985, 1986). It is homicide to those who believe that human life, with all its need for protection, is present from the moment of conception (or, with a twist, under the Victorian Infertility, Medical Procedures, Act of 1984, from the moment of syngamy). It is logical nonsense to most secular philosophers (Kuhse & Singer, 1982) and to some theological ones (Dunstan, 1984; McCormick, 1989). But a non-issue, unfortunately, it still is not.

As a result, in the 16 years that have now elapsed since the world's first birth following conception *in vitro*, substantively no more has been learned about the nutritional needs of fertilized human oocytes than was known then. Scientists have had to mark time while others have developed moral, ethical and political positions to determine the immediate future of human embryo research. The clinical applications of IVF-related reproductive technology have been advanced, to be sure, but the chance of birth after two or three days' development after fertilization of oocytes *in vitro* has been kept low by woolly thinking on whose humanness needs protecting in IVF laboratories.

Embryos develop in stages, whatever moralists and overzealous statutory authorities have to say on the matter. For longer than it can generally survive *in vitro,* a human embryo consists of a loosely arranged group of totipotent cells that are mostly destined to become supporting membranes and afterbirth for the fetus. No purely embryonic cells are definable until a week from fertilization, at about the time that the embryo (i.e. the 'pre-embryo') normally implants in the uterus. Several weeks pass before neurological differentiation might imply the beginnings of sentience, which is given weight by philosophers as a determinant of the fetus's human or moral status (Duhse & Singer, 1982). In a world that still exhibits infanticide, homicide and genocide, an observer on the moon would be forgiven for thinking that the Protestant moral position that would allow embryo research to the stage of implantation, and the Roman Catholic position that life with all its needs for absolute protection exists from the moment of conception, are close enough to accommodate embryo research for a few days after fertilization. Far from it. The clarity of conviction that condemns as a mortal threat to human values a mere several days of oocyte life after fertilization *in vitro* is testament to the lasting power of superstition over secular ethics.

Also unconvincing is the brave argument of some secular ethicists that non-human but 'sentient' animals have greater claim to protection than neurologically undeveloped human fetuses or embryos do. To speak of the *rights* of sentient animals that have no intelligent power over their environment is to put the cart before the horse. Consider, for a moment, the morality of killing mice and rats. *Rodenticide* is a practice that is sprinkled through human social history in the form of village rat catchers, store-bought mousetraps and modern agricultural wheat-silo-maintenance-procedures. The moral simplicity with which vermin mice have been, or are, exterminated by farmers and others contrasts with the understandable and growing difficulty of killing mice in the course of medical or cosmetic research. Think too of the human, if fleeting, tragedy that the death of someone's pet mouse can bring. Are the ethics of rodenticide immutable? Or are the moral circumstances of these three settings different? However inconsistent it is for mice, morality for most of we who write or read these ideas equates with how our own notions of humanity are affected by a mouse's death. Animal rights require human sensibilities first, human duties or obligations second; without them, mice have no rights. So it is with preimplantational human embryos.

Embryo research is unequivocally necessary for women fully to exercise choice in their reproduction (Dunstan, 1986). It is plain, however, that there are still some people who perceive their and others' humanity to be threatened by the idea. They find the thought of placing fertilized human eggs in culture for scientific curiosity instead of for the immediate good of the particular embryos that result to be abhorrently dehumanising. (These perceptions sometimes, but not reliably, change, either when more information is made available – this is all it took for British Lords and MPs – or when the dehumanising experience of infertility happens close to home.) While moral positions on embryo research are as divided as those are of the Archbishop of York (in favour) and the Cardinal Archbishop of Westminster (against) (Walton, 1990), consensus is impossible and more debate will probably just polarize opinion further. At Sydney IVF before embryo freezing was made available as a clinical option, 18 to 19 of every 20 women undergoing gamete intrafallopian transfer procedures requested *in vitro* fertilization of unused eggs purely for the information it would provide, knowing that the resulting embryos would then simply and inevitably be discarded (Jansen, 1991). One might ask the question, what kind of society would legislate against such informed opinion? Unfortunately the answer is: too many.

It seems it will be some time in Denmark (Holm, 1988), Germany (Dickson, 1988; Beier & Beckman, 1991), probably Austria (Kramser, 1992), most states of Australia and the United States, and of course Ireland, before it becomes the moral beliefs of the couple concerned, the provider of oocyte and sperm, that prevail in such research. In each of these states, embryo research of the type that first made IVF possible is now illegal. Western society *will*, none the less, eventually embrace deliberate, unabashed embryo research *in vitro*, not because of cogent logic, papal revision or essays such as this one, but because the importance of such research for advancing human health will outlive those who believe they should oppose it.

It needs to be made well known, meanwhile, that what happens in IVF laboratories does not dehumanize or brutalize the people, mostly women, who carry out research on oocytes and spermatozoa. Our experience with newcomers to embryo laboratories is that the opposite happens. IVF, embryo research, and knowing the couples whose hopes are present *in vitro*, increase one's awe of, and respect for, that which is human.

Oocytes kept: altruism, commerce and confusion

A man's genetic destiny, or at least his interest in it, is taken for granted. A sense of genetic destiny among women independent of that of the men they marry needs, however, to overcome millenia of patriarchy and to surface, let alone to blossom. There is still not much sign of it in our society, although the growing retention of a woman's 'maiden' name for reasons other than professional recognition may represent a first glimpse. Generally, too, women, unlike men, have such a large biological and psychological endowment vested in the processes of gestation and giving birth that an underlying sense of genetic destiny can be hard to distinguish (Annas, 1992).

This section uses the oocyte's destiny to explore the present interplay between women and society in giving women power over that destiny.

The family: its cultural evolution continues

The ideal nuclear family of the late twentieth century in the west provides a man and a woman with mutual affection, love, sexual satisfaction, personal fulfilment, prosperity, a chosen number of children, and companionship for many years after the child or children have left home. Longevity and certainty in the number of children have been made possible by modern hygiene, medicine, contraception and reproductive technology. Modern social devices such as divorce enable second choices to be made if our first choice of partner turns out to have been wrong.

The ancient tensions that make the ideal the lucky exception persist. What is good for the individual can be destructive to the family; what preserves the family can be harsh on the expression of the individual (Wilson, 1975). This principle is as true for animal societies since life on earth began as it is a feature of human society and human families into the twenty-first century. It is a sociological and historical fact that women subjugate their individuality in favour of the family more often than men do. Whether this is a good or a fair thing is generally a personal matter for the couple themselves to resolve. The rising frequency of divorce reveals the rarity of the perfect resolution.

Two sides of the modern notion of family need to be looked at in considering the more socially disruptive reproductive technologies associated with oocyte donation and 'surrogacy'. First, we should examine how permanent a thing the concept of *family* really represents. Secondly, we should start to consider the values that might be aspired to by the people composing such a family or families, principally for their own good, in the face of the new reproductive technologies.

The modern period

In a scholarly account of the cultural development of the family, sex and marriage in England during the modern period, historian L. Stone identifies several stages that differ considerably from the nuclear family we treasure in Western societies today (Stone, 1977). I will draw on Stone's work in this section to set the stage for the innovations of family structure we are seeing today.

Love and companionship, as England came out of the Middle Ages, were not observed independently of sex based on lust, according to Stone. None of these three values, lust, love and companionship, had much to do with marriage. Marriage was mostly arranged through ties to ancestors and to living kin. Neither personal autonomy nor privacy were respected as desirable ideals; happiness could be expected in the next world but not in this; and sex was not so much a pleasure as a sinful necessity, justified by the need to propagate the race. Life was cheap, death came easily and often, and it was imprudent to become emotionally dependent upon anyone. Relations within the family – between husband and wife, and between parents and children – were not much closer than those between neighbours. Neighbours and relations moved freely in and out of the household. Stone calls this the *open lineage family*.

Family relationships were characterized by interchangeability. The probability of surviving childhood was small. Children were commonly given the same name as a dead brother or sister; in mediaeval times, several children could share the same name, expecting that few would survive. Before the age of about two, infants were not regarded by upper-class parents as fully human. The children who did survive left home at a young age, between seven and fourteen, and generally for good, to work, to serve, or rarely to go to school. The period for bonding between parent and child was brief, and not much bonding took place.

In the sixteenth century, the Reformation led to a new appreciation of individual moral accountability and redemption, and to better bonding within the family. Loyalty to lineage, kin and local community declined as the Church and the state further encouraged patriarchy. Why? The Church wished to reinforce accountability to God; the state needed to discipline a society inadequately policed or controlled.

The demand by the Puritan theologians for 'holy matrimony' encompassed lust and procreation as reasons for having sex, but affection was rare and it was usually ambiguous. Religious zeal was intensifying the way the community interfered morally in intimate domestic matters, including stricter definitions of what constituted marriage. This resulted in a decline in allegiance to kinship, with a corollary growth of loyalty outward to the state and to religion, and inward to the family. Stone calls this the *restricted patriarchal nuclear family*. The authoritarian family and the authoritarian nation state were the solutions to a general sense of anxiety and a deep yearning for order in society. The husband, as the head of the household, was, Stone writes, typically and legally a tyrant within the home. Wives maltreated by their husbands were now less able to turn to their kin for help. Married life was brutal, often hostile, and legally indissoluble. It would have taken a woman gifted with great strength of character, independence of mind and tactical skill to be the one to make important decisions. Children, individually ephemeral, remained a commodity.

After 1660 in England, with a decline of religious, social, economic and political tensions, the need for authoritarianism within the family relaxed. The eighteenth century family was unprecedentedly private, domestic and emotionally bonded. Stone calls this the *closed domesticated nuclear family*. Personal autonomy – for this was The Enlightenment, The Age of Reason – called for growing introspection and interest in individual personality, as well as respect of self-expression and privacy. Forks and handkerchiefs were invented. Houses for the first time were built with halls and corridors so that some rooms of the house could be private. At least among the aristocracy, there was more recognition and acceptance of sensuality; eroticism could be expressed openly within marital, and especially extramarital, relations. Stone finds historical evidence that the female orgasm was regarded as both medically desirable and morally legitimate. Pornography, dildos and sheep-gut condoms (used more as venereal prophylactics than contraceptives) were advertised in pamphlets and in the press. Homosexuality, sexual deviations and perversions were generally tolerated, though legally they were still capital offences.

Children, for the first time, were identified as a group with special status, to be educated and to be protected from knowing prematurely about sex and death. This worldly secularism, literacy, the pursuit of happiness, humanitarianism, physical and bodily privacy, and personalized death became common to the whole of Western culture. Stone calls it the rise of *effective individualism*. With it came the development of the 'companionate marriage', as men and women with foresight realized the need for personal affection, companionship and friendship in choice of a husband or wife, a calculated assessment of the chance of long-term compatibility, based on the fullest possible knowledge of the moral, intellectual and psychological qualities of the prospective partner. In England and America, generally in advance of continental Europe, there was a shift of power over the choice of mate from parents to children – a first sign of the exercise of modern reproductive choice. None the less patriarchy and the well-known double standard of sexual experience for men but not for women meant that a successful marriage depended, as it had always done, on the docility and adaptability of the woman. Women reacted to humiliation by turning their affections toward their children, who in turn generally benefited. But, in a pre-contraceptive, pre-antibiotic, pre-divorce society, sexual permissiveness for both men and women carried a high price.

Rising dissatisfaction among women with their role as biological reproductive machines and their demand for freedom from the tyranny of constant child-bearing coincided with an appreciation by men that their material comfort and their endowment to their descendants were helped by restricting the number of children their wives should bear. Even theologians permitted the thinking that poverty might be a reason for limiting the number of children, and admitted the legitimacy of *coitus reservatus,* or sexual intercouse without ejaculation; *coitus interruptus,* with withdrawal just prior to ejaculation, was still condemned as the sin of Onan (Genesis 38: 9-10). Not much distinction was made between contraception, deliberate acts to abort the fetus, and infanticide at or immediately after birth.

A new wave of moral repression began in England in 1770, was spreading fast by 1810, and reached its apogée in the mid-Victorian period. The Puritan leadership of the early seventeenth century was reborn in the early nineteenth under Methodist and Evangelical leadership. Sunday Schools and other agencies had helped to create a diligent, thrifty and sober labour force, mobile in relation to parents, but centred around the family to exploit society's rapid industrialization. A drive to reform the morals first of the poor, then of the rich, was seen in parliamentary legislation, in the revival of societies for the suppression of vice, and in other (probably more effective) organs of social control such as the family, the Church, schools and the courts of petty sessions. Flogging and transportation supplemented death sentences as legal punishments in England for ordinary misdemeanours and crimes.

The key institution upon which this new moralism centred was the family, and the device again used by Church and state was the encouragement of paternal authority. The status of women inevitably declined. The new ideal of womanhood involved, according to Stone, total abnegation, making the wife a slave to convention, to propriety, and to her husband. Inevitably this could only be achieved, if at all, at high psychic costs, particularly at a time when divorce was not available, and wives and husbands were living longer. Suicide grew more common. Formality was revived as a device for distance. Punishment became once again severe and frequent. Children were flogged at school and deprived at home. It was normal to lock a child for hours or even days in a dark room or closet on a limited diet of bread and water. A child's will had to be broken.

Victorian England and Puritan New England also saw a general hostility towards sexuality. Despite efforts to clear the streets of prostitutes, their number increased, the cause of the surge having changed from a supply-led abundance of women who could find no other livelihood in the eighteenth century to a nineteenth century demand that was led by men who found no sexual satisfaction within marriage. Already-fragile ladies, according to Stone, were taught to be frail and sickly. Prudery reached extraordinary heights, as newspaper and ordinary conversation eschewed not only the Anglo-Saxon words for sexual and excretory organs but of all mention of these bodily functions. For the first time in Western history, there was a strong body of opinion that denied the existence of the sexual drive in the majority of women. A female who showed too much ardour or desire was said to risk sterility. Masturbation became a peril. Surgical mutilation of the clitoris and the use of chastity belts were customs that were not rare. The most treasured value was respectability, which took the form of moral asceticism, buttressed by Evangelical piety and reinforced by patriarchy.

Stone argues that reticence, sobriety and thrift, punctuality, self-discipline and industry, chastity, prudery and piety are all qualities that had been predominant among some sections of the middling ranks in society uninterruptedly since the late sixteenth century – as they remain today. These values bloomed in Britain, America and Europe in the nineteenth century to affect large numbers of both the upper landed and professional élite, and also the respectable end of the labouring classes.

The new age of reason

Since the late nineteenth century there have been several increasing waves of liberalism, coinciding with female emancipation, the development of effective contraception, hygiene, antibiotics, privacy and divorce. Freudianism has discouraged the inhibition of sexuality in child-rearing. The women's liberation movement has intensified the pressure for change. The decades that followed the invention of the oral contraceptive pill, the 1960s and 1970s, saw a rise in sexual permissiveness that was at last unshackled from a corresponding risk of unwanted pregnancy. Abortion received widespread sanction in the 1970s. Only in the 1980s did the spectre of untreatable venereal diseases from viruses begin to slow down the gathering popularity of premarital and extramarital sexual liaisons.

In summary, although moral standards have appeared to wax and to wane, there are secular changes that have taken place inexorably since the early sixteenth century. These have been improved technology, improved health and longevity, personal freedoms, and – very conspicuously – an increase in the individual value placed on children.

The present position is that survival is taken for granted from infancy to old age, that command of contraception and, recently, conception make reproduction, for the first time, truly a matter of choice. Children are regarded, sometimes overly so, as society's most important members, with the popular claim that in matters of reproduction the wellbeing of the child is paramount. Today's family in Western societies is, as a result of this cultural evolution, intensely self-centred, inwardly turned, emotionally bonded, sexually liberated, child-orientated ... and often temporary. The separate ambitions of parents detach both of them from the home and from their dependence on each other. The guilt felt over depriving children of adequate family life is countered by focusing too much on their personal achievements, leading to their isolation within the family and, for their socialisation, by emphasizing their peer groups instead of the family (Stone, 1977; Reddy, 1992). Modern families, especially it seems in America and Scandinavia, are more loosely structured and are less emotionally and sexually cohesive than has been the case for centuries. To an Indian social anthropologist, used to close relations within his own extended family, a modern European family lacks spirituality, overly emphasizes individualism, and has children brought up isolated and lonely (Reddy, 1992). Such a family type has an impermanence that recalls past centuries. It has not taken reproductive technology for the traditional family as ideal to be threatened.

There is little reason to suppose that today's typical Western family will be more lasting than its predecessors, or that today's Western model has a special claim to be the best. It has been called ethnocentric to assume that any one form of the family is crucial to the survival of a society (Whiteford, 1989). Secondary though my sources for this section have been, this is the context in which we should examine gamete donation, embryo donation and surrogacy. Cultural evolution, like biological evolution, works best if it allows the realization of preadaptations that come from successful diversity. There needs to be room to widen our concept of the family, to extend the notion of parenthood, to broaden our social options.

Donors and recipients

Oocyte donation and receipt

To satisfy the biological urge for motherhood and the social urge to have a family, the women who have received donated eggs (a) may themselves have depleted their oocyte reserves and thus suffer ovarian failure (Leeton *et al.*, 1983), (b) have oocytes that are genetically unsuitable, such as with X-linked genetic diseases, or (c) have oocytes that are simply inaccessible. Changes have taken place in the distribution of these three reasons for receiving donated oocytes. Transvaginal aspiration of follicles for IVF has put an end to oocyte donation for one of its original indications, namely inaccessible ovaries at laparoscopy. On the other hand, more and more older women, premenopausal or postmenopausal, are receiving donated oocytes, as it is realized that the limits to human fertility with age stem from oocyte ageing and depletion, and not from senescence of the reproductive tract (Serhal & Craft, 1989).

Oocyte donation, like sperm donation, can be driven by sympathy for infertile women, known or anonymous, or by money (Leeton & Harman, 1987; Robertson, 1989; Sauer & Paulson, 1990; Braverman and Ovum Donor Task Force, 1993). Obtaining oocytes, unlike obtaining sperm, is necessarily an intrusive procedure, although the intrusion may be part of another surgical operation and so be incidental. Because of its usual physical difficulty, one would expect the emotional compensation and the financial compensation needed for egg donation to be greater than it is for sperm donation – and so it seem to be. A survey of 51 oocyte donation programmes by Sauer and Paulson in the United States showed that 30 (59%) used only donors designated and provided to them by the recipient couples, implying that there was a personally identified sympathy for the infertility of a close relation; the donors were usually sisters (Sauer & Paulson, 1992). Sauer and Paulson also found that among commercial arrangements the donor's compensation varied from US $500 to US $2000 per aspiration, a price that in 1992 lay between that paid for a sperm donation (US $50 to $100) and a surrogate gestating a pregnancy (US $10 000 to $15 000). Payment for eggs can also take the form of discounting the cost of IVF services for infertile patients who agree to make some of their eggs available for fertilization by a prospective recipient's husband (Braverman and Ovum Donor Task Force, 1993). In at least one centre in France, the voluntary, anonymous donation of one oocyte, should at least 7 eggs be obtained, and two oocytes with more than 10, finds acceptance among 58% of couples having IVF (Plachot, 1989). Unlike sperm donors, these infertile oocyte donors risk knowing that another woman may be pregnant while the donor herself remains infertile – an uncomfortable piece of news for a doctor to present to a patient.

Oocyte donation, and hence oocyte receipt, differs from that of sperm donation in other ways. Whereas new legislation has generally been necessary fully to ensure the husband's legal paternity in cases of donor insemination, it seems unlikely, except perhaps in cases of contractual surrogacy (e.g. Annas, 1992), that the connection between giving birth and legal maternity will require special legislative attention. In a further distinction from sperm donation, Leeton and Harman (1987) found that both known and anonymous oocyte donors were unlikely to agree to make eggs available to single women. A study at Hammersmith, however, found that 72% of women resting after their own embryo transfer would have agreed to donate eggs to infertile recipients, and 51% would have approved donation to single women. Women, even more than men, may be willing to be made known to their otherwise anonymous offspring, an observation that makes the 1991 recommendations of Britain's then IVF Interim Licensing Authority, that oocyte donation should ordinarily be anonymous, look awkward (Templeton, 1991).

For a woman to get pregnant and then to donate either her embryos or her baby to an infertile couple is the epitome of reproductive generosity. There is much evidence that women take a less proprietorial view of their gametes, and their offspring, than men do. Conversely, however, women generally have a greater wish than men to know and to be known by the recipients and, especially in the case in which they part with a baby, to *remain* known, and in touch.

Embryo donation and receipt

In the case of embryo donation after eggs have been fertilized *in vitro*, the couple who donate spare embryos after their own procreative needs have been met does not put the woman at special physical risk. There seem to have been many examples of its occurrence utilising embryos placed in cryostorage after IVF. From the point of view of both the genetic parents, however, there are similarities to adopting a baby out. The genetic parents' curiosity and possible wish to stay in touch are, in 1995, essentially unresearched. As with sperm and egg donation, recipients may expect increasing interest from embryo donors to be a part of their child's family and, if they are told or find out, increasing interest from their children to know their genetic parents.

Embryo donation can also follow impregnation of a woman with the semen of an infertile woman's husband by artificial insemination, followed by recovery of embryos by lavaging the uterus at the time when the blastocyst is free in the cavity, just before implantation (Bustillo *et al.*, 1984). The procedure carries medical as well as ethical hazards (Jansen, 1987c), including translocation of the embryos to the tubes, resulting in ectopic pregnancy. Ethics committees outside the United Stages have generally not condoned such 'womb flushing' for embryo donation (e.g. National Health and Medical Research Council, 1985). As IVF programmes became prevalent in the United States during the 1980s, fewer and fewer clinical circumstances required uterine lavage and embryo donation for treatment, so even there the method did not become popular. There are now no obvious circumstances where oocyte donation and IVF is not a better alternative for the prospective donor, ethically and medically.

Altruistic surrogacy

It is no new thing for a woman to conceive and to give birth to a baby she then gives away, though the giving has no doubt ever been easy. The custom by which an infertile wife could 'give' her maid to her husband for sexual intercourse and then claim the child as her own is as ancient as Genesis (Chapter 16 (1–6), *New Oxford Annotated Bible*, Revised Standard Version). Nowadays, the surrogate is more likely to be inseminated artificially. The other difference is that it is only in relatively modern times that Western society has developed the legal machinery that reinforces marriage and legitimacy of children – to the point where there are now formidable legal obstacles to recognizing as mother a woman other than the woman who gives birth.

Although altruistic surrogacy is thus not novel, and in no need of special reproductive technology, the surrogate carries the biological risks of impregnation and gestation, and the emotional risks of giving up both her genetic and gestational motherhood. Through history the compensation for the surrogate has come from her sense of generosity, supplemented usually by a continuing association with the child, even if at some distance. But it is worth recalling that Hagar, the surrogate in Genesis 16, looked with contempt on her infertile mistress, Sarai, who in turn dealt so harshly with Hagar, that Hagar had to flee.

Commercial surrogacy

In commercial surrogacy an infertile couple commissions a woman to have a baby for them, usually, in America, under the brokerage of a surrogacy agency, which typically retains about half of the fee paid. A legal or quasi-legal contract is signed, which to a substantial extent limits the right of the pregnant surrogate to make decisions for herself concerning medical and social matters while pregnant, and seeks to compel her to give up the baby at delivery. The United States of America is the one country in which the practice of commercial surrogacy is accepted.

Today, two forms of surrogacy need to be distinguished. In the first and still in 1994 probably the most prevalent form, artificial insemination is used for the surrogate to conceive. The oocyte, in other words, is the surrogate's own. She is selling her egg first, leasing her body for the gestation second, and third she is giving up a baby who differs from one in normal reproductive circumstances only by her not having chosen her mate; genetically and biologically the baby is the surrogate's before and after she sells it. Today, this *genetic-plus-gestational surrogacy* is referred to as 'traditional surrogacy'. The first such surrogate to try to have her contract overturned in the American courts was Mary Beth Whitehead (The Washington Post, April 1, 1987, p. A8). She was unsuccessful.

In the second form that surrogacy can take, the surrogate receives an embryo fertilized *in vitro* using the egg and sperm from the infertile couple. She sells the use of her body for its gestational function, much in the way that wet-nurses in the seventeenth century sold their mammary function. This is *gestational surrogacy*. Inarguably, the baby is genetically that of the commissioning parents. Inarguably too, the surrogate mother is the gestational mother. Who the biological mother is is now confused, but because there is little recent social precedent for not regarding the woman who gives birth to a baby to be other than its natural mother, the law in most countries would leave her the legal mother too, at least until adoption processes transfer the guardianship. Nevertheless, in the first such case in America in which the gestational mother attempted to have her contract overturned in the courts, the woman, Anna Johnson, like Mary Beth Whitehead before her, was also unsuccessful (Annas, 1992). This finding, in which the intentions of the parties in conceiving a child were held to determine parenthood, has at the time of writing been confirmed on appeal to the California Supreme Court (Oxman, 1993). Newspapers at the time of the first judgement generally appeared content in their commentaries to regard the genetic parents as the biological parents.

It is when the commissioning woman has no uterus, or when for some reason pregnancy would be exceptionally hazardous, that surrogacy remains medically necessary for an infertile couple to secure genetic offspring. The commercial development in the United States in the 1970s of genetic-plus-gestational surrogacy was an alternative to IVF, before IVF became effective and available. In this respect it resembled the ill-fated commercialization in America of uterine flushing or lavage to obtain embryos for sale. The developing practice of oocyte donation or sale accompanied by IVF in America should, in the future, diminish the medical needs for the traditional genetic-plus-gestational surrogacy to very low levels. Demand for it, I expect, will, like the demise of wet-nursing in the seventeenth century, be further depressed by a rising price for it as the true emotional costs the surrogate bears come to be appreciated better.

By 1993 several legislatures inside and outside America had begun responding to public opinion that has consistently favoured allowing altruistic surrogacy (e.g. Ramsay, 1993). This move recognizes that, when a relative or close friend is agreeable to gestating an IVF embryo for a woman without a uterus of her own, there is exhibited a supreme act of generosity that is capable, in carefully considered circumstances, of benefiting everyone involved. The legislation envisaged will facilitate parental orders, in which a court can order, upon agreement of all concerned, that a child's birth certificate record the commissioning mother instead of the birth mother, thus obviating the need for lengthy adoption procedures to complete the surrogacy arrangement.

Exploitation and autonomy

The criticism that commercial surrogacy promotes the exploitation of women and infertile couples confuses the messenger (the surrogacy broker) with the message (the need of infertile couples and the readiness of third parties to fill this need). The fear that commercial surrogacy leads to 'the dehumanization of babies' is at odds with history. The interpretation we might give on a couple commissioning a child from a surrogate when all else has failed (Davies, 1985) is perfectly consistent with the historical trend towards ascribing more and more individual value to children. It is not the child but the autonomous surrogate herself who risks the experience of being 'dehumanized' – a paid means to a lonely end. How can we estimate this hapless dehumanization?

One measure of exploitation in the selling of body parts – whether blood, gametes, embryos, babies or body organs – is the size of the broker's commission in relation to his or her efforts, and, conversely, how much of the payment reaches the donor. In each case, the people who commission the service are likely to be relatively wealthy, the person commissioned relatively poor. In none of these cases is it clear, however, that what an outsider might call exploitation is particularly important to the people who opt to be so commissioned (e.g. Wight, 1991). In general, it can be difficult to devise ways of dealing with the problem of exploitation without seeming to wish to lock people into poverty (Angell, 1990). Arguments that society has an obligation to better the economic position of the potentially exploited to the point where they would not be tempted by the money or coerced or forced through their personal situation to accept the role are not strong, because such a betterment might simply bring a higher price for the donation. None the less it was the rising price of wet-nursing that contributed to its decline in popularity 300 years ago. Society naturally aims to reduce the unfortunate circumstances in which people have little alternative to sell a part of themselves, but in the meantime to make the practices illegal may simply not work and, worse, may make it more difficult to police those whose duty it should be to provide fair compensation.

Voluntariness is the key to ethical donations of tissues and organs, whether the recipient is personally known to the donor or not, and whether or not the donor is paid. Nevertheless it is clear from the distress of Mary Beth Whitehead and Anna Johnson that bearing a child and reliquishing it can be extremely difficult. An agreement to do so is not like other commercial contracts (Angell, 1990) any more, say, than was Shylock's pound of flesh in *The Merchant of Venice* (La Puma, Schiedermayer & Grover, 1989). The general unease that something so natural has become so unnatural (Angell, 1990) – the key to the dehumanizing side of surrogacy – lies not with reproductive technology but with the giving away of a child. The fact remains that forewarning, payment and notions of autonomy are poor compensation for loneliness and the loss of a baby. This loss will be more frequent with the rigidity of predominantly commercial surrogacy, in which I predict an escalating price will need to be paid for privacy (to buy-off the gestational mother), in comparison with the usually more flexible circumstances of a surrogacy agreement that from the beginning is more obviously altruistic.

Several writers on ethics have argued convincingly that two conditions emerge as a way of protecting those involved in traditional, genetic-plus-gestational surrogacy (Wood & Singer, 1988; Whiteford, 1989). The first is to provide a period of grace for the surrogate mother during which she would be free to decide whether or not to surrender the child. The second condition is to establish reasonable compensation. To these I would add the need for a plain protocol for selecting the path to follow should a congenital abnormality result and, preferably, a way in which the gestational mother can stay in contact with the child and with those she has helped.

There is a potential dark side to surrogacy arrangements. A woman without a partner can pretend agreement as a ruse to become pregnant and then seek to keep the baby. This possibility entangles traditional, gestational-plus-genetic surrogacy particularly. For gestational surrogacy, where the birth mother is not the child's genetic mother but disputes the surrogacy agreement, it is not obvious that giving the surrogate the legal option of keeping the child will always be the safe or most reasonable course.

Just how morally hazardous the practice of commercial surrogacy is, I expect will continue to be revealed. There will be the occasional sad eventuality of a baby born with an undiagnosed abnormality, wanted by no one. More often the hazards will be revealed by the high price that successful parents will pay to keep their privacy from the relinquishing surrogate, however miserable she may be.

Brave new world: towards empirical ethics

Looking into a future with test-tube babies has brought many writers to recall Aldous Huxley's *Brave New World,* written in the 1930s, and to be fearful of a slippery slope into it. Sanity is a rare phenomenon in public life, according to Huxley in a new preface to the book in 1946, and it was prizing stability over true popular will by world governments that would drive those governments to totalitarian ends. The sinister feature of the future in Huxley's prophecies was not what was possible with IVF and life in test-tubes: it was the control the Utopian government had over people's lives.

Our concern today should not be to limit reproductive technology. Still less should we be urging our governments to constrain or to over-regulate it. If we leave matters of morals in reproductive decisions in the hands of the couple who provide the egg and the sperm that make up the embryo, we will probably see a social advance that will truly rival the development of effective contraception and of safe childhood in giving couples in general, and women in particular, control over their reproductive destiny and in exercising their reproductive choice. For Huxley, too, the antidote for his *Brave New World* lay in decentralizing control over technology, not in simply limiting it.

While it is appealing to say that children should not be conceived unless there is a loving family to receive them (e.g. Ryan, 1989), history tells us that we should not define such families too rigidly. Reproductive ethics is a subject that needs to be studied empirically, respecting and researching the medical and emotional interests of the people who have to live with the consequences of their own medical and moral decisions, so that others will do better.

For our society to be robust we should understand and tolerate diversity. With caution we should allow sociological innovations to take place when there is clear popular support for them, though we may expect problems and we may try to anticipate what they will be. This way we can learn the true ethical consequences instead of imagining them, often wrongly. When we consider such social experiments, which while not dependent on reproductive technology are facilitated by it – egg and sperm donation, surrogacy, commerce in human tissues, and homosexual marriage and child-raising – then it is better not to ban them, but to observe them and to learn from them.

References

AIH National Perinatal Statistics Unit & Fertility Society of Australia. *Assisted conception. Australia and New Zealand. 1989*. Sydney, AIH NPSU, 1991: p. 29.

Angell M. New ways to get pregnant. *N Engl J Med* 1990; **323**: 1200–2.

Annas GJ. Using genes to define motherhood – the California solution. *N Engl J Med* 1992; **326**: 417–20.

Anonymous. Chinese communists blood stained. *The Economist* 1992; July 18: 88.

Beier HM, Beckman JO. German Embryo Protection Action (October 14th, 1990: Gesetz zum Schutz bon Embryonen (Embryonenschutzgesetz-ESchG). *Hum Reprod* 1991; **6**: 605–6.

Biggers JD. *In vitro* fertilization and embryo transfer in human beings. *N Engl J Med* 1981; **304**: 336–42.

Bongaarts J. Infertility after age 30: a false alarm. *Fam Plann Persp* 1982; **14**: 75–8.

Braverman AM, Ovum Donor Task Force. Survey results on the current practice of ovum donation. *Fertil Steril* 1993; **59**: 1216–20.

Bustillo M, Buster JE, Freeman AG *et al*. Nonsurgical ovum transfer as a treatment for intractable infertility: what effectiveness can be realistically expected? *Am J Obstet Gynecol* 1984; **149**: 371–5.

Clutton-Brock TH. *The evolution of parental care*. Princeton, NJ: Princeton University Press, 1991: 352 pp.

Davies I. Contracts to bear children. *J Med Ethics* 1985; **11**: 61–65.

Dawkins R. *The Selfish Gene*. 2nd edn. Oxford: Oxford University Press, 1989: 234–66.

DeCherney AH, Berkowitz GS. Female fecundity and age. *N Engl J Med* 1982; **306**: 424–6.

D'Hooge TM, Bambra CS, Cornillie FJ, Isahakia M, Koninckx PR. Prevalence and laparoscopic appearance of spontaneous endometriosis in the baboon (*Papio anubis, Papio cynocephalus*). *Biol Reprod* 1991; **45**: 411–16.

Dickson D. Europe split on embryo research (News & Comment). *Science* 1988; **242**: 1117–18.

Dunstan GR. The moral status of the human embryo: a tradition recalled. *J Med Ethics* 1984; **10**: 38–44.

Dunstan GR. *In vitro* fertilization: the ethics. *Hum Reprod* 1986; **1**: 41–44.

Dwyer C. Agony and ecstasy. *The Bulletin* 1992; May 19: 48–50.

Fildes VA. *Wet Nursing as a Social Institution, In: Breasts, Bottles and Babies. A History of Infant Feeding.* Edinburgh: Edinburgh University Press, 1986: 152–67.

Fleagle JG. *Primate Adaptation and Evolution.* San Diego, CA: Academic Press, 1988: 203–29.

Frisch RE. Body fat, menarche, fitness and fertility. *Hum Reprod* 1987; **2**: 521–33.

Gwynne DT. Weighing up the costs. *Nature, London,* 1991; **353**: 118.

Hammond MG, Jordan S, Sloan CS. Factors affecting pregnancy rates in a donor insemination program using frozen semen. *Am J Obstet Gynecol* 1986; **155**: 480–5.

Holm S. New Danish law: human life beings at conception. *J Med Ethics* 1988; **14**: 11–8.

Hughes E. *The Sociological Eye.* Chicago: Aldine, 1971: 305.

Jansen R. The clinical impact of *in vitro* fertilization. I. Results and limitations of conventional reproductive medicine. *Med J Aust* 1987a; **146**: 342–53.

Jansen R. The clinical impact of *in vitro* fertilization. II. Regulation, money and research. *Med J Aust* 1987b; **146**: 362–6.

Jansen R. Ethics in infertility treatment. In: Pepperell R, Wood C, Hudson B. eds. *The Infertile Couple.* Edinburgh: Churchill Livingstone, 1987c: 346–87.

Jansen R. *Mouse tales and embryo research. In: Proceedings of the First Annual Conference of the Australian Bioethics Association.* Melbourne: Australian Biotechnics Association, 1991: 97–101.

Jansen RPS. Minimal endometriosis and reduced fecundability: prospective evidence from and AID program. *Fertil Steril* 1986; **46**: 141–3.

Jansen RPS. Relative infertility: modeling clinical paradoxes. *Fertil Steril* 1993; **59**: 1041–5.

Jansen RPS. Ovulation and the polycystic ovary syndrome. Aust. NZ. *J Obstet Gynaecol.* 1994;**34**: 277–85.

Jones GS. Update on *in vitro* fertilization. *Endocr Reb* 1984; **5**: 62–75.

Kavanagh M. *A Complete Guise to Monkeys, Apes and Other Primates.* London: Jonathan Cape, 1983: 175–208.

Keverne EB. Reproductive behaviour. In: Austin Cr, Short RV. eds. *Reproduction in Mammals. Book 4: Reproductive fitness.* Cambridge: Cambridge University Press, 1984: 133–75.

Klein R. Resistance: from the exploitation of infertility to an exploration of infertility. In: Klein RD. ed. *Infertility. Women Speak Out About Their Experiences of Reproductive Medicine.* London: Pandora Press, 1989: 229–95.

Kolate G. Wet-nursing boom in England explored. *Science* 1987; **235**: 745–7.

Krasmer A. Austria: restrictions on infertility treatments. *Lancet* 1992; **339**: 1531.

Kuhse H, Singer P. The moral status of the embryo. In: Walters W, Singer P. eds. *Test-tube Babies.* Melbourne: Oxford University Press, 1982: 57–63.

Lamb EJ, Leurgans S. Does adoption affect subsequent fertility? *Am J Obstet Gynecol* 1979; **138**: 139–44.

La Puma J, Schiedermayer DL, Grover J. Surrogacy and Shakespeare: The Merchant's contract revisited. *Am J Obstet Gynecol* 1989; **160**: 59–62.

Leeton J, Harman J. The donation of oocytes to known recipients. *Aust NZ J Obstet Gynaecol* 1987; **27**: 248–50.

Leeton J, Trounson A, Conti A, Gianaroli L, Wood C. Pregnancy established in an infertile recipient patient after transfer of a donated embryo fertilized *in vitro* [abstract]. *Fertil Steril* 1983; **39**: 414–15.

Levine RJ, Bordson BL, Mathew RM, Brown MH, Stanley JM, Starr TB. Deterioration of semen quality during summer in New Orleans. *Fertil Steril* 1988; **49**: 900–7.

Levran D, Ben-Rafael Z, Ben-Shlomo I, Nebel L, Dor J, Mashiach S. Ageing of endometrium and oocytes: observations on conception and abortion rates in an egg donation model. *Fertil Steril* 1991; **56**: 1091–4.

Lippi J, Turner M, Jansen RPS. Pregnancies after *in vitro* fertilization by sperm microinjection into the perivitelline space. *Fertil Steril* 1990; **54**: s29.

Lofts B. Amphibians. In: Lamming GE. ed. *Marshall's Physiology of Reproduction. Volume I. Reproductive Cycles of Vertebrates.* Edinburgh: Churchill Livingstone, 1984: 127–205.

McClure HM, Ridley JM, Graham CE. Disseminated endometriosis in a rhesus monkey (*Macaca mulatta*) [ITAL]. *J Med Assoc Ga* 1971; **60**: 11–13.

McCormick RA. *The Critical Calling. Reflections on Moral Dilemmas Since Vatican II.* Washington DC: Georgetown University Press, 1989: 329–52.

Mahmood TA, Templeton A. The relationship between endometriosis and semen analysis: a review of 490 consecutive laparoscopies. *Hum Reprod* 1989; **4**: 782–5.

Majerus MEN, O'Donald P, Weir J. Female mating preference is genetic. *Nature, London* 1982; **300**: 521–3.

Maynard Smith J. *Evolutionary Genetics.* Oxford: Oxford University Press, 1989: 257–70.

Mazure CM, Greenfeld DA. Psychological studies of *in vitro* fertilization/embryo transfer participants. *J In Vitro Fert Embryo Transf* 1989; **6**: 242–56.

Moller AP. Ejaculate quality, testes size and sperm condition in primates. *J Hum Evol* 1988; **17**: 479–88.

Morris D. *The Illustrated Naked Ape.* London: Jonathan Cape, 1986: 14–73.

National Health and Medical Research Council. *Embryo Donation by Uterine Flushing: Interim Reprot on Ethical Considerations May 1985.* Canberra: Australian Government Publishing Service, 1985: 1–8.

National Perinatal Statistics Unit, Fertility Society of Australia. *IVF and GIFT Pregnancies. Australia and New Zealand. 1988.* Sydney: National Perinatal Statistics Unit, 1990: 14.

Olive DL, Lee KL. Analysis of sequential treatment protocols for endometriosis- associated infertility. *Am J Obstet Gynecol* 1986; **154**: 613–19.

Oxman RB. California's experiment in surrogacy. *Lancet* 1993; **341**: 1468–9.

Plachot M. Discussion on ethical and judicial aspects of embryo research. *Hum Reprod* 1989; **4**: 206–8.

Ramsay S. New surrogacy regulations? *Lancet* 1993; **341**: 1274.

Reddy P. *Saadan er Danskerne ('Danes are like that').* Aarhus: Grevas Forlag, 1992:

Reid BL, French P, Singer A, Hagan BE, Coppleson M. Sperm basic proteins in cervical carcinogenesis: correlation with socio-economic class. *Lancet* 1978; **ii**: 60.

Robertson JA. Ethical and legal issues in human egg donation. *Fertil Steril* 1989; **52**: 353–63.

Rowland R. *In: Living Laboratories. Women and Reproductive Technologies.* Sydney: Sun Australia, 1992: 1–14, 273–303.

Ryan KJ. Ethics on obstetrics and gynecology. *Am J Obstet Gynecol* 1985; **151**: 840–3.

Ryan KJ. Ethical issues in reproductive endocrinology and infertility. *Am J Obstet Gynecol* 1989; **160**: 1415–17.

Sauer MV, Paulson RJ. Human oocyte and preembryo donation: an evolving method for the treatment of infertility. *Am J Obstet Gynecol* 1990; **163**: 1421–4.

Sauer MV, Paulson RJ. Understanding the current status of oocyte donation in the United States: what's really going on out there? *Fertil Steril* 1992; **58**: 16–18.

Senate Select Committee on the Human Embryo Experimentation Bill 1985. *Human*

Embryo Experimentation in Australia. Canberra: Australian Government Publishing Service, 1986: 1–158.

Serhal PF, Craft IL. Oocyte donation in 61 patients. *Lancet* 1989; **1**: 1185–7.

Short RV. Sexual selection and its component parts, somatic and genital selection, as illustrated by man and the great apes. *Adv Stud Behav* 1979; **9**: 131–58.

Short RV. Species differences in reproductive mechanisms. In: Austin CR, Short RV. eds. *Reproduction in Mammals. Book 4: Reproductive Fitness*. Cambridge: Cambridge University Press, 1984: 24–61.

Silber SJ. *Why are humans so Infertile? In: How to Get Pregnant with the New Technology*. New York: Warner Books, 1990: 27–45.

Simpson JL, Elias S, Malinak LR, Buttram VC Jr. Heritable aspects of endometriosis. I. Genetic studies. *Am J Obstet Gynecol* 1980; **137**: 327–31.

Small MF. *Female Choices. Sexual Behavior of Female Primates*. Ithaca: Cornell University Press, 1993.

Stone L. *The Family, Sex and Marriage in England 1500–1800*. London: Weidenfeld and Nicolson, 1977.

Templeton A. Gamete donation and anonymity. *Br J Obstet Gynaecol* 1991; **98**: 343–50.

Tulandi T, Mouchawar M. Treatment-dependent and treatment-independent pregnancy in women with minimal and mild endometriosis. *Fertil Steril* 1991; **56**: 790–1.

Veeck L. *Atlas of the Human Embryo*. 1991; Baltimore: Williams & Wilkins.

Walton. Embryo research - why the Cardinal is wrong. *J Med Ethics* 1990; **16**: 185–6.

Watt WB, Carter PA, Donohue K. Females' choice of 'good genotypes' as mates is promoted by an insect mating system. *Science* 1986; **233**: 1187–90.

Whiteford L. Commercial surrogacy: social issues behind the controversy. In: Whiteford Lm, Poland ML. eds. *New Approaches to Human Reproduction. Social and Ethical Dimensions*. Boulder, CO: Westview Press, 1989: 145–69.

Wight JP. Ethics, commerce, and kidneys. *Br Med J* 1991; **303**: 110.

Wilson EO. *Sociobiology. The New Synthesis*. Cambridge MA: Harvard University Press, 1975: 4.

Wood EC, Singer P. Whither surrogacy? *Med J Aust* 1988; **149**: 426–30.

Wyshak G, Frisch RE. Evidence for a secular trend in age of menarche. *N Engl J Med* 1982; **306**: 1033–5.

Index

Printed in the United States
By Bookmasters